Study Guide for

Basic Pharmacology for Nurses

Fourteenth Edition

Valerie O'Toole Baker, APRN, BC
Assistant Professor
Villa Maria School of Nursing
Ganon University
Erie, Pennsylvania

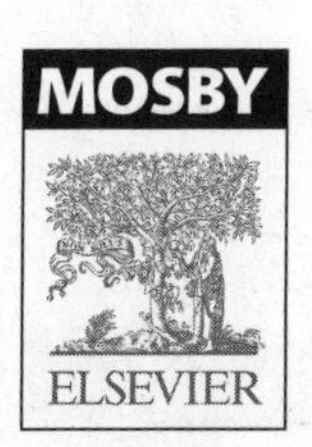

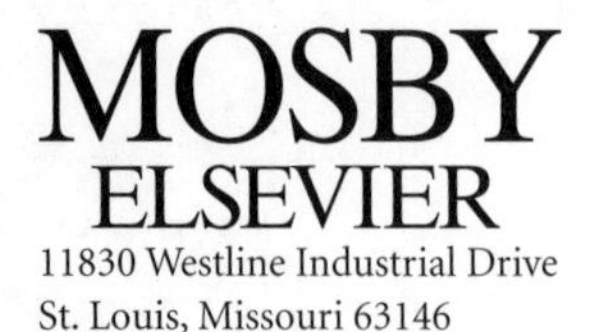

11830 Westline Industrial Drive
St. Louis, Missouri 63146

Study Guide for Basic Pharmacology for Nurses, Fourteenth Edition ISBN-13 978-0-323-03559-0
ISBN-10 0-323-04147-7

Notice

Pharmacology is an ever-changing field. Standard safety precautions must be followed but as new research and clinical experience broaden our knowledge, changes in treatment and drug therapy may become necessary or appropriate. Readers are advised to check the most current product information provided by the manufacturer of each drug to be administered to verify the recommended dose, the method and duration of administration, and contraindications. It is the responsibility of the treating physician, relying on experience and knowledge of the patient, to determine dosages and the best treatment for each individual patient. Neither the Publisher nor the author assumes any liability for any injury and/or damage to persons or property arising from this publication.

The Publisher

ISBN-13 978-0-323-03559-0
ISBN-10 0-323-04147-7

Senior Acquisitions Editor: Lee Henderson
Senior Developmental Editor: Rae L. Robertson
Publishing Services Manager: Gayle May
Senior Project Manager: Mary Stueck
Publishing Services: Lisa Hernandez

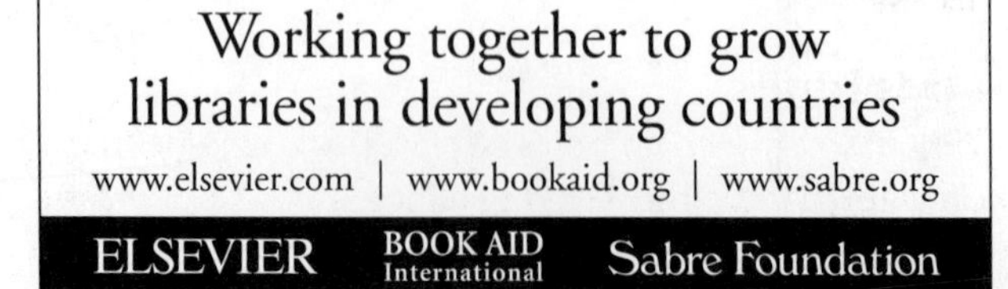

Printed in USA.

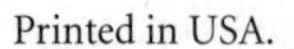

To the Student

This study guide was created to assist you in achieving the objectives of each chapter in *Basic Pharmacology for Nurses, Fourteenth Edition*, and establishing a solid base of knowledge in nursing pharmacology. Completing the exercises in each chapter in this guide will help to reinforce the material studied in the textbook and learned in class. Such reinforcement also helps students to be successful on the NCLEX-PN.

STUDY HINTS FOR ALL STUDENTS

Ask Questions!

There are no stupid questions. If you do not know something or are not sure, you need to find out. Other people may be wondering the same thing but may be too shy to ask. The answer could mean life or death to your patient. That is certainly more important than feeling embarrassed about asking a question.

Chapter Objectives

At the beginning of each chapter in the textbook are objectives that you should have mastered when you finish studying that chapter. Write these objectives in your notebook, leaving a blank space after each. Fill in the answers as you find them while reading the chapter. Review to make sure your answers are correct and complete. Use these answers when you study for tests. This should also be done for separate course objectives that your instructor has listed in your class syllabus.

Key Terms

At the beginning of each chapter in the textbook are key terms that you will encounter as you read the chapter. The key terms are in color the first time they appear significantly in the chapter. Phonetic pronunciations are provided for terms that students might find difficult to pronounce. The terms that were assigned simple phonetic pronunciations were selected because they are either (1) difficult medical, nursing, or scientific terms or (2) other words that may be difficult for students to pronounce. The goal is to help the student reader with limited proficiency in English to develop a greater command of the pronunciation of scientific and nonscientific English terminology. It is hoped that a more general competency in the understanding and use of medical and scientific language may result.

Key Points

Use the Key Points at the end of each chapter in the textbook to help with review for exams.

Reading Hints

When reading each chapter in the textbook, look at the subject headings to learn what each section is about. Read first for the general meaning. Then reread parts you did not understand. It may help to read those parts aloud. Carefully read the information given in each table and study each figure and its caption.

Concepts

While studying, put difficult concepts into your own words to see if you understand them. Check this understanding with another student or the instructor. Write these in your notebook.

Class Notes

When taking lecture notes in class, leave a large margin on the left side of each notebook page and write only on right-hand pages, leaving all left-hand pages blank. Look over your lecture notes soon after each class, while your memory is fresh. Fill in missing words, complete sentences and ideas, and underline key phrases, definitions, and concepts. At the top of each page, write the topic of that page. In the left margin, write the key word for that part of your notes. On the opposite left-hand page, write a summary or outline that combines material from both the textbook and the lecture. These can be your study notes for review.

Study Groups

Form a study group with some other students so you can help one another. Practice speaking and reading aloud. Ask questions about material you are not sure about. Work together to find answers.

References for Improving Study Skills

Good study skills are essential for achieving your goals in nursing. Time management, efficient use of study time, and a consistent approach to studying are all beneficial. There are various study methods for reading a textbook and for taking class notes. Some methods that have proven helpful can be found in *Saunders Student Nurse Planner: A Guide to Success in Nursing School.* This book contains helpful information on test taking and preparing for clinical experiences. It includes an example of a "time map" for planning study time and a blank form that the student can use to formulate a personal time map.

ADDITIONAL STUDY HINTS FOR ENGLISH AS SECOND-LANGUAGE (ESL) STUDENTS

Vocabulary

If you find a nontechnical word you do not know (e.g., *drowsy*), try to guess its meaning from the sentence (e.g., *With electrolyte imbalance, the patient may feel fatigued and drowsy*). If you are not sure of the meaning, or if it seems particularly important, look it up in the dictionary.

Vocabulary Notebook

Keep a small alphabetized notebook or address book in your pocket or purse. Write down new nontechnical words you read or hear along with their meanings and pronunciations. Write each word under its initial letter so you can find it easily, as in a dictionary. For words you do not know or for words that have a different meaning in nursing, write down how they are used and sound. Look up their meanings in a dictionary or ask your instructor or first-language buddy. Then write the different meanings or usages that you have found in your book, including the nursing meaning. Continue to add new words as you discover them. For example:

primary
- of most importance; main: *the primary problem or disease*
- the first one; elementary: *primary school*

secondary
- of less importance; resulting from another problem or disease: *a secondary symptom*
- the second one: *secondary school (in the United States, high school)*

First Language Buddy

ESL students should find a first-language buddy – another student who is a native speaker of English and who is willing to answer questions about word meanings, pronunciations, and culture. Maybe your buddy would like to learn about your language and culture as well. This could help in his or her nursing experience as well.

Quick Review of Drug Classifications

ACE inhibitors Prevent the synthesis of angiotensin II, a potent vasoconstrictor; used to treat hypertension and heart failure

Acetylcholinesterase inhibitors Promote the accumulation of acetylcholine, resulting in prolonged cholinergic effects

Adrenergic Produce effects similar to the neurotransmitter norepinephrine; see Chapter 13

Adrenergic blocking agents Inhibit the adrenergic system, preventing stimulation of the adrenergic receptors

Aldosterone receptor antagonists Block stimulation of mineralocorticoid receptors by aldosterone, thus reducing high blood pressure by reducing sodium reabsorption

Aminoglycosides Gentamicin, tobramycin, and related antibiotics; particularly effective against gram-negative microorganisms; noted for potentially dangerous toxicity

Amylinomimetic agents Used to reduce elevated postprandial hyperglycemia in patients with type 1 or type 2 diabetes mellitus

Analgesics Narcotic and nonnarcotic; relieve pain without producing loss of consciousness or reflex activity

Androgens These steroid hormones produce masculinizing effects

Angiotensin II receptor antagonists Also known as ARBs (angiotensin receptor blockers); act by binding to angiotensin II receptor sites, preventing angiotensin II (a very potent vasoconstrictor) from binding to receptor sites in vascular smooth muscle, brain, heart, kidneys, and adrenal gland, thus blocking the blood pressure–elevating and sodium-retaining effects of angiotensin II

Anesthetics For example, local anesthesia, general anesthesia; cause a loss of sensation with or without a loss of consciousness

Antacids Reduce the acidity of the gastric contents

Antianginals Used to prevent or treat attacks of angina pectoris; most common is nitroglycerin

Antianxiety Used to treat anxiety symptoms or disorders; also known as minor tranquilizers or anxiolytics, although the term *tranquilizer* is avoided today to prevent the misperception that the patient is being tranquilized

Antibiotics Used to treat infections caused by pathogenic microbes; the term is often used interchangeably with antimicrobial agents

Anticholinergic Block the action of acetylcholine in the parasympathetic nervous system; also known as cholinergic blocking agents, antispasmodics, and parasympatholytic agents

Anticoagulants Do NOT dissolve existing blood clots, but do prevent enlargement or extension of blood clots

Anticonvulsants Suppress abnormal neuronal activity in the CNS, preventing seizures

Antidepressants Relieve depression

Antidiabetics Also known as hypoglycemics; include insulin (used to treat type 1 diabetes mellitus) and oral hypoglycemic agents (used in the treatment of type 2 diabetes mellitus)

Antidiarrheals Relieve or control the symptoms of acute or chronic diarrhea

Antidysrhythmics Used to correct cardiac arrhythmias (any heart rate or rhythm other than normal sinus rhythm)

Antiemetics Used to prevent or treat nausea and vomiting

Antifungals Used to treat fungal infections

Antiglaucoma Used to reduce intraocular pressure

Antigout Used in the treatment of active gout attacks or to prevent future attacks

Antihistamines Used to treat allergy symptoms; may also be used to treat motion sickness, insomnia, and other nonallergic reactions

Antihypertensives Used to treat elevated blood pressure (hypertension)

Antilipemics Used to reduce serum cholesterol and/or triglycerides; most common are statins

Antimicrobials Chemicals that eliminate living microorganisms pathogenic to the patient; also called antibiotics or antiinfectives

Antineoplastics Also called chemotherapy agents; used alone or in combination with other treatment modalities such as radiation, surgery, or biologic response modifiers for the treatment of cancer

Antiparkinson's Used in the treatment of Parkinson's syndrome and other dyskinesias

Antiplatelets Prevent platelet clumping (aggregation), thereby preventing an essential step in formation of a blood clot; most common are aspirin and clopidogrel

Antipsychotics Used in the treatment of severe mental illnesses; also known as major tranquilizers or neuroleptics, although the term *tranquilizer* is avoided today to prevent the misperception that the patient is being tranquilized

Antipyretics Used to reduce fevers associated with a variety of conditions; most common are aspirin and acetaminophen

Antispasmodics Actually anticholinergic agents

Antithyroid Used to treat the symptoms of hyperthyroidism; also known as thyroid hormone antagonists

Antituberculins Used to prevent or treat an infection caused by *Mycobacterium tuberculosis*

Antitussive Used to suppress a cough by acting on the cough center of the brain

Antiulcer agents These drugs, such as histamine-2 antagonists, decrease the volume and increase the pH of gastric secretions

Antivirals Used to treat infections caused by pathogenic viruses

Bronchodilators Stimulate receptors within the tracheobronchial tree to relax and dilate the airway passages, allowing a greater volume of air to be exchanged and improving oxygenation

Beta blockers Inhibit the activity of sympathetic transmitters, norepinephrine, and epinephrine; used to treat angina, dysrhythmias, hypertension, and glaucoma

Calcium channel blockers Also called calcium ion antagonists, slow channel blockers or calcium ion influx inhibitors; inhibit the movement of calcium ions across the cell membrane; used to decrease dysrhythmias, slow rate of contraction of the heart, and cause dilation of blood vessels

Carbapenems Antibiotics (imipenem, ertapenem, meropenem) that have a broad spectrum of activity against gram-positive and gram-negative bacteria; they act by inhibiting cell wall synthesis

Carbonic anhydrase inhibitors Interfere with the production of aqueous humor, thereby reducing intraocular pressure associated with glaucoma

Cell-stimulating agents Improve immune function by stimulating the activity of various immune cells

Cholinergic Also known as parasympathomimetics; produce effects similar to those of acetylcholine

Cholinesterase inhibitors These enzymes destroy acetylcholine, the cholinergic neurotransmitter

Coating agent This drug, sucralfate, forms a complex that adheres to the crater of an ulcer, protecting it from aggravation from gastric secretions

Colony-stimulating factors Stimulate progenitor cells in bone marrow to increase numbers of leukocytes, thereby improving immune function

Corticosteroids These hormones are secreted by the cortex of the adrenal gland

Cycloplegics Anticholinergic agents that paralyze accommodation of the iris of the eye

Cytotoxics Agents that cause direct cell death; often used for cancer chemotherapy

Decongestants Reduce swelling in the nasal passages caused by a common cold or allergic rhinitis, usually by vasoconstriction

Digestants Combination products containing digestive enzymes used to treat various digestive disorders and to supplement deficiencies of natural digestive enzymes

Digitalis glycosides A class of drugs, also known as cardiac glycosides, that increase the force of contraction and slow the heart rate, thereby improving cardiac output

Diuretics Act to increase the flow of urine

Emetics Used to induce vomiting

Estrogens Steroids that cause feminizing effects

Expectorants Liquefy mucus by stimulating the natural lubricant fluids from the bronchial glands

Fluoroquinolones Ciprofloxacin and related agents; widely used broad-spectrum antibiotics

Gastric stimulants Used to increase stomach contractions, relax the pyloric valve, and increase peristalsis in the gastrointestinal tract; result in a decrease in gastric transit time and more rapid emptying of the intestinal tract

Glucocorticoids Also known as adrenocorticosteroids; are used to regulate carbohydrate, fat, and protein metabolism

Gonadal hormones Hormones produced by the testes in the male and ovaries in the female

Herbals Plant products usually sold as food supplements; may have pharmacologic effects that are not evaluated or regulated by the FDA

Histamine (H_2) antagonists Decrease the volume and increase the pH of gastric secretions both during the day and at night

HMG-CoA reductase enzyme inhibitors Also known as the statins; antilipemic agents that inhibit hydroxymethyl-glutaryl coenzyme A (HMG-CoA) reductase enzyme, the enzyme that stimulates the conversion of HMG-CoA to mevalonic acid, a precursor in the biosynthesis of cholesterol, thus reducing the potential for atherosclerosis

Hyperuricemics Used to decrease the production and increase the excretion of uric acid

Hypnotics Used to produce sleep

Incretin-mimetics Used to reduce basal glucose concentrations and elevated post-prandial glucose concentrations; used to treat diabetes mellitus

Insulins Hormone required for glucose transport to the cells

Lactation suppressants Used to prevent physiologic lactation

Laxatives Act by a variety of mechanisms to treat constipation

Low molecular weight heparins Derivatives of heparin; anticoagulants for the prophylactic treatment of pulmonary thromboembolism and deep vein thrombosis

Macrolides Erythromycin, azithromycin, and related antibiotics

MAO inhibitors Agents that block monoamine oxidase, thereby preventing the degradation and prolonging the action of norepinephrine and serotonin

Mineralocorticoids Steroids that cause the kidneys to retain sodium and water

Miotics Cause constriction of the iris

Mucolytics Reduce the thickness and stickiness of pulmonary secretions by acting directly on the mucus plugs to dissolve them

Muscle relaxants Relieve muscle spasms

Mydriatics Cause dilation of the iris

Neuromuscular blockers Skeletal muscle relaxants used to produce muscle relaxation during anesthesia; reduce the use and side effects of general anesthetics; used to ease endotracheal intubation and prevent laryngospasm

Nitrates Metabolize to nitric oxide, a potent vasodilator used to treat angina

Nonsteroidal antiinflammatory drugs (NSAIDs) These “aspirin-like” drugs are chemically unrelated to the salicylates but are prostaglandin inhibitors

Opioids Centrally acting analgesic agents related to morphine

Oral contraceptives Used for birth control; administered orally

Oral hypoglycemics Used in type 2 diabetes mellitus to improve glucose metabolism and lower blood glucose levels

Progestins Steroids regulating endometrial and myometrial function; used alone or in combination with estrogen for oral contraception

Protease inhibitors Saquinavir, ritonavir, indinavir, and related drugs; block the maturation of human immunodeficiency virus; used to treat HIV infections

Salicylates Effective as analgesics, antipyretics, and antiinflammatory agents

Sedatives Given to an individual to produce relaxation and rest; do not necessarily produce sleep

Selective serotonin reuptake inhibitors (SSRIs) Antidepressants that act by specifically blocking the reuptake of serotonin, thus prolonging its action

Serotonin antagonists Used to block serotonin; prevent emesis induced by chemotherapy, radiation therapy, and surgery

Statins (HMG-CoA reductase inhibitors) Agents that block the synthesis of cholesterol

Stool softeners or fecal softeners Draw water into the stool, thereby softening it

Sympatholytics Interfere with the storage and release of norepinephrine

Sympothomimetics Mimic the action of dopamine, norepinephrine, and epinephrine

Thrombolytics A specific group of drugs (alteplase, anistreplase, streptokinase, or urokinase) given to dissolve existing blood clots

Thyroid hormone antagonists Used to counteract or block the action of excessive formation of thyroid hormones

Thyroid hormones Used when thyroid hormones are not being produced or are not produced in sufficient quantities to meet the body’s physiologic needs

Tricyclic antidepressants Inhibit the reuptake of norepinephrine and serotonin (include doxepin, amitriptyline, and imipramine)

Uricosuric agents Act on the tubules of the kidneys to enhance the excretion of uric acid

Urinary analgesics Produce a local anesthetic effect on the mucosa of the ureters and bladder to relieve burning, pain, urgency, and frequency associated with urinary tract infections (UTIs)

Urinary antimicrobials Substances excreted and concentrated in the urine in sufficient amounts to have an antiseptic effect on the urine and the urinary tract

Uterine relaxants Used to primarily prevent preterm labor and delivery

Uterine stimulants Increase the frequency or strength of uterine contractions

Vaccines Suspensions of either live, attenuated, or killed bacteria or viruses administered to induce immunity against infection by specific bacteria or viruses

Vasodilators Relax the arteriolar smooth muscle, causing dilation of the blood vessels

Contents

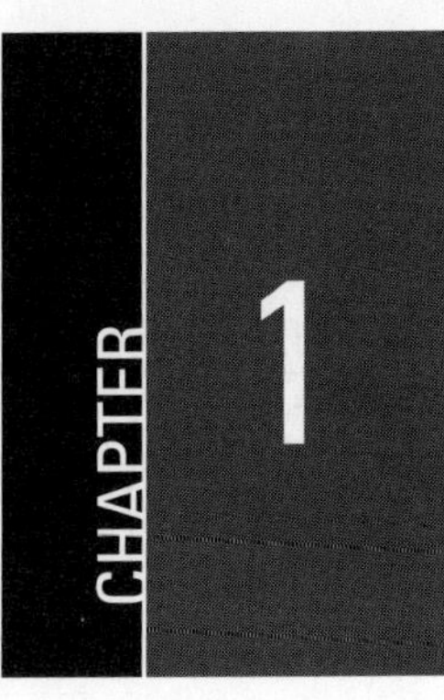

Definitions, Names, Standards, and Information Sources

Review Sheet

The QUESTION column and the ANSWER column have been offset so that you can cover the answer while reading the question, allowing you to assess your knowledge.

Question

1. Define *pharmacology.*
2. Define *drugs.*
3. Define *medicine.*
4. What is the chemical name of a drug?
5. What is the generic or nonproprietary name of a drug?
6. What is the official name of a drug?
7. What is the trademark, brand, or proprietary name of a drug?
8. What are some of the drug standards or official sources of American drug standards?
9. Summarize the Controlled Substances Act of 1970.
10. Summarize the steps of new drug development in the United States.

Answer

1. Pharmacology deals with the study of drugs and their actions on living organisms.
2. Drugs are chemical substances that have an effect on living organisms.
3. Therapeutic drugs are often called *medicines*; they are drugs used in the prevention and treatment of disease.
4. The chemical name of a drug is the chemical constitution of the drug and the exact placing of its atoms or molecular groupings. This name is most meaningful to the chemist.
5. Before a drug becomes official, it is given a generic name or common name. A generic name is simpler than the chemical name.
6. The official name of a drug is the name under which the drug is listed by the U.S. Food and Drug Administration.
7. This is the name of the drug that is registered and used by the owner of the drug who is usually the manufacturer.
8. Refer to the text for a review of these publications.
9. This Act repealed almost 50 other laws written since 1914 that relate to the control of drugs. The new composite law was designed to improve the administration and regulation of manufacturing, distributing, and dispensing of drugs that have been found necessary to be controlled. The Drug Enforcement Administration (DEA) was organized to enforce the Act. The basic structure of the Act consists of five classifications or schedules of controlled substances. Refer to the text for a detailed explanation of these five schedules.

10. *Preclinical research*: Begins with discovery, synthesis, and purification of the drugs. The goal at this stage is to use laboratory studies to determine whether the experimental drug has therapeutic value and whether the drug appears to be safe in animals.
    Clinical research and development: The "testing in humans" stage is subdivided into three phases. Phase 1 studies determine an experimental drug's pharmacologic properties, such as its pharmacokinetics, metabolism, and potential for toxicity at certain dosage. Phase 2 uses a smaller population of patients who have the condition the drug was designed to treat, and in phase 3 an even larger patient population is used to ensure statistical significance of the results.
    New Drug Application: When sufficient data have been collected to demonstrate that the experimental drug is both safe and effective, a New Drug Application is submitted to the FDA formally requesting approval to market a new drug for human use.
    Postmarketing surveillance: After the manufacturer decides to market the drug, this phase consists of an ongoing review of adverse effects of the new drug, as well as periodic inspection of the manufacturing facilities and products.

CHAPTER 1

Student Name ____________________

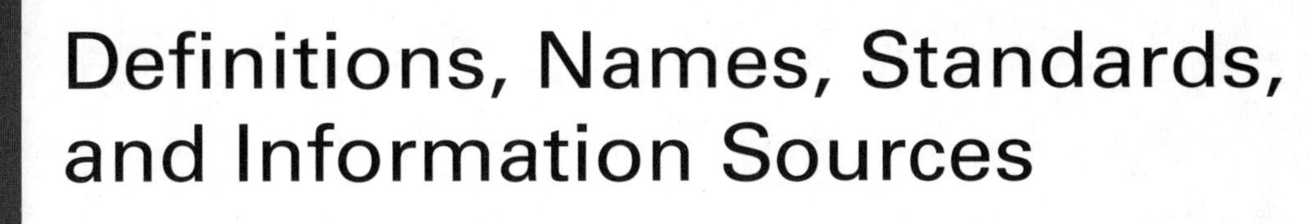

Definitions, Names, Standards, and Information Sources

Learning Activities

FILL-IN-THE-BLANK

Finish each of the following statements using the correct term.

1. Therapeutic drugs, often called ______________, are those drugs used in the prevention or treatment of diseases.
2. Before a drug becomes official, it is given a(n) ______________ name or common name. This name may be used in any country and by any manufacturer.
3. ______________ drugs, sometimes referred to as *recreational drugs*, are drugs or chemical substances used for nontherapeutic purposes.
4. The study of drugs and the actions they have in the human body is ______________.
5. The actual substance that causes the response in a living organism is a(n) ______________.

MATCHING

Using the textbook and other resources, match the drug with the corresponding DEA schedule. Schedules may be used more than once.

_____ 6. Darvocet N

_____ 7. Percodan

_____ 8. Tylox capsules

_____ 9. LevoDromoran

_____ 10. Diazepam

_____ 11. Flurazepam

_____ 12. Morphine sulfate

_____ 13. Meperidine

_____ 14. Tylenol with codeine no. 2

_____ 15. Tylenol with codeine no. 3

_____ 16. Tylenol with codeine no. 4

a. Schedule I
b. Schedule II
c. Schedule III
d. Schedule IV

TRUE OR FALSE

Mark "T" for true and "F" for false for each statement. Correct all false statements.

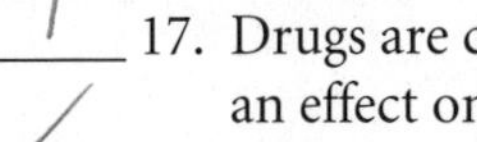

_____ 17. Drugs are chemical substances that have an effect on living organisms.

_____ 18. The Controlled Substances Act was passed by Congress in 2000.

_____ 19. The basic structure of the Controlled Substances Act consists of five classifications, or schedules, of controlled substances.

CHAPTER 1

Student Name ______________________________

Definitions, Names, Standards, and Information Sources

Practice Questions for the NCLEX Examination

_____ 1. Those patients who participate in "testing in humans" are part of which phase of new drug development?
1. Preclinical research and development stage
2. Clinical research and development stage
3. New drug application review
4. Postmarketing surveillance

_____ 2. Which of the following is the drug name used in the United States under which the drug is listed by the U. S. Food and Drug Administration (FDA)?
1. Chemical name
2. Generic name
3. Official name
4. Trademark name

_____ 3. Which of the following are considered to be therapeutic methods for the treatment of illness? (Select all that apply.)
1. Drug therapy
2. Diet therapy
3. Physiotherapy
4. Psychologic therapy

_____ 4. According to the Controlled Substances Act of 1970, drugs with a high potential for abuse that have no current accepted medical use in the United States and that have a lack of accepted safety for use under medical supervision are classified under which schedule?
1. Schedule I
2. Schedule II
3. Schedule III
4. Schedule IV

_____ 5. Which of the following are acceptable sources of drug information when seeking information about prescription medications? (Select all that apply.)
1. *American Drug Index*
2. *Physician's Drug Reference*
3. *American Hospital Formulary Service, Drug Information*
4. *Drug Interaction Facts*

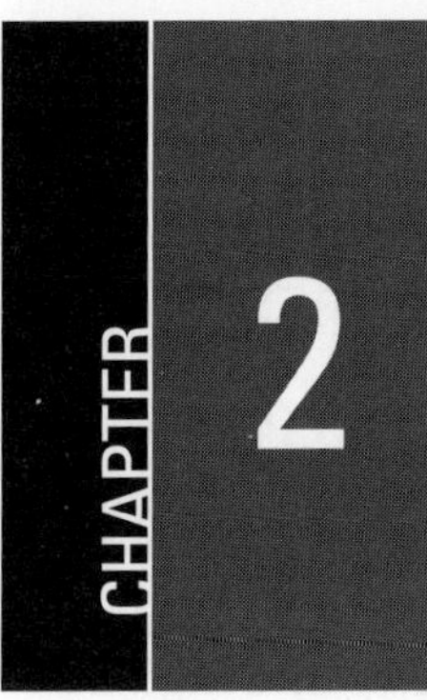

Principles of Drug Action and Drug Interactions

Review Sheet

Note: Understanding the vocabulary associated with the study of pharmacology is fundamental to understanding the remaining information presented in the textbook. Therefore, the first step is to define and memorize the vocabulary. The second step is to apply the vocabulary learned during the pharmacology course. The third step in learning pharmacology is to apply the vocabulary during the actual clinical practice of nursing.

The QUESTION column and the ANSWER column have been offset so you can cover the answer while reading the question, allowing you to assess your knowledge. Define the following vocabulary.

Question

1. Pharmacodynamics
2. Receptors
3. Agonists
4. Antagonists
5. Partial agonists
6. ADME
7. Pharmacokinetics
8. Absorption
9. Enteral
10. Parenteral
11. Percutaneous
12. Distribution

Answer

1. The study of drug interactions including the drug receptors and the series of events that culminates in a pharmacologic response.
2. Sites on the cells where chemical bonding of drugs occurs are receptors.
3. Drugs that stimulate a response at a receptor site are agonists.
4. Drugs that attach to receptor sites but do NOT stimulate a response are antagonists.
5. Drugs that interact with a receptor to stimulate a response and concurrently inhibit other responses are partial agonists.
6. ADME is an abbreviation for the four stages of drug processing: absorption, distribution, metabolism, and excretion.
7. Pharmacokinetics is the study of the mathematical relationship among the absorption, distribution, metabolism, and excretion of medicines.
8. Absorption is the process by which a drug is made available to the body fluids for distribution.
9. The enteral route of drug administration is placing the drug directly into the gastrointestinal tract by oral, rectal, or nasogastric routes.
10. Parenteral routes of drug administration are subcutaneous, intramuscular (IM), or intravenous (IV) injection.
11. Percutaneous drug administration is done via inhalation, sublingual, or topical routes.

13. Drug blood level
14. Biotransformation (metabolism)
15. Excretion
16. Half-life
17. Desired action
18. Side effects
19. Adverse effects
20. Idiosyncratic reaction
21. Allergic reactions
22. Urticaria (hives)
23. Carcinogenicity
24. Teratogen
25. Placebo

12. The term *distribution* refers to the ways in which drugs are transported by the circulating body fluids to the sites of action (receptors) for metabolism and excretion.
13. The drug blood level measures the amount of a drug present in the blood to determine if it is within the therapeutic range, below the range (subtherapeutic), or above the range (toxic).
14. *Metabolism* and *biotransformation* are defined as the process by which a drug is inactivated (broken down). The terms are used interchangeably.
15. Excretion of a drug is the elimination of the active drug or its metabolites from the body.
16. The time required for one-half, or 50%, of the drug administered to be excreted from the body.
17. Desired action is the achievement of the expected response to the drug administered.
18. Most side effects are predictable responses seen when a specific drug is administered. (The drug monographs throughout the textbook will give suggested nursing actions that can make these anticipated reactions more tolerable to the patient.)
19. Adverse effects are side effects that are more serious and require reporting to the HCP for further orders on how to manage these reactions. These are sometimes referred to as *drug toxicity reactions*. Adverse effects are labeled "side effects to report" throughout this textbook. See also World Health Organization definition on p. 19.
20. Idiosyncratic reactions are reactions that are not predictable; they are unusual or abnormal responses to the drug administered.
21. An allergic reaction, also called a *hypersensitivity reaction*, occurs in an individual who has previously taken the drug and is sensitized to it. With repeated administration of the drug, antibodies formed when the drug was first given respond to the repeated exposure, producing an undesirable response such as severe itching, urticaria (hives), or in more severe cases, collapse of the respiratory and cardiovascular systems, known as *anaphylactic reaction* or *anaphylaxis*, a life-threatening situation.
22. Urticaria or hives are elevated, irregular, patchlike rashes on the skin accompanied by itching.
23. Carcinogenicity is the ability of a drug to cause living cells to be altered (mutate) and become cancerous.
24. A drug that causes birth defects is a teratogen.

26. Tolerance
27. Drug dependence
28. Drug accumulation
29. Drug interaction
30. Unbound drug
31. Additive effect
32. Synergistic effect
33. Antagonistic effect
34. Displacement
35. Interference
36. Incompatibility

25. A placebo is a drug dosage form that contains no active ingredients.
26. Tolerance occurs when higher doses of a drug are required to achieve the same effects that a lower dose once achieved.
27. Drug dependence, also called *addiction* or *habituation*, occurs when the individual is no longer able to control the ingestion of the drug.
28. Drug accumulation occurs when there is an excess amount of a drug in the body due to a number of possible physiologic variables. This can result in drug toxicity.
29. Drug interaction occurs when one drug being administered changes the action of other drugs being used at the same time.
30. Unbound or free drug is the active amount of drug available to achieve the desired physiologic response.
31. Additive effect occurs when two drugs with similar actions have an increased effect.
32. Synergistic effect occurs when the combined effect of two drugs is greater than the effect of each drug given alone.
33. Antagonistic effect occurs when one drug interferes with the action of another.
34. Displacement occurs when one drug is moved from the protein binding sites by a second drug. This usually increases the activity of the first drug because it is now unbound.
35. Interference occurs when one drug inhibits the metabolism or excretion of a second drug, causing increased activity of the second drug.
36. Incompatibility occurs when one drug is chemically incompatible with another drug, resulting in deterioration of the drug.

CHAPTER 2

Student Name ______________________________

Principles of Drug Action and Drug Interactions

Learning Activities

FILL-IN-THE-BLANK

Finish each of the following statements using the correct term.

1. Drugs that interact with a receptor to stimulate a response are known as ______________.

2. The study of the mathematical relationships among the absorption, distribution, metabolism, and excretion of individual medicines over time is called ______________.

3. ______________ is the process by which a drug is transferred from its site of entry into the body to the circulating fluids of the body for distribution.

4. ______________ or ______________ is a skin reaction to antibodies that is most commonly manifested as raised irregularly shaped patches on the skin with severe itching.

5. ______________ is the ability of a drug to induce living cells to mutate and become cancerous.

6. A drug interaction that produces an increased action is known as a(n) ______________ effect.

7. Two drugs with similar actions that produce an effect substantially greater than either drug administered alone are said to be ______________.

8. When one drug moves the original drug administered from a binding site to produce an increased drug effect, this is known as ______________.

9. Drug ______________ is defined as one drug chemically destroying a second drug if mixed together prior to administration.

TRUE OR FALSE

Mark "T" for true or "F" for false for each statement. Correct all false statements.

_____ 10. Drugs that attach to a receptor but do not stimulate a response are called *antagonists*.

_____ 11. In the enteral route, the drug bypasses the gastrointestinal tract.

_____ 12. Drugs that interact with a receptor to stimulate a response but inhibit other responses are called *partial agonists*.

_____ 13. A drug that induces a birth defect is known as a *teratogen*.

_____ 14. Drug dependence occurs when a person begins to require a higher dosage to produce the same effects that a lower dosage once provided.

_____ 15. Percutaneous route is the administration of drugs by subcutaneous, intramuscular, or intravenous injection.

_____ 16. Enteral route is the administration of drugs to the gastrointestinal tract.

_____ 17. Agonists stimulate a response at a receptor site on the cells.

_____ 18. Partial agonists stimulate some responses while inhibiting others at a receptor site on the cells.

F 19. Parenteral route is the administration of drugs by inhalation, sublingual, or topical methods.

T 20. Receptors are specific sites within the body where a drug acts.

F 21. Antagonists cause a drug response at a receptor site.

T 22. *Absorption* refers to the ability of a drug to be integrated into the body fluids.

F 23. Metabolism is the activation of a drug for use by the body. deactivation?

T 24. Distribution is the transportation of a drug by the body fluids for utilization within the body.

T 25. Excretion of a drug is the elimination of a drug from the body.

F 26. *Biotransformation* is another term for excretion of a drug.

T 27. Drug blood level is a measurement of the amount of drug present in the blood at the specific time of the blood draw.

CHAPTER 2

Student Name______________________________

Principles of Drug Action and Drug Interactions

Practice Questions for the NCLEX Examination

_____ 1. The primary routes for drug excretion are:
1. skin and lungs.
2. gastrointestinal tract and skin.
3. renal tubules and GI tract.
4. lungs and renal tubules.

_____ 2. Drug distribution occurs by:
1. decreasing body protein levels.
2. transporting in blood and lymphatic systems.
3. keeping the drug at toxic levels.
4. increasing the amount of adipose tissue.

_____ 3. When a combination of two drugs will provide a greater effect than the sum of the effect of each drug if given alone, this is called a(n):
1. additive effect.
2. synergistic effect.
3. antagonistic effect.
4. displacement.

_____ 4. A partial agonist is a drug that:
1. stimulates action at receptor sites within the circulating blood.
2. stimulates one response and inhibits another response.
3. inhibits response when attached to a receptor site.
4. stimulates a response at a receptor site.

_____ 5. Another name for an idiosyncratic reaction is a(n):
1. allergic reaction.
2. unexpected reaction.
3. teratogenic reaction.
4. drug overresponse.

_____ 6. The literature states that the half-life of a particular drug is 8 hours. This means _____% of the drug will have been excreted in this time period.
1. 25
2. 30
3. 50
4. 75

_____ 7. A *desired* drug action is:
1. the predictable/usual response to the drug.
2. an unusual or idiosyncratic response to a drug.
3. capable of inducing cell mutations.
4. the development of symptoms that should be reported to the prescribing physician.

_____ 8. Mr. Y. now requires a higher dose of a pain medication to produce the same effect that a lower dose of the medication once provided. The nurse identifies this phenomenon as:
1. placebo effect.
2. tolerance.
3. drug dependence.
4. drug accumulation.

_____ 9. The term used to describe the effect of a first drug inhibiting metabolism or excretion of a second drug, causing increased activity of the second drug, is:
1. interference.
2. incompatibility.
3. displacement.
4. reaction.

_____ 10. Nurses working with patients who have disease of the ________ are at an increased risk of developing toxicity to the drug because most drugs are eliminated through this organ system.

1. lungs
2. pancreas
3. heart
4. kidneys

_____ 11. The nurse identifies which of the following factors as affecting pharmacokinetics? (Select all that apply.)

1. Age
2. Disease
3. Dehydration
4. Psychological factors
5. Drug tolerance
6. Smoking and alcohol use

_____ 12. When obtaining a trough level of a drug to assess serum drug levels, most trough levels of drugs are drawn usually ______ minutes before the next dose.

1. 10
2. 20
3. 30
4. 45

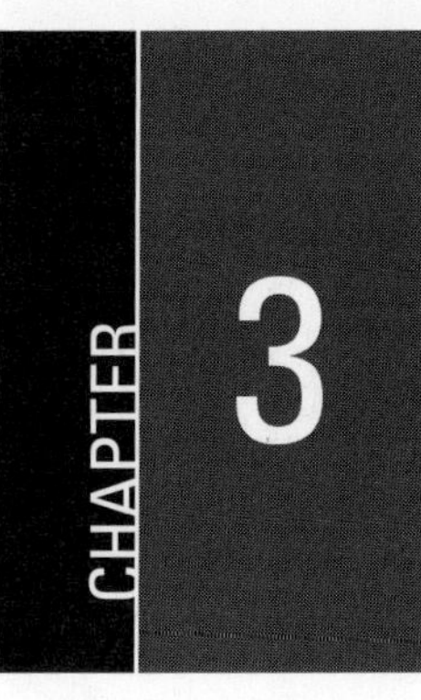

Drug Action Across the Life Span

Review Sheet

The QUESTION column and the ANSWER column have been offset so you can cover the answer while reading the question, allowing you to assess your knowledge.

Question

1. What are common terms used to refer to individuals of different ages up to 5 years old?
2. What is the meaning of *gender-specific medicine*?
3. What are the underlying rationales for the erratic absorption of intramuscular (IM) drugs in both the neonate and the geriatric population?
4. Define *passive diffusion*. (Research other sources.)
5. Define *carrier-mediated diffusion*. (Research other sources.)
6. Define *active transport*. (Research other sources.)
7. State two factors that influence drug absorption from the gastrointestinal tract.

Answer

1. Fewer than 38 weeks = premature, 0–1 months = newborn or neonate,
   1–24 months = infant or baby, 1–5 years = young child.
2. Gender-specific medicine is a new area of pharmacology that studies the differences in the response of females and males to prescribed drugs.
3. The underlying rationales for the erratic absorption of IM drugs are differences in muscle mass and blood flow to muscles and muscular inactivity in the bedridden patient.
4. Passive diffusion is the most common mechanism associated with drug absorption. It requires no cellular energy and involves the movement of a drug from an area of high concentration to an area of low concentration.
5. Carrier-mediated diffusion, or facilitated transport or diffusion, occurs when the drug molecules combine with a carrier substance such as an enzyme or other protein. An example is glucose combining with insulin to be carried from the bloodstream into the cell, moving from an area of high concentration (the bloodstream) to an area of low concentration (the cell). In other words, the drug needs help to pass across the cell membrane and the insulin passively provides the transport. This passive process requires no cellular energy.
6. Active transport involves the movement of drug molecules from an area of low concentration to an area of high concentration. This process requires cellular energy to accomplish the movement.

8. Compare the gastric pH in a premature infant, newborn, infant, adult, and older adult.
9. Compare gastric emptying time in a premature infant, adult, and older adult.
10. Look up the term *hydrolysis* in a dictionary.
11. In the newborn, what factor affects the absorption of drugs during the process of hydrolysis?
12. If gastric emptying time increases, what happens to the speed of absorption of a drug?
13. What is the purpose of performing therapeutic drug monitoring?
14. What effect does the route of drug administration have on drug absorption?
15. List accurate methods of measuring oral liquid medications.
16. What nursing actions are appropriate when "off-label use" of medications is prescribed?
17. Why is transdermal absorption of a drug in an older adult difficult to predict?

7. Passive diffusion and gastric emptying time influence the absorption of drugs in the intestinal tract. Both passive diffusion and gastric emptying time are dependent on pH.
8. The gastric pH values are:

premature	6–8
newborn	6–8; decreases to 2–4 in 24 hrs
infant	1–3
adult	1–3
older adult	pH is increased due to decreasing number of acid-secreting cells

9. Premature infants and geriatric patients have slower gastric emptying time; therefore, the drug is in contact with the absorptive tissue longer. This may result in more absorption and a higher serum concentration of the drug in the blood.
10. Hydrolysis is the chemical alteration or decomposition of a compound with water.
11. In an infant, the absence of enzymes needed for hydrolysis of certain drugs influences the ability of the drug to be absorbed.
12. The faster the gastric emptying time, the less time the drug has to be absorbed; therefore, drug absorption is decreased.
13. Assays measure blood levels of specific drugs, providing a means to identify needed dosage adjustments.
14. In general, drug absorption is affected by: dosage form (e.g., liquid versus enteric-coated tablets); route of drug administration (e.g., oral, intramuscular, inhalation); solubility of the drug; gastrointestinal function; the condition of the absorptive surface (e.g., inflamed, open skin area versus intact skin); and blood flow to and from the site.
15. Use medicine cups, droppers provided with a specific medication, or oral syringes to measure liquid forms of oral medications accurately.
16. "Off-label use" of medications is legal; however, nurses should check reliable references or with the pharmacist for further information. In all cases, monitor the patient carefully for side effects or adverse effects whenever the medicine is administered.

18. What factors affect drug distribution?
19. Examine Table 3-1 on p. 27 of the text. Compare the total percentage of body water in a premature infant, a full-term infant, a 1-year-old infant, and a male adult. What conclusion(s) did you reach?
20. What effect will a higher percentage of total body water have on drug absorption?
21. Research the meaning of *lipid-soluble* and *water-soluble.*
22. Define *protein binding.*
23. What happens to the concentration of albumin in the body after the age 40?
24. What happens to the rate of drug metabolism in older adults?
25. How functional is the renal filtration system of preterm infants and of full-term newborns when compared to that of an adult?
26. What effect do age and renal function have on drug dosages?
27. What test is used as the best predictor to estimate renal function in older adults?
28. Define *polypharmacy.*

17. In an older adult, there is decreased dermal thickness that may increase drug absorption; however, there may be drying, wrinkling, and decreased hair follicles that decrease absorption. There is often decreased cardiac output, which results in decreased blood flow to the tissues (decreased tissue perfusion), which results in decreased drug absorption.
18. Distribution is dependent on pH, body water concentration (intracellular, extracellular, and total body water), presence and quantity of fat tissue, protein binding, cardiac output, and regional blood flow.
19. The younger the individual, the higher the percentage of the total body water.
20. A higher percentage of total body water means drugs that are water-soluble will be more rapidly distributed and the individual may require a higher dose of these drugs. Conversely, fat-soluble drugs would be poorly absorbed.
21. Water-soluble drugs have an affinity for body fluids and are quickly absorbed and excreted through the kidneys; therefore, water-soluble drugs often have a shorter half-life. Lipid-soluble drugs have an affinity for fat tissue in the body and will often have a longer half-life.
22. Protein binding occurs when a drug binds to proteins in the body, such as albumin. When "bound," the drug is not "free" or actively available for use at the receptor sites for action.
23. Total albumin concentration decreases after age 40, while other proteins increase. This results in an increase in unbound drug making more free drug available for action and metabolism.
24. The number of functioning hepatic cells and the blood flow decreases with aging, resulting in slower drug metabolism. As drug metabolism decreases, drug doses must be reduced to prevent accumulation of the drug, producing toxicity.
25. At birth, preterm infants have approximately 15% of the renal capacity of an adult and full-term infants have approximately 35%.
26. Drug doses must be adjusted so an adequate, therapeutic serum blood concentration is maintained. Increased age and decreased renal function often require a reduced dosage.
27. The urine creatinine test is used to estimate renal function in older adults.

29. Describe the safest method of initiating newly prescribed medications to a geriatric patient.
30. Identify principles of drug administration that are specifically applicable to a pregnant patient.

28. Polypharmacy is the use of multiple drugs concurrently.

29. Drug dosage should be initiated at 1/3 to 1/2 the normal adult dose and, whenever available, therapeutic drug monitoring should be completed.
30. Take a thorough drug history of all prescribed and over-the-counter medications and "street drugs" being taken. Ask specifically about any herbal remedies or nutritional supplements being taken. Ask about the use of alcohol, tobacco, and herbal products during pregnancy. Refer to Tables 3-6 and 3-7, pp. 33-34 in the textbook.

CHAPTER 3

Student Name ____________________

Drug Action Across the Life Span

Learning Activities

FILL-IN-THE-BLANK

Finish each of the following statements using the correct term.

1. ____________________ medicine is a developing science that studies the differences in the normal function of men and women and how people of each sex perceive and experience disease.
2. At ____________________ year(s) of age, the child's stomach pH approximates that of an adult.
3. Drugs that are relatively insoluble are transported in the circulation by being bound to ____________________ proteins.
4. Certain medicines require that blood be drawn twice to assess both subtherapeutic levels and the potential for toxicity. One of the levels is drawn at 30 minutes before the next dose is to be administered to obtain the ____________________ or lowest blood level of medicine, and another is drawn at 20 minutes after the medicine has been administered intravenously to obtain the ____________________ or highest blood level.
5. ____________________ is the term used to describe patients requiring multiple drug therapy.

TRUE OR FALSE

Mark "T" for true and "F" for false for each statement. Correct all false statements.

F 6. Transdermal administration of drugs to the geriatric population is often difficult to predict because dermal thickness increases with aging.

F 7. Medicines given intramuscularly are usually erratically absorbed in both neonates and older adults.

T 8. Men and women respond to medications differently.

_____ 9. Therapeutic drug monitoring is the measurement of a drug's concentration in biologic fluids to correlate the dosage administered and the level of medicine in the body with the pharmacologic response.

T 10. Drug metabolism is the process by which the body inactivates medicines.

_____ 11. The older adult population includes people 65 years and older.

F 12. Absorption of drugs administered intramuscularly is consistent and predictable.

T 13. Transdermal drug absorption has a predictable rate.

T 14. Enteric-coated and sustained-release tablets are absorbed erratically if crushed.

_____ 15. Passive diffusion requires cellular energy.

T 16. The gastric emptying time of an older adult and a premature infant are slow and result in increased drug absorption.

_____ 17. Hydrolysis involves the chemical breakdown of a compound, such as a drug, in water.

_____ 18. The older adult patient has a greater percentage of total body fluid than an infant.

_____ 19. Drug elimination is affected by the number of functional renal tubules.

_____ 20. Albumin is a protein to which drugs bind for transport.

_____ 21. "Unbound" drug is the active portion of the drug dose available for the desired drug action.

_____ 22. "Bound" drug is the portion of the drug causing the desired drug action.

_____ 23. The term *infant* is used to signify babies 0–1 month of age.

_____ 24. Gender-specific medicine studies how disease differences affect normal functions of men and women.

_____ 25. The pH environment of the gastrointestinal tract affects passive diffusion and gastric emptying time.

_____ 26. Some drugs such as erythromycin, prednisolone, diazepam, and verapamil are metabolized more rapidly in men than in women.

_____ 27. Saliva assays may be used for therapeutic drug monitoring of some types of medications.

_____ 28. "Peak" and "trough" laboratory values should be communicated promptly to the prescribing health care provider.

_____ 29. Household teaspoons provide a safe, reliable measurement for drug doses.

_____ 30. Many drugs, in addition to street drugs, may be teratogenic.

CHAPTER 3

Student Name ______________________________

Drug Action Across the Life Span

Practice Questions for the NCLEX Examination

_____ 1. Which one of the following statements is correct when considering specific needs of pediatric patients receiving medications?
1. Infants and young children have a lower total body water content than adults.
2. Many medicines are not approved by the FDA for use in children.
3. Salicylates are most effective when administered to pediatric patients from infancy through their teenage years.
4. Administration of ibuprofen to children is a common cause of Reye's syndrome.

_____ 2. When administering medications to a 2-year-old child, which is the most likely to cause an allergic reaction?
1. Digoxin
2. Acetaminophen
3. Penicillin
4. Dilantin

_____ 3. A 76-year-old patient has just completed a teaching session with the nurse on safe medication administration. Which of the following statements by the patient causes the nurse to conclude that more teaching is needed?
1. "I should not start any type of pills including those from the health food store unless I first clear it with my primary health care provider."
2. "I will go to the laboratory as directed to have my blood levels of drugs measured as indicated."
3. "I will get rid of any old pills I was taking to avoid confusion with the current pills I am taking."
4. "I will take all of my pills at the same time each day to avoid having to take them throughout the day."

_____ 4. When teaching a group of pregnant patients about the use of medications during pregnancy, the nurse would include which one of the following statements?
1. "Because of the potential for injury to the developing fetus, drug therapy during pregnancy should be avoided if at all possible."
2. "It is all right to drink alcohol during pregnancy as long as you keep it to just wine."
3. "If you smoke, you should cut back to just five cigarettes a day. That way you are guaranteed of having no problems."
4. "You can use any herbal medicine you like because they are natural and will not hurt the baby."

_____ 5. The nurse is teaching a postdelivery patient about breastfeeding, including information on drug administration with breastfeeding mothers. Which of the following statements by the patient indicates that more teaching is needed?

1. "It is safe for me to take all of my prescription medications because my doctor would not order anything that isn't all right."
2. "If I need to take medicine, I will take it immediately after my baby has finished breastfeeding."
3. "I will discuss the use of any herbal products with my primary care provider before I take them because they can affect my baby."
4. "I know that many drugs are known to enter breast milk, so I will be sure to ask my primary care provider about any drugs before I take them."

_____ 6. When administering drugs to older adult patients, distribution and subsequent effects of the drugs on these patients are different than those expected in the adult population, because older adults: (Select all that apply.)

1. have an increased metabolism.
2. have a slower circulation.
3. often have factors such as diabetes and liver or renal failure which make them more prone to experience toxic effects necessitating dosage adjustments.
4. have an increased hepatic blood flow.

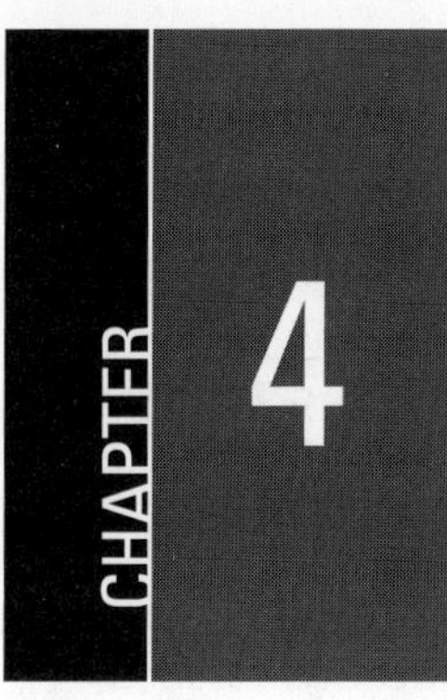

The Nursing Process and Pharmacology

Review Sheet

The QUESTION column and the ANSWER column have been offset so that you can cover the answer while reading the question, allowing you to assess your knowledge.

Question	Answer
1. Identify the purpose of nursing classification systems.	
2. Define *nursing diagnosis.*	1. Nursing classification systems provide a standardized language for recording and analysis of individualized nursing care delivery.
3. State the five steps of the nursing process.	2. A nursing diagnosis is a clinical judgment about individual, family, or community responses to actual or potential health problems/life processes.
4. Explain the purpose of the assessment phase of the nursing process.	3. The five steps of the nursing process are assessment, nursing diagnosis, planning, implementation, and evaluation.
5. What are defining characteristics?	4. Assessment is an ongoing data-gathering process that starts with the admission of the patient and continues until the patient is discharged from care. It is the problem-identifying phase of the nursing process used to identify existing (actual) patient problems and/or to identify patient problems that may be evolving.
6. How does a medical diagnosis differ from a nursing diagnosis?	5. Defining characteristics are existing signs and symptoms that help define the presence of a patient problem. They provide clinical evidence of an existing or developing patient problem.
7. What is a collaborative problem?	6. A medical diagnosis is a statement relating to a disease's or disorder's effect on the individual's physiological functioning. A nursing diagnosis usually refers to the patient's ability to function in activities in daily living (ADLs) in relation to the impairment induced by the medical diagnosis. It identifies the individual's or group's response to the illness and defines a patient problem in which the nurse can intervene.
8. Why is a focused assessment beneficial to the nurse?	7. Collaborative problems require both medical or dental prescriptive orders and nursing interventions to monitor and evaluate the existing condition.

9. Differentiate among actual, risk, possible, wellness, and syndrome nursing diagnoses.
10. Explain the intent of using critical pathways.
11. What are the four phases of the planning process used to prepare to provide patient care?
12. Use Maslow's hierarchy of needs on p. 44 of the text to label and prioritize the following individual needs:
    a. need for family visitors,
    b. need to avoid falls while ambulating,
    c. need for basic care to prevent skin breakdown,
    d. need for praise for learning about self-care.
13. Which of the following are nursing actions?
    a. giving a bed bath
    b. forcing fluids
    c. taking vital signs
    d. developing a medical diagnosis statement
14. Label the following nursing actions as "D" for dependent, "I" for interdependent, and "ID" for independent:
    a. administering a tube feeding
    b. administering PRN medications
    c. positioning patient for comfort
    d. providing oral hygiene
    e. monitoring respiratory function between treatments by respiratory therapist
15. Develop a short-term goal for a patient receiving Maalox.
16. Explain why a drug history may be beneficial.

8. After establishing that a patient problem may or does exist, a focused assessment allows the nurse to concentrate the data collection process on a specific area that would help to define, validate, or negate the existence of a specific nursing diagnosis.
9. See definitions in textbook, pp. 39-40.
10. Critical pathways provide a sequential, detailed plan for clinical interventions within a specified time period for a particular disease or disorder.
11. Planning encompasses: a) setting priorities, b) developing measurable goal statements, c) formulating nursing interventions, and d) developing anticipated therapeutic outcomes as a basis for evaluating the patient's status.
12. During a period of ambulation, these needs would be in the following order: b, c, a, d. The priority may vary depending on variables present.
13. a, b, and c are nursing actions.
14. Items a and b are dependent, c and d are independent, and e is interdependent. Note: d could be dependent if the oral hygiene was specifically ordered by the HCP.
15. Multiple possible answers. One example is: The patient will be able to state the correct schedule for self-administration of Maalox on Tuesday, (date).

17. Label the following statements "S" for subjective data or "O" for objective data.
    a. "My medication makes me dizzy."
    b. "Yesterday the pain medication gave me good pain relief."
    c. One hour after administration of chemotherapy the nurse charts, "Patient vomited 4 ounces greenish-tinged, watery vomitus."
18. Turn to a drug classification section in the textbook. Find the area labeled Nursing Diagnosis. Explain the difference between indications and side effects when used to designate the nursing diagnoses associated with drug therapy.
19. Develop a statement for the therapeutic intent of a sedative for a patient having surgery tomorrow morning.
20. Differentiate between side effects to expect and side effects to report.
21. List common laboratory studies used to evaluate liver (hepatic) function and those used to evaluate kidney (renal) function.
22. When are culture and sensitivity (C&S) tests taken?
23. What changes in the baseline CBC report should be reported to the HCP?
24. Why are serum drug levels monitored?
25. What patient education should be done prior to discharge for all patients with medications prescribed?

16. A drug history can be used to identify current drugs, OTC, and herbal products being taken or problems relating to drug therapy and to evaluate the need for medications.
17. Items a and b are subjective; c is objective.
18. Indications are nursing diagnosis statements that exist as a result of patient problems being experienced due to disruption of normal functioning by a disease process or disorder. Side effects are patient problems that have evolved as a result of drug therapy.
19. Therapeutic intent is to "provide rest and relaxation prior to surgery."
20. Side effects to expect are those that can generally be anticipated when the drug therapy is prescribed. It is important for the nurse to teach the patient steps he/she can take to minimize the side effects to make the drug therapy more tolerable. Side effects to report, also known as adverse drug effects, are those that require notification of the physician regarding the drug's action.
21. Hepatic function tests include AST, ALT, alkaline phosphatase, LDH, and GGT. Renal function tests include serum creatinine, creatinine clearance, blood urea nitrogen (BUN), and urinalysis.
22. C&S specimens (e.g., throat culture) are usually obtained prior to initiation of antibiotic therapy for an infection.
23. Elevated WBCs, bands, "segs," and/or lymphocytes should be reported.
24. Serum drug levels are monitored to establish whether the serum blood level of the specific drug is too low or in the nontherapeutic range, within the normal range and therapeutic, or too high and toxic to the patient.

26. List a minimum of five drugs that can be monitored by a blood draw.

25. Patient education before discharge should include drug name, dosage, route, and specific time(s) of administration; reason for taking the drug (therapeutic outcome or intent); side effects to expect and ways these can be minimized or eliminated; side effects to report; what to do if a dose is missed; and how to have the medication prescription filled.
26. Digoxin, theophylline, gentamicin, tobramycin, lithium, lidocaine, phenytoin, procainamide, quinidine, vancomycin, cyclosporine, and chloramphenicol can be monitored by a blood draw.

CHAPTER 4

Student Name ______________________________

The Nursing Process and Pharmacology

Learning Activities

FILL-IN-THE-BLANK

Complete the following statements using the correct term.

1. A(n) ____________________ diagnosis is a statement of the patient's alterations in structure and function, and results in a diagnosis of a disease or disorder that impairs normal physiologic function.

2. A(n) ____________________ nursing diagnosis is a clinical judgment about an individual, group, or community in transition from a specific level of wellness to a higher level of wellness.

3. A(n) ______________ ______________ ______________ is a standardized care plan derived from "best practice" patterns, enabling the nurse to develop a treatment plan that sequences detailed clinical interventions to be performed over a projected amount of time for a specific case type or disease process.

4. Mary tells you she developed nausea and vomiting 4 hours after taking the first dose of her newly prescribed antibiotic. This would be an example of (subjective, objective) data.

5. The nursing instructor tells the student nurse to collect further data relating to Mary's case. The collection of patient data is known as the ____________________ phase of the nursing process.

6. Further inquiry reveals that Mary took the antibiotic on an empty stomach. In addition to gaining further information about the nausea and vomiting, the student nurse also asks Mary to tell her of all other medications being taken, both prescription and nonprescription. This is known as taking a(n) ______________ ______________. Mary indicates that she does not regularly take any other medicine.

7. After collecting the data, the student reviews the drug monograph on the antibiotic. It states that nausea and vomiting are side effects to expect if taken on an empty stomach. The student nurse compares the signs and symptoms present with the ______________ ______________ listed in a nursing diagnosis resource book to establish the actual ______________ ______________.

8. Rescheduling of the time the medication is taken is an example of a nursing ____________________. The student nurse suggests that Mary take the next dose of the medication with food.

9. Mary will self-administer the prescribed antibiotic with food at 6 AM, 12 noon, 6 PM, and midnight starting with the next dose. This is a(n) ______________ ______________ statement.

10. When a culture and sensitivity is ordered on a patient, it is important to be sure the test is performed ____________________ the first dose of medication is administered.

11. Nursing diagnosis statements dealing with a patient with a family history of a disease who is likely to develop the disease would be called ____________________ nursing diagnosis statements.

12. An example of a phase of the nursing process called ____________________ is the periodic review of goals/outcomes of care.

13. A nursing minimum data set is an example of a(n) ______________ ______________ ______________.

TRUE OR FALSE

Mark "T" for true and "F" for false for each statement. Correct all false statements.

_____ 14. The nursing process is the foundation for the clinical practice of nursing.

_____ 15. Nurses should familiarize themselves with the nurse practice act in the state where they practice, to identify the educational and experiential qualifications necessary to perform physical assessment and develop nursing diagnoses.

_____ 16. A risk/high-risk nursing diagnosis is a clinical judgment that an individual, family, or community is more susceptible to the problem than others in the same or similar situation.

_____ 17. The measurable goal statements start with the specific amount of time allotted for attainment of a certain behavior followed by the nursing actions to be followed.

_____ 18. Evaluation of the expected outcomes of the patient's behavior is the final step of the nursing process.

CHAPTER 4

Student Name ____________

The Nursing Process and Pharmacology

Practice Questions for the NCLEX Examination

_____ 1. The nurse identifies which of the following as the proper sequence of the nursing process?
1. Planning, intervention, evaluation, assessment
2. Nursing diagnosis statement, assessment, planning, intervention, evaluation
3. Assessment, nursing diagnoses statement, planning, intervention, evaluation
4. Planning, nursing diagnosis statement, intervention, evaluation

_____ 2. In which phase of the nursing process does the nurse set priorities, develop written outcome statements, formulate nursing interventions, formulate anticipated therapeutic outcomes, and integrate outcomes/classification system into critical pathways and/or care plans?
1. Implementation
2. Evaluation
3. Nursing diagnosis
4. Planning

_____ 3. The nurse identifies which one of the following as the priority ranking of Maslow's subcategory of human needs?
1. Personal growth and maturity
2. Love and affection
3. Protection from physical harm
4. Oxygen, circulation

_____ 4. When incorporating the nursing process into medication administration, the nurse would follow which of the following practices in obtaining a drug history? (Select all that apply.)
1. Report any weight loss associated with use of the drug but not weight gain as this is an expected side effect of medication administration.
2. Ask the patient about drugs currently being taken as well as those drugs which the patient has taken in the past year.
3. Ask the patient about any drug allergies and the specifics about the reaction that occurs as well as treatments used for the reaction.
4. Record any over-the-counter medications the patient states are being taken into the clinical record.

_____ 5. Which of the following pieces of information are necessary when obtaining a medication history of a patient? (Select all that apply.)
1. Use of herbal medicines or vitamins
2. Use of illegal drugs
3. Diet
4. Use of over-the-counter medications
5. Sexual activity
6. Exercise

_____ 6. Which of the following are components of the planning phase of the nursing process? (Select all that apply.)
1. Set priorities
2. Formulate nursing diagnosis statements
3. Provide for patient safety
4. Formulate nursing interventions

_____ 7. Which of the following are nursing diagnoses approved by the North American Nursing Diagnosis Association? (Select all that apply.)
1. Congestive heart failure
2. Hypertension
3. Anxiety
4. Diarrhea

_____ 8. Using Maslow's subcategories, rank the following human needs in order of highest to lowest priority.
1. Personal growth and maturity
2. Dignity
3. Love and affection
4. Comfort

CHAPTER 5

Patient Education and Health Promotion

Review Sheet

The QUESTION column and the ANSWER column have been offset so that you can cover the answer while reading the question, allowing you to assess your knowledge.

Question

1. Explain the *cognitive domain.*
2. Explain the *affective domain.*
3. Explain the *psychomotor domain.*
4. When preparing to teach the patient and family health-related information, how is the process best started?
5. What is the most effective way to ensure mastery of psychomotor skills being taught?
6. Before initiating a teaching plan, what is most important for the nurse to do first?
7. What must the nurse take into consideration when assessing a child's readiness to learn?

Answer

1. The cognitive domain is the level at which basic knowledge is learned and stored. It is the thinking portion of the learning process and incorporates a person's previous experience and perceptions.
2. The affective domain is the most intangible portion of the learning process. Affective behavior is conduct that expresses feelings, needs, beliefs, values, and opinions.
3. The psychomotor domain involves the learning of a new procedure or skill. It is often referred to as the "doing" domain.
4. Glean what information is essential, then consider what the patient wants to know. It is best to begin with the patient's questions and proceed from there. Otherwise, you may be explaining things the patient is not interested in knowing, and the individual may not be focused on the presentation.
5. Reciprocal demonstrations are particularly useful for ensuring mastery. It helps to allow the learner to practice the task several times. Giving the person immediate feedback on skills mastered, and then giving time to practice the skills that are more difficult allows the learner to improve in manual dexterity and master the sequencing of the procedure.
6. The nurse must be certain that the patient is able to focus and concentrate on the tasks and material to be learned. The patient's basic needs such as food, oxygen, and pain relief must be met before he or she is able to focus on learning.

8. What must the nurse take into consideration when teaching the older adult?

9. Summarize Herberg's description of the three ways people explain life events.

10. How would you develop a plan to teach a patient how to take a medication?

7. Psychosocial, cognitive, and language abilities must be considered. Cognitive and motor development, as well as the learner's language usage and understanding, must be assessed. Age definitely influences the type and amount of self-care activities the child is capable of learning and executing independently.
8. The older adult needs additional assessment before health teaching is implemented. Assess vision, hearing, and short- and long-term memory. If a task is to be taught, assess fine and gross motor abilities. When teaching an older adult patient, it is prudent to slow the pace of the presentation and limit the length of each session to prevent overtiring. Older adults can learn the material, but often they process things more slowly than younger people because their short-term memory may be more limited.
9. Herberg described three ways people explain life events. The scientific biomedical paradigm states that all disease has a cause. The magicoreligious paradigm views the world and its inhabitants as being under the control of supernatural, mystical forces. The holistic paradigm recognizes harmony between the body, mind, and spirit.
10. Refer to Box 5-1 in the text.

CHAPTER 5

Student Name____________________

Patient Education and Health Promotion

Learning Activities

FILL-IN-THE-BLANK

Complete the following statements using the correct term.

1. The ____________________ domain is the level at which basic knowledge is learned and stored.

2. The ____________________ domain involves the learning of a new procedure or skill; it is often referred to as the *doing domain*.

3. ____________________ is the assumption that one's culture provides the right way, the best way, and the only way to live.

TRUE OR FALSE

Mark "T" for true and "F" for false for each statement. Correct all false statements.

_____ 4. Affective behavior is conduct that expresses feelings, needs, beliefs, values, and opinions.

_____ 5. When providing patient teaching, it is best to begin with the information that the nurse feels is most important to be taught.

_____ 6. The holistic paradigm views the world and its inhabitants as being under the control of supernatural, mystical forces.

_____ 7. Explaining the various self-care needs to an individual and exploring his or her prior knowledge is an example of the affective domain learning.

_____ 8. Establishing an environment that is conducive to learning is essential to the overall learning process.

_____ 9. Deciding what to teach and how much to teach is essential to the learning process.

_____ 10. Utilizing an established teaching plan that all nurses can build on is important to the continuity of health teaching.

_____ 11. Health teaching is valued by all individuals equally.

_____ 12. Children may need adaptations in prepared learning materials based on their age, learning capabilities, and development.

_____ 13. It is best to explain all of the information needed for self-care so the teaching plan on the chart documents that all the health teaching was accomplished prior to discharge.

_____ 14. The magicoreligious belief system stresses that humans are under control of supernatural forces.

_____ 15. The scientific-biomedical belief system emphasizes health promotion and restoration.

_____ 16. Illness may not have the same meaning for all individuals.

CHAPTER 5

Student Name________________________________

Patient Education and Health Promotion

Practice Questions for the NCLEX Examination

_____ 1. A nurse is preparing to teach a patient the subcutaneous insulin administration process. The nurse will be working with the patient in which of the following domains of leaning?
1. Cognitive
2. Psychomotor
3. Affective
4. Effective

_____ 2. The nurse is preparing to teach a group of adults about the transmission and prevention of illness. Which of the following teaching techniques is most likely to accommodate the learning styles of most of the participants? (Select all that apply.)
1. Pamphlets
2. Video
3. Charts
4. Computer software

_____ 3. When teaching patients psychomotor skills, the nurse identifies which of the following as most useful in ensuring mastery of content taught?
1. Written test
2. Asking the patient if he or she understands the process, and moving on if they say yes
3. Reciprocal demonstrations
4. Patients should not be placed under stress; the nurse will know whether they got the information based on their interaction with the patient.

_____ 4. A nurse is preparing to teach a patient about the care of her dressings from a laparotomy and colon resection after discharge from the hospital. Before the nurse starts, it is most important for the nurse to:
1. schedule enough time to complete the teaching.
2. plan when the next teaching session should take place.
3. take the patient to a private room.
4. ensure that the patient's basic needs, such as pain relief, are met before initiating a teaching plan.

_____ 5. When conducting patient education using an interpreter, which of the actions by the nurse is considered to be inappropriate?
1. Looking directly at the interpreter when conversing.
2. Sometimes supplementing pictures when interacting with the patient.
3. Using pantomime when interacting with the patient.
4. Keeping the questions brief, and asking them one at a time to the interpreter.

_____ 6. The assumption that one's culture provides the right way, the best way, and the only way to live is known as:
1. ethnography.
2. scientific biomedical paradigm.
3. ethnocentrism.
4. magicoreligious paradigm.

_____ 7. Identify the correct sequence of the following steps that the nurse should follow when teaching a patient about his inhaled medication regimen.
1. Determine if the patient is able to take the medication as he was taught to do.
2. Determine the patient's current level of knowledge and understanding of how to take the medication.
3. Demonstrate the correct method of taking the medication.
4. Determine mutual realistic and measurable goals or outcomes for the teaching.

_____ 8. Which of the following belief systems about health and illness is part of the holistic paradigm to explain life events?
1. Fate is under the control of supernatural forces.
2. Health is a reward from God.
3. Life is controlled by physical and biochemical processes.
4. Everything in the universe has a place and role according to laws that maintain order.

CHAPTER 6

Student Name ________________________________

A Review of Arithmetic

Learning Activities (Part 1)

EQUIVALENTS AND CONVERSION

Memorize the equivalents listed in Chapter 6, then answer the following questions.

Household Equivalents

1. 4 cups = _____ quarts
2. 1 tablespoon = __5__ teaspoons
3. 8 ounces = _____ cup(s)
4. 1 pint = _____ cup(s)

Metric Equivalents

5. 1 mL = __100__ cc
6. 1 liter = __1000__ mL
7. 1 milligram (mg) = __1000 000__ micrograms (mcg)
8. 1 gram (g) = __1000__ milligrams (mg)

Conversion Rules

9. To convert milligrams to grams:

STOP! IF YOU HAVE NOT MEMORIZED THE EQUIVALENTS AND THE CONVERSION RULES, YOU SHOULD NOT PROCEED UNTIL YOU HAVE DONE SO.

CHAPTER 6

Student Name _______________

A Review of Arithmetic

Learning Activities (Part 2)

Roman Numerals

Convert the following Arabic numerals to Roman numerals.

1. 5 = _____
2. 7½ = _____
3. 4 = _____
4. 15 = _____
5. 20 = _____
6. 24 = _____

Fractions, Decimals, and Percents

Which of the following fractions is the largest? Circle your answer.

7. 1/8 or 1/16
8. 2/3 or 3/4
9. 1/100 or 1/200
10. 1/4 or 1/3
11. 3/8 or 7/8
12. 1/150 or 1/90

Reduce the following fractions.

13. 4/16 = _____
14. 12/24 = _____
15. 4/8 = _____
16. 36/48 = _____
17. 1 12/18 = _____
18. 3 34/85 = _____
19. 1 6/8 = _____
20. 12 6/8 = _____
21. 2 30/60 = _____
22. 3/9 = _____

Write the following fractions as decimals. When applicable, carry the decimal to thousandths and round to hundredths.

23. 7/8 = _____
24. 5/6 = _____
25. 1 3/4 = _____
26. 2/3 = _____
27. 15/16 = _____
28. 1/3 = _____
29. 5/8 = _____
30. 7/9 = _____
31. 1/16 = _____
32. 1/2 = _____

Identify the numerator or denominator for each of the following fractions as indicated.

33. 1/5 numerator is _____
34. 2/3 numerator is _____
35. 3/8 numerator is _____
36. 1 1/2 denominator is _____
37. 9/10 denominator is _____
38. 2 2/5 numerator is _____

39. 6/10 denominator is _____

40. 1 1/3 denominator is _____

Multiply the following fractions. Reduce answers to lowest terms.

41. 1/3 × 1/4 = _____

42. 2/3 × 3/8 = _____

43. 7/8 × 1/2 = _____

44. 3/4 × 7/8 = _____

45. 1/2 × 4/7 = _____

46. 7/8 × 2/3 = _____

47. 1 1/2 × 3/4 = _____

48. 2 2/3 × 4/5 = _____

Divide the following. As appropriate, carry to hundredths and round to tenths.

49. 2/3 ÷ 7/8 = _____

50. 1/3 ÷ 1/2 = _____

51. 5/9 ÷ 1/4 = _____

52. 21.78 ÷ 1.23 = _____

53. 756 ÷ 12.3 = _____

54. 32 ÷ 1.78 = _____

55. 112 ÷ 0.06 = _____

56. 1.22 ÷ 0.32 = _____

57. 3.789 ÷ 0.112 = _____

Change the following percents to decimals and the fractions to percents.

58. 56% = _____

59. 1/150 = _____%

60. 2/3 = _____%

61. 75% = _____

62. 1/2% = _____

63. 3/4 = _____%

64. 7/8 = _____%

65. 123% = _____

Change the following decimals to fractions and the fractions to decimals.

66. 0.3 = _____

67. 0.003 = _____

68. 0.03 = _____

69. 4/10 = _____

70. 4/100 = _____

71. 4/1000 = _____

Change the following percents to ratios.

72. 75% = _____

73. 60% = _____

74. 1/2% = _____

Convert the following using equivalency tables.

75. 1 quart = _____ cup(s)

76. _____ ounces = 1 pint

77. 3 teaspoons = _____ tablespoon(s)

78. 0.125 g = _____ mg

79. 250 mg = ____ g

80. 1 teaspoon = _____ mL

81. 6 lbs = _____ kg (round to hundredths)

82. 165 lbs = _____ kg

CHAPTER 6

Student Name ____________________

A Review of Arithmetic

Practice Questions for the NCLEX Examination

1. Order: Motrin 0.8 g PO
   Supply: Motrin 400 mg
   _____ tablets are needed for each dose

2. Order: Depakene 0.75 g PO
   Supply: 250 mg per 5 mL
   _____ mL are needed for each dose

3. Order: Coumadin 15 mg PO
   Supply: 10 mg tablets
   _____ tablets are needed for each dose

4. Order: 120 mg furosemide IM
   Supply: 10 mg/mL
   _____ mL should be administered

5. Order: Haldol 4 mg IM
   Supply: 5 mg/mL
   _____ mL should be administered

6. Order: Administer 1000 mL of D5W every 8 hours IV. The drop factor is 15 gtt/mL. How many drops per minute should the IV rate be?
   _____ gtt/min

7. Order: 600 mL of solution over 12 hours IV. The drop factor is 20 gtt/mL. How many gtt/min will the nurse administer?
   _____ gtt/min

8. A child who weighs 55 pounds weighs _____ kilogram(s).

9. A patient takes aldomet, 500 mg tablets, 3 to 4 times per day. She is advised not to exceed a daily dose of 3 grams or _____ tablets.

10. A patient's temperature of 100°F converts to _____ °C.

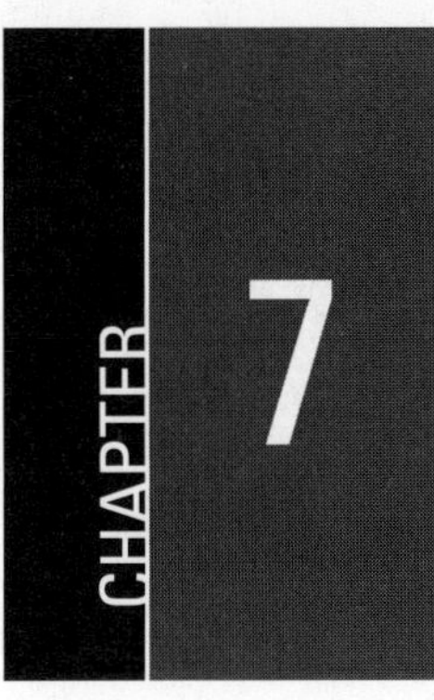

Principles of Medication Administration

Review Sheet

The QUESTION column and the ANSWER column have been offset so you can cover the answer while reading the question, allowing you to assess your knowledge.

Question

1. What is the nurse practice act?
2. What are the Standards of Care in relationship to nursing?
3. Can an employing agency write policies that require the nurse to exceed the standards established by the state board of nursing/nursing licensing agency?
4. What types of medications may have restrictions regarding the qualifications of an individual to administer the medicine?
5. What information is the nurse expected to know about a specific drug before administering it?
6. What information should be recorded whenever a "PRN" medicine is to be administered?
7. What role do critical pathways have on the delivery of clinical care?

Answer

1. The nurse practice act establishes the rules and regulations for the practice of nursing at the various entry levels within a practice area within each state.
2. Guidelines for the practice of nursing are defined by the nurse practice act of each state, by state and federal laws regulating health care facilities, the Joint Commission on Accreditation of Healthcare Organizations, as well as by professional organizations such as the American Nurses Association and other speciality nursing organizations such as the Intravenous Nurses Society, Inc.
3. No. Policies of the employing agency can authorize less than, but not more than, the established maximum standards.
4. Antineoplastic medicines, magnesium sulphate, lidocaine, Imferon, RhoGAM, allergy extracts, and heparin are administered in accordance with specific limitations of the employing agency. Most policies require doses of heparin and insulin to be checked by two qualified individuals. Additional policies are developed to identify guidelines within a particular clinical site for the administration of intravenous therapy.
5. See textbook, pp. 85-86, two paragraphs above the information on patient charts.
6. Before administration of any PRN medication, the patient's chart should be checked to ensure that someone else has not administered the drug, and that the specified time interval has passed since the medication was last administered. When a PRN medication is given, it should be charted immediately. Record the response to the medication.

8. Examine the sections on a medication administration record (MAR) to identify the categories used.
9. Where would information regarding a patient's possible allergies be found?
10. Explain the differences among the ward stock, computer-controlled ordering and dispensing system, individual prescription order, and unit dose drug distribution (acute and long-term care) systems.
11. Identify procedures for the electronic transmission of patient orders.
12. What are adverse drug events (ADEs)?
13. Referring to the controlled substance inventory form, Figure 7-12 in the textbook, list some controlled narcotic drugs routinely used in the acute care setting.
14. What information is recorded on the controlled substance inventory form when a controlled substance is administered?
15. Explain the differences between a stat order, standing order, PRN order, verbal order, and fax order.
16. How is a drug order verified and transcribed?
17. What are the six "rights" of drug administration?
18. What tests are used to identify hepatic and renal function?
19. What methods are used to ensure correct identification of a patient prior to drug administration? (Discuss adults, children, and inpatient and outpatient settings.)

7. Critical pathways are a multidisciplinary plan used by all health care providers to track the individual's progress toward expected outcomes within a specified time period.
8. Medication administration records are usually divided into five sections: scheduled section, parenteral section, stat section, preoperative orders, and PRN medication section.
9. Information about a patient's allergies is recorded in the history and physical section of the chart, the Kardex, the MAR, the patient's chart holder, and on the patient's allergy bracelet.
10. See textbook pp. 98-101 under Drug Distribution Systems.
11. Faxed orders must be signed within a specified time, often 24 hours.
12. See textbook p. 103 information under Medication Errors.
13. Diazepam (Valium), meperidine, morphine, Tylenol with codeine.
14. The date, time, name of medicine administered, patient's name, amount wasted (if any), and the number of dosage containers (such as unit dose tablets or ampules) remaining after the drug is removed are recorded on the form. The nurse administering the medicine signs the record as well as the qualified witness if any medicine is wasted.
15. See textbook p. 103, information under Types of Medication Orders.
16. See textbook p. 104, information under Nurse's Responsibilities.
17. The six "rights" of drug administration are: right drug, right time, right dose, right patient, right route, and right documentation.
18. Liver function tests include aspartate aminotransferase (AST), alanine aminotransferase (ALT), alkaline phosphatase, lactic dehydrogenase (LDH), and gamma glutamyl transferase (GGT). Renal function tests include serum creatinine, creatinine clearance, blood urea nitrogen (BUN), and urinalysis.

20. Review error-prone abbreviations, symbols, and dose designations to be avoided in written communications to prevent medication errors.

19. See textbook, pp. 106-107, information under Right Patient.

20. See Appendix A, Prescription Abbreviations.

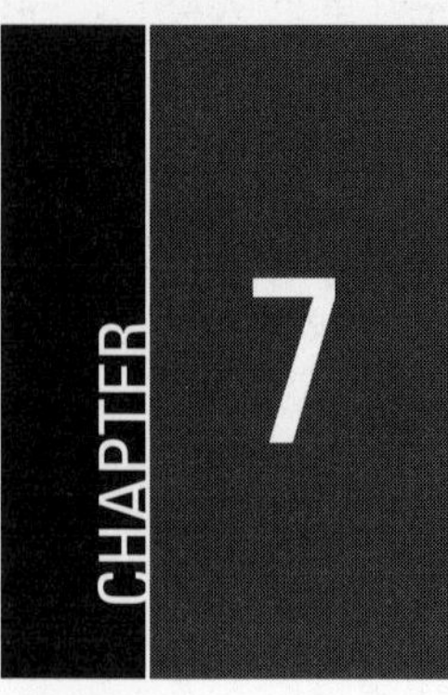

Student Name ______________________

Principles of Medication Administration

Learning Activities

FILL-IN-THE-BLANK

Finish each of the following statements using the correct term.

1. A component of the patient's chart includes the ____________ form which grants permission to the health care facility and physician to provide treatment.

2. A component of the patient's chart includes the ____________ pathways which are standardized outcomes and timetables which require health care providers to assess the patient's progress towards the goals of discharge while maintaining quality care.

3. The MAR or medication administration record lists all medications to be administered, and provides the pharmacist and the nurse with identical medication profiles for the patient.

4. ____________ ____________ ____________ is the drug distribution system that uses single-unit packages of drugs dispensed to fill each dose requirement as it is ordered.

5. A(n) stat order is generally used on an emergency basis; it means that the drug is to be administered as soon as possible, but only once.

MATCHING

Match the definition with the corresponding term. Definitions may be used more than once and some may not be used.

D 6. PRN medications

A 7. physician's order form

E 8. MAR

C 9. "stat"

F 10. Kardex

a. Check this section of the patient chart when questioning details of a drug order on the MAR.
b. Give around-the-clock.
c. Give immediately.
d. Administer as required or necessary within defined limits of the drug order.
e. Record scheduled drugs administered here.
f. Section of the patient record containing the care plan.
g. Controlled substances are recorded here when administered.

TRUE OR FALSE

Mark "T" for true and "F" for false for each statement. Correct all false statements.

T 11. Standards of care are guidelines developed for the practice of nursing that are defined by the nurse practice act of each state, by state and federal laws regulating health care facilities, by the Joint Commission on Accreditation of Healthcare Organizations, as well as by professional organizations such as the American Nurses Association and other specialty nursing organizations.

______ 12. The graphic record is an example of manual recording of temperature, pulse, respirations, and blood pressure.

______ 13. When a medication is ordered PRN, the nurse identifies this as meaning the patient should receive this medication every night before bedtime.

______ 14. A standing order must be written and signed by the physician before the nurse can continue to administer the medication.

______ 15. Medication errors can result in serious complications known as *adverse drug events.*

______ 16. A student nurse may accept a verbal drug order.

CHAPTER 7

Student Name______________________________

Principles of Medication Administration

Practice Questions for the NCLEX Examination

_____ 1. It is 0900, and the nurse reads the patient's chart. The physician has written diazepam 10 mg IV stat. The nurse interprets this as meaning:
1. the patient will receive 10 mg of diazepam IV every morning at 0900.
2. 10 mg of diazepam IV will be administered at this time, but only once.
3. the nurse will administer the diazepam with the next group of medicines scheduled to be administered.
4. Because the patient doesn't have an IV started, the nurse will double the dose of the diazepam to 20 mg and administer it orally.

_____ 2. When preparing to administer a medication to a patient, the nurse is not able to verify that the medication as ordered is appropriate. The nurse should act in which of the following ways? (Select all that apply.)
1. Document the reasons for refusal to administer the drug in accordance with the policies of the employing institution.
2. Contact the physician who prescribed the drug.
3. If the physician who prescribed the drug cannot be contacted, notify the nursing supervisor on duty.
4. Administer the medication because it went through pharmacy, and they would have caught a problem if there was one.

_____ 3. A patient has developed nausea and has been vomiting off and on for the past 20 minutes in reaction to the multiple medications she is taking for Crohn's disease and a heart condition. In this situation, the nurse should:
1. place a nasogastric tube into the patient and administer the medications via that route.
2. tell the patient that she really needs to take the medicines and administer them.
3. contact the physician and discuss alternative mediation orders, since the parenteral or rectal route may be preferred.
4. contact the pharmacy, have the medicines sent back to you in rectal form, and administer via that route.

_____ 4. The nurse identifies which of the following statements with proper documentation of medication administration? (Select all that apply.)
1. Record when a drug is not administered and why.
2. Record medication administration before it is administered.
3. Do not record in the nurse's notes that an incident report has been completed when a medication error has occurred.
4. Record and promptly report any adverse symptoms concerning medication administration.

_____ 5. When working with pediatric patients, the most effective method the nurse should use for identification of the patient for medication administration is:
1. asking the child his or her name.
2. asking a family member the child's name.
3. checking the identification bracelet.
4. checking the room assignment and bed the child is in.

_____ 6. 6 AM in military time is
1. 0600.
2. 1200.
3. 1800.
4. 2200.

_____ 7. 2 PM in military time is:
1. 0200.
2. 0600.
3. 1200.
4. 1400.

_____ 8. The inventory control record is completed when the:
1. patient asks for a controlled substance.
2. controlled substance is removed.
3. medication is administered.
4. degree of pain relief is assessed.

_____ 9. The PRN medication record is completed:
1. when the patient asks for a controlled substance.
2. when the controlled substance is removed.
3. immediately after administering the drug.
4. when the degree of pain relief is assessed.

_____ 10. The narcotic control count is performed by:
1. the charge nurse.
2. the nurse going off duty.
3. the nurse coming on duty.
4. two nurses; one from shift going off duty and one from shift coming on duty.

_____ 11. A drug on a scheduled order is given:
1. as many times as needed.
2. at prescribed/designated intervals.
3. one time only.
4. immediately.

_____ 12. When a verbal order is taken, it must be co-signed and dated by the physician within:
1. 3 days.
2. 2 days.
3. 24 hours.
4. 12 hours.

_____ 13. The person responsible for the transcription of the drug order is the:
1. nurse's aide.
2. unit secretary/ward clerk.
3. physician.
4. nurse.

_____ 14. When "wasting" a portion of a dose of narcotic, the nurse must have this witnessed by:
1. the prescribing physician.
2. the charge nurse.
3. a second qualified nurse.
4. the medication aide.

_____ 15. When measuring a fractional dose of a medication with a volume of less than 1 mL, the most accurate method would be to use a:
1. medicine cup.
2. tuberculin syringe.
3. teaspoon.
4. medicine dropper.

_____ 16. The most reliable method of calculating pediatric drug doses is using:
1. body surface area (BSA).
2. Clark's rule.
3. a fraction of the adult dose.
4. Pyxis system of measurement.

_____ 17. A client has a new drug ordered bid. This means the drug will be administered:
1. once daily.
2. two times per day.
3. three times per day.
4. four times per day.

_____ 18. The Pyxis system refers to a(n):
1. narcotic inventory system.
2. individual prescription order system.
3. unit dose system used primarily in long-term care.
4. electronic medication dispensing system.

_____ 19. The medication administration record (MAR) in a long-term care setting is designed to be used for:
1. 8 hours.
2. 24 hours.
3. 1 week.
4. 1 month.

_____ 20. Faxed medication orders are usually signed by the health care provider within:
1. 8 hours.
2. 12 hours.
3. 24 hours.
4. 48 hours.

_____ 21. Electronic database charting systems may vary, but they must comply with the guidelines/requirements of the _______ while incorporating standards of care.
1. American Nurses Association
2. Joint Commission on Accreditation of Healthcare Organizations
3. Intravenous Nurses Society
4. National League of Nurses

_____ 22. Unit dose systems in a long-term care setting supply enough medication containers for a(n) _______ period.
1. 8-hour
2. 24-hour
3. 48-hour
4. one-week

_____ 23. Which of the following are common contents of patient charts in health care facilities? (Select all that apply.)
1. Consent forms
2. Nursing care plans
3. Medication administration records
4. Patient education records

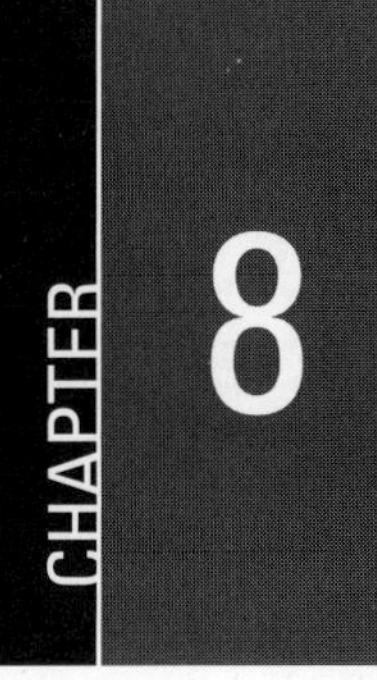

Percutaneous Administration

Review Sheet

The QUESTION column and the ANSWER column have been offset so you can cover the answer while reading the question, allowing you to assess your knowledge.

Question

1. What factors affect the absorption of topical medications?
2. What is the major advantage of the percutaneous route for drug administration?
3. Explain the differences among a cream, lotion, ointment, and wet dressing, and cite the methods used to apply each.
4. What health teaching should be given to a patient using a topical form of medication?
5. What is the purpose of patch testing?
6. Describe the method used to apply allergens and read results.
7. List commonly used symbols for reading of reactions to allergen testing.
8. Describe the specific method used to apply nitroglycerin ointment and a nitroglycerin transdermal disk.
9. Why is it important for the nurse to wear gloves when applying a topical ointment or transdermal patch?

Answer

1. Factors affecting the absorption of topical medications include drug concentration, the length of time the medication is in contact with the skin, size and depth of affected area, and thickness and hydration of the skin.
2. The action of the drug is primarily limited to the site of application, thereby decreasing the systemic side effects.
3. See textbook, pp. 110-111.
4. Patients receiving topical medications should receive the following health teaching: personal hygiene measures to treat/improve underlying condition, methods of application, ways to avoid touching affected areas, and prevention of spread of infection when present.
5. Patch testing is used to identify specific sensitivity to allergens.
6. See textbook, pp. 112-114.
7. Commonly used symbols for reading allergen patch test reactions include (see also p. 114):

+	1+ no wheal, 3 mm flare
++	2+ 2–3 mm wheal with flare
+++	3+ 3–5 mm wheal with flare
++++	4+ > 5 mm wheal

8. See textbook, pp. 114-116.

10. What types of medications are available in transdermal patch form?
11. Why is it important to discard transdermal medication patches safely after removal?
12. What schedule is used for the administration of the estrogen transdermal system Ortho-Evra patch?
13. Where are sublingual and buccal forms of medication administered?
14. What is the primary advantage of the sublingual route?
15. Describe the correct techniques for administering eye drops, eye ointments, and eye disks, including patient teaching.
16. Compare the correct technique of administering an ear (otic) drug to a child and to an adult.
17. Explain the procedure for instilling nose drops/nasal sprays into an adult and a child; include health teaching.
18. Why shouldn't oily preparations be administered by inhalation?
19. Explain how to give medications by inhalation.
20. What is a metered-dose inhaler?
21. Explain how to teach a patient to administer a medication using an inhaler.
22. Explain the correct technique for inserting a vaginal suppository and proper hygiene measures used during the course of treatment.

9. The nurse should wear gloves when administering a topical ointment or transdermal patch to avoid inadvertent absorption of the medication by the nurse through the skin.
10. Nitroglycerin, clonidine, estrogen, nicotine, scopolamine, fentanyl, and Ortho-Evra are available in transdermal patch forms.
11. Used transdermal patches must be safely discarded because the patch may still contain some medication that could be harmful to individuals or pets for whom it is not prescribed.
12. Ortho-Evra transdermal system is worn continuously for 3 weeks, with week 4 patch-free.
13. Sublingual medications are administered under the tongue; buccal medications are administered in the back cheek area of the mouth.
14. In addition to being easy to access, the sublingual area provides rapid absorption and onset of action of the drug because the drug passes directly into the systemic circulation with no immediate pass through the liver, where extensive metabolism usually takes place.
15. See textbook, pp. 119-121.
16. See textbook, p. 121.
17. See textbook, pp. 122-124.
18. Oily preparations should not be administered by inhaler because oil droplets would be carried to the lungs and initiate a lipid pneumonia.
19. See textbook, pp. 124-125.
20. A metered-dose inhaler is an aerosolized, pressurized inhaler that delivers a measured amount of medication with each depression of the device.
21. See textbook, pp. 125-126.
22. See textbook, pp. 127-128.

CHAPTER 8

Student Name ______________________________

Percutaneous Administration

Learning Activities

FILL-IN-THE-BLANK

Finish each of the following statements using the correct term.

1. ______________ are semisolid emulsions containing medicinal agents for external application.

2. ______________ tablets are designed to be placed under the tongue for dissolution and absorption through the vast network of blood vessels in this area, and ______________ tablets are designed to be held between the cheek and molar teeth for absorption from the blood vessels of the cheek.

3. Medications that are labeled "ophthalmic" are meant for administration to the ______________.

4. When administering ear drops to a child under the age of 3 years, the nurse should restrain the child, turn the head to the appropriate side, and gently pull the earlobe ______________ and ______________.

5. Bronchodilators and corticosteroids may be administered by oral inhalation through the mouth using an aerosolized, pressurized ______________ ______________ ______________.

TRUE OR FALSE

Mark "T" for true and "F" for false for each statement. Correct all false statements.

_____ 6. It is now recognized that a major principle in wound healing is the need for a moist environment to propagate epithelization of the wound.

_____ 7. Patch testing is a method used to identify a patient's sensitivity to contact materials.

_____ 8. After applying the prescribed amount of nitroglycerin ointment to the skin, the nurse should rub the ointment into the skin until it can no longer be seen.

_____ 9. Aerosols use a flow of air or oxygen under pressure to disperse the drug throughout the respiratory tract.

_____ 10. Douching is not recommended during pregnancy.

CHAPTER 8

Student Name______________________________

Percutaneous Administration

Practice Questions for the NCLEX Examination

_____ 1. Which of the following actions would the nurse take when applying a wet dressing to a patient?
1. Leave about one-half of the previous dressing in place to promote epithelization and wound healing.
2. Wring out wet dressing to prevent dripping and apply the gauze in a single layer directly to the wound surface.
3. Do not pack deep wounds, lightly place gauze over them.
4. After the wound is dressed, pour the liquid onto the top of the dressing and leave it open to air.

_____ 2. The nurse is working in an allergy clinic. Which of the following should be taken into consideration by the nurse when administering allergy testing to patients? (Select all that apply.)
1. Ensure that emergency equipment is in the immediate area in case of an anaphylactic response.
2. Position the patient so that the surface where the test material is to be applied is horizontal.
3. Administer antihistamine and antiinflammatory agents immediately before the test.
4. Cleanse the area where the allergens are to be applied with an alcohol pledget and allow the area to dry before starting testing

_____ 3. When administering nitroglycerin percutaneously to a patient, the nurse should:
1. wear gloves.
2. apply wax paper over the site of the nitroglycerin to enhance absorption of the drug.
3. ensure that the drug is on the patient 24 hours a day, 7 days a week to avoid complications.
4. always place the nitroglycerin ointment over the left chest to provide the most effective route of drug delivery to the heart.

_____ 4. When administering eye drops to a patient, the nurse follows which of the following practices? (Select all that apply.)
1. Have the patient look upward over your head.
2. Drop the specified number of drops into the conjunctival sac.
3. After instilling the drops, apply gentle pressure using a cotton ball to the outer corner of the eye for 30 seconds.
4. When more than one type of eye drop is ordered for the same eye, wait 1 to 5 minutes between instillation of the different medications.

_____ 5. When teaching a patient how to administer a medication for oral inhalation via a metered dose inhaler without the use of a spacer, the nurse should inform the patient to perform which of the following actions? (Select all that apply.)
1. If the medication is a suspension, shake the canister before administration.
2. Close the mouth around the canister when administering the medication.
3. Activate the metered dose inhaler and instruct the patient to inhale deeply over 10 seconds to ensure that airways are open and that the drug is dispersed as deeply as possible.
4. If the inhaled medication is a corticosteroid, instruct the patient to rinse the mouth with water when administration is complete.

_____ 6. Eye medications may be administered by which of the following methods? (Select all that apply.)
1. Irrigation
2. Drops
3. Ointment
4. Patch

_____ 7. When administering ear medication to an adult, the pinna should be pulled:
1. up.
2. up and back.
3. down.
4. down and back.

_____ 8. When administering ear medication to a child, the pinna should be pulled:
1. up.
2. back and up.
3. down.
4. back and down.

CHAPTER 9

Enteral Administration

Review Sheet

The QUESTION column and the ANSWER column have been offset so you can cover the answer while reading the question, allowing you to assess your knowledge.

Question

1. When an individual is unable to swallow or has had oral surgery, an alternative route of administration is the __________ route.
2. A major advantage of using the rectal route for drug administration is __________.
3. List the composition and advantages of the following dosage forms: capsules, timed-release capsules, lozenges, tablets, elixirs, emulsions, suspensions, and syrups.
4. Why is it important to use the medicine dropper that accompanies a medication?
5. Why is an oral syringe preferred over a household teaspoon for administering a medication?
6. List the five "rights" of medication administration.
7. What is the sixth "right" of medication administration and why is it important?
8. What are the primary principles of giving a solid form and liquid form of a medication?
9. Discuss the proper method(s) of checking NG tube placement prior to the administration of a drug or an enteral formula.
10. Identify the color and pH values of gastric, intestinal, and pleural secretions, both with and without the administration of H_2 blockers (antagonists).
11. Name four general categories of enteral formulas.

Answer

1. Nasogastric
2. Bypass the digestive enzymes and avoid irritation to the esophagus and stomach.
3. See textbook, pp. 130-131, information under Dose Forms.
4. The dropper has been specifically made to correspond with the viscosity of the drug to deliver the correct volume of medication.
5. An oral syringe is more accurate.
6. The five rights of drug administration are: RIGHT patient, RIGHT drug, RIGHT dosage, RIGHT time of administration, and RIGHT route of administration.
7. RIGHT documentation explains not only what was administered but also the patient's response.
8. See textbook, pp. 135 and 137, information under General Principles of Solid-Form Oral Medication and General Principles of Liquid-Form Oral Medication.
9. Verify NG location after initial placement using x-ray verification BEFORE administering any drug or enteral formula for the first time. (See textbook, pp. 138-139.
10. See textbook, p. 138, Method 1: pH and color testing of gastric contents to check for tube placement.

12. How long can an enteral formula be left standing open with refrigeration?
13. Review the procedure for NG administration of enteral formulas using bolus and continuous infusion techniques.
14. State the positioning used for a patient when he or she is receiving an NG feeding using the bolus and using a continuous delivery method.
15. How are rectal suppositories inserted?
16. What position is the patient placed in to administer a disposable enema?

11. Four general types of enteral formulas are: intact (polymeric) nutrient, elemental, disease- or condition-specific, and modular nutrients.
12. An open enteral formula can be kept refrigerated up to 24 hours. The tubing and formula receptacle used for a continuous method of delivery such as the Kangaroo also should be changed every 24 hours.
13. See textbook, pp. 140-141.
14. Place the patient in semi-Fowler's position with head of bed (HOB) elevated 30 degrees for 30 minutes before and at least 1 hour after a bolus feeding. Most patients with a continuous feeding are maintained at a 30 to 45 degree elevation of the HOB.
15. Apply a glove or finger cot, have suppository in a solid form, use water-soluble lubricant or plain water to moisten, then insert suppository about one inch past the internal sphincter in the rectum.
16. To administer a disposable enema, place the patient on the left side.

CHAPTER 9

Student Name ____________________

Enteral Administration

Learning Activities

FILL-IN-THE-BLANK

Finish each of the following statements using the correct term.

1. The three routes of drug administration can be classified into the following categories: enteral, parenteral, and percutaneous
2. ____________ are small, cylindrical gelatin containers that hold dry powder or liquid medicinal agents.
3. ____________ are dispersions of small droplets of water in oil or oil in water, and are often used to mask bitter tastes or provide better solubility to certain drugs.
4. When using the metric system, one teaspoon equals ______ mL.
5. After a patient receives a suppository, the nurse should instruct the patient to remain lying on the side for ______ to ______ minutes to allow melting and absorption of the medication.
6. Elixirs are drugs dissolved in ____________ and ____________.
7. Syrups are drugs dissolved in concentrated ____________ with ____________.
8. On the medicine cup, 1 oz (fl oz) equals ______ tbsp.
9. On the medicine cup, 1 tsp equals ______ mL.

TRUE OR FALSE

Mark "T" for true and "F" for false for each statement. Correct all false statements.

______ 10. The oral route is safe, most convenient, and relatively economical, and dose forms are readily available for most medications. The major disadvantage of this route is that it has the slowest and least dependable rate of absorption, and thus onset of action, of the commonly used routes of administration.

T 11. Enteric-coated tablets must not be crushed or chewed, or the active ingredients will be released prematurely and be destroyed in the stomach.

T 12. When a liquid medication is poured into a medicine cup, a meniscus forms in the cup. The amount of medication in the cup should be read at the lowest point of the concave curve of the meniscus.

T 13. Suppositories are intended only for rectal administration.

F 14. Patients receiving an enema should be placed in the right lateral position, unless the knee-chest position has been specified.

______ 15. The oral dropper that accompanied a specific drug is lost. The nurse should substitute a dropper from another medication for the lost one.

_____ 16. To validate the correct placement of an NG tube prior to administering a medication or enteral feeding, it is acceptable to aspirate gastric contents and check the pH and color.

_____ 17. When flushing an NG tube, do not clamp the tube until all the solution has time to reach the stomach.

_____ 18. When documenting an enteral feeding, the amount administered is charted on the intake and output sheet and then is included in the intake total for each shift.

_____ 19. Intermittent tube feedings require that the unused formula mixed and dispensed by the pharmacy be discarded every 48 hours.

_____ 20. The head of the bed (HOB) is elevated 30 minutes before and 30 minutes to 1 hour after administering an intermittent tube feeding.

_____ 21. Rectal suppositories are generally inserted with the patient positioned in the Sims' position.

_____ 22. A disposable enema is administered with the patient positioned on the right side.

_____ 23. When testing gastric pH for a person NOT taking an H_2 blocker such as ranitidine, the gastric contents would have a pH of 1.0–4.0.

_____ 24. When testing gastric pH for a person who is taking an H_2 blocker such as ranitidine, the gastric contents would have a pH > 4.0.

_____ 25. Aspirated intestinal fluid should be a clear- to straw-colored secretion.

_____ 26. Auscultation is an accurate method of checking NG tube placement.

CHAPTER 9

Student Name ______________________________

Enteral Administration

Practice Questions for the NCLEX Examination

_____ 1. When administering a liquid form of an oral medication to an infant, the nurse would perform which one of the following activities?
1. Be certain that the infant is alert.
2. Position the infant so that the head is lowered.
3. Place the syringe or dropper at the tip of the infant's tongue.
4. Inject the medicine rapidly to facilitate swallowing of the medicine.

_____ 2. When administering medications to an adult via a nasogastric tube, the nurse should:
1. crush timed-released capsules before administration via the nasogastric tube to prevent clogging of the tube.
2. flush the nasogastric tube with at least 30 mL of sterile water before and after administration of the medicine.
3. flush between each medication with 50 mL of water (when more than one medication is to be administered at about the same time).
4. check for correct placement of the nasogastric tube after the medications are instilled.

_____ 3. When checking for correct placement of a nasogastric tube, the nurse aspirates yellow fluid from the nasogastric tube. Based on the color of the aspirate, the nurse identifies the fluid as most likely being of which type?
1. Gastric
2. Intestinal
3. Pleural
4. Tracheobronchial

_____ 4. When working with patients receiving enteral feedings via gastrostomy or jejunostomy tube, the nurse should perform which of the following actions? (Select all that apply.)
1. Check the residual volume before each feeding.
2. Check to ensure the presence of bowel sounds.
3. Check the position of the tube to ensure that it is still in the stomach.
4. Discard unused portions every 8 hours.

_____ 5. Which of the following actions should the nurse take when administering an enema to an adult patient?
1. Encourage the patient to hold the solution for about 5 minutes before defecating.
2. Tell the patient not to flush the toilet until you return and can see the results of the enema.
3. Insert one inch of the lubricated rectal tube into the rectum.
4. Heat the enema to 101° F to ensure comfort in administration.

_____ 6. Before administering a medication, the nurse should check which of the following? (Select all that apply.)
1. Dose
2. Drug
3. Time of administration
4. Route of administration
5. Patient identification

7. An order for 1 teaspoonful of a medication converts to _____ mL.

_____ 8. Before administering medication via a nasogastric tube, the nurse checks for correct tube placement. Which of the following findings indicate that the tube is in the correct location? (Select all that apply.)
1. Aspiration of clear fluid from the nasogastric tube
2. Recent x-ray verification of tube placement
3. Gastric pH result of 3.0
4. Auscultation of air over the right upper quadrant of the abdomen.

CHAPTER 10

Parenteral Administration: Safe Preparation of Parenteral Medications

Review Sheet

The QUESTION column and the ANSWER column have been offset so that you can cover the answer while reading the question, allowing you to assess your knowledge.

Question

1. Define *parenteral.*
2. What are the major advantages of parenteral medication administration?
3. Cite specific nursing actions required during medication administration to provide for accurate, safe drug delivery to the patient.
4. Discuss established policies and procedures used for checking and transcribing medication orders and for preparing, administering, recording, and monitoring of therapeutic responses to drug therapy in clinical sites where assigned.
5. List the parts of a syringe and the method of reading the measuring scale on the tuberculin, 3-mL, and insulin syringes.
6. What volume can safely be injected at one site for intradermal, subcutaneous, IM, and IV medications?
7. Identify the types of tips found on syringes.
8. Examine calibrations found on different types of syringes.
9. What are common manufacturers' names for prefilled syringes?
10. Name the parts of an "insulin pen."
11. What medication is contained in an Epi-Pen® and what is the intended use for this device?

Answer

1. Parenteral medication administration routes are intradermal, intramuscular (IM), and intravenous (IV) injections.
2. See textbook, p. 145.
3. 1) Knowledge of individual drugs ordered, prepared, and administered; 2) awareness of symptoms for which the drug is prescribed as well as baseline evaluation of desired therapeutic outcomes; 3) understanding of nursing assessments needed to detect, prevent, or ameliorate adverse events; and 4) the nurse must exercise clinical judgment when drug orders are changed, new drugs are ordered, drug doses are missed, or when substitution of therapeutically equivalent medicines are made by the pharmacy.
4. Instructor needs to assist the student to identify policies developed by the school and by individual clinical sites relative to this question.
5. See Figures 10-1, 10-2, 10-5, 10-8.
6. See Table 10-1, p. 151.
7. See Figure 10-4 A, B.
8. See Figure 10-2, 10-5, 10-8.
9. Tubex, Carpuject
10. See Figure 10-10.

12. The inner diameter of a needle is known as ____________.
13. Why are different length needles available for intramuscular and subcutaneous injections?
14. What do the terms *package integrity* or *package continuity* mean?
15. What are the provisions of the Needlestick Safety and Prevention Act of 2000?
16. What is the purpose of a filter needle?
17. Research safety devices developed for syringes and needles.
18. Identify the location of the OSHA-approved sharps containers on the clinical unit where assigned.
19. Differentiate between an ampule, a vial, and a Mix-O-Vial. Read the section on removal of medications from these containers.
20. Practice the procedures involved in the removal of a drug from an ampule, vial, and Mix-O-Vial.

11. Epinephrine, p. 150. It is used in emergencies caused by allergy to insect stings, foods, or drugs.
12. Gauge: the larger the number, the smaller the diameter.
13. Provides a means of depositing the prescribed medication into the correct location/depth for maximum drug response in individuals of different build and age.
14. The terms *package integrity* or *package continuity* mean inspecting the container to ensure sterility of the contents has been retained.
15. The Act requires OSHA to develop and revise standards for blood-borne pathogens, monitoring and reporting of needlestick injuries, and the development of safety equipment to protect health care providers.
16. A filter needle is used to screen out glass particles that may have inadvertently fallen into the ampule during removal of its top. *Note:* After medication is removed from the ampule, remove filter needle, apply appropriate gauge and length needle for drug administration, and measure the amount of drug prescribed.
17. Under new OSHA regulations, needleless systems are required for the collection of body fluids, or the withdrawal of body fluids after initial venous or arterial access is established, the administration of medication or fluids and any other procedure involving the potential for occupational exposure to blood-borne pathogens as a result of percutaneous injuries from contaminated sharps. Another new delivery system under development is a jet injection system that delivers subcutaneous injections of liquid medications such as insulin and vaccine through the skin without use of a needle. See information on blunt access devices.
18. Ask your instructor.
19. See Figures 10-20, 10-21, and 10-22.
20. See Figures 10-23, 10-24, and 10-25.

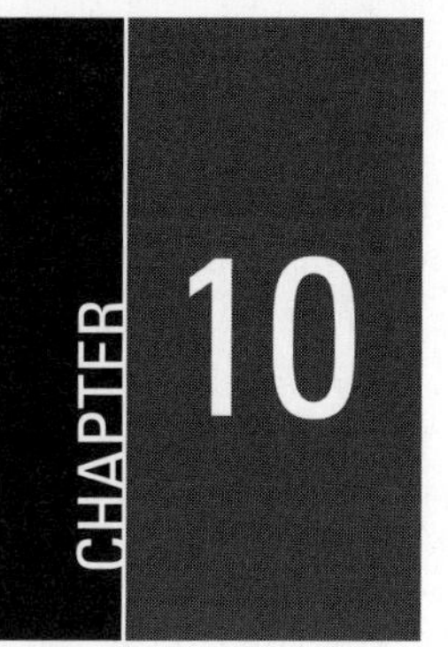

Student Name ____________________

Parenteral Administration: Safe Preparation of Parenteral Medications

Learning Activities

FILL-IN-THE-BLANK

Finish each of the following statements using the correct term.

1. The Occupational Safety and Health Administration reports that more than 5 million workers in the health care industry and related occupations are at risk for occupational exposure to blood-borne pathogens, including such devastating diseases as ____________ ____________ virus, ____________ virus, and ____________ virus.

2. The syringe has three parts: the ____________________ is the outer portion on which the calibrations for the measurements of drug volume are located, the ____________________ is the inner cylindrical portion that fits snugly into the barrel, and the ____________________ is the portion that holds the needle.

3. The needle ____________________ is the diameter of the hole through the needle.

4. The proper gauge for an intradermal injection is _____ to _____ g, and the appropriate length of the needle is _____ to _____ inch.

5. The proper needle gauge for blood administration is _____ to _____ g.

In the blanks provided, write the volume of a drug that can be injected at one site by the following methods.

6. Intradermal: _____ mL

7. Subcutaneous: _____ mL

8. Intramuscular: _____ mL

   Divided dose is: _____

9. Intravenous fluid: _____ mL

LABELING

Label the syringe below.

10.

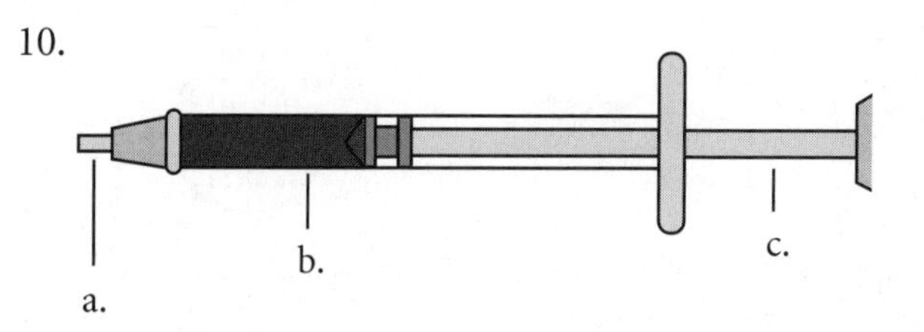

Read the following syringes.

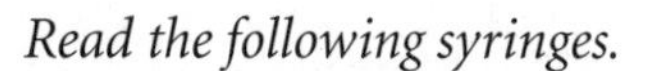

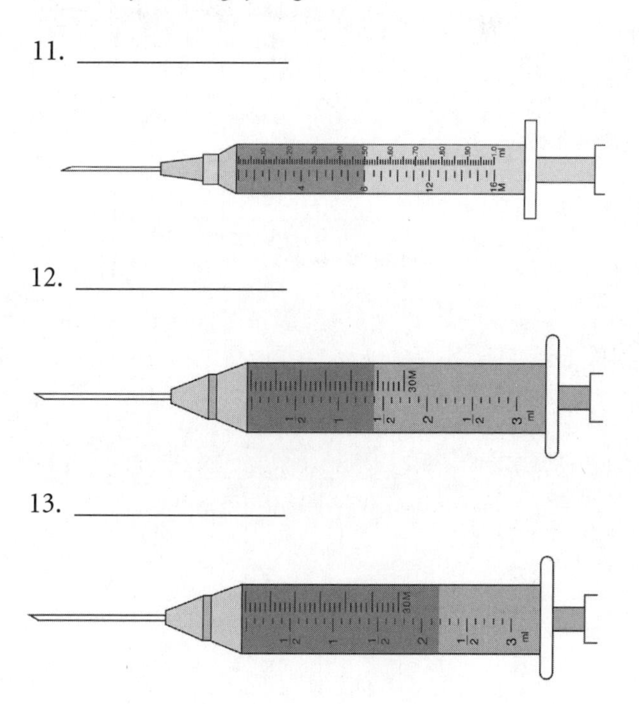

11. ________________

12. ________________

13. ________________

14. ______________

15. ______________

16. ______________

17. ______________

18. ______________

19. ______________

20. ______________

21. ______________

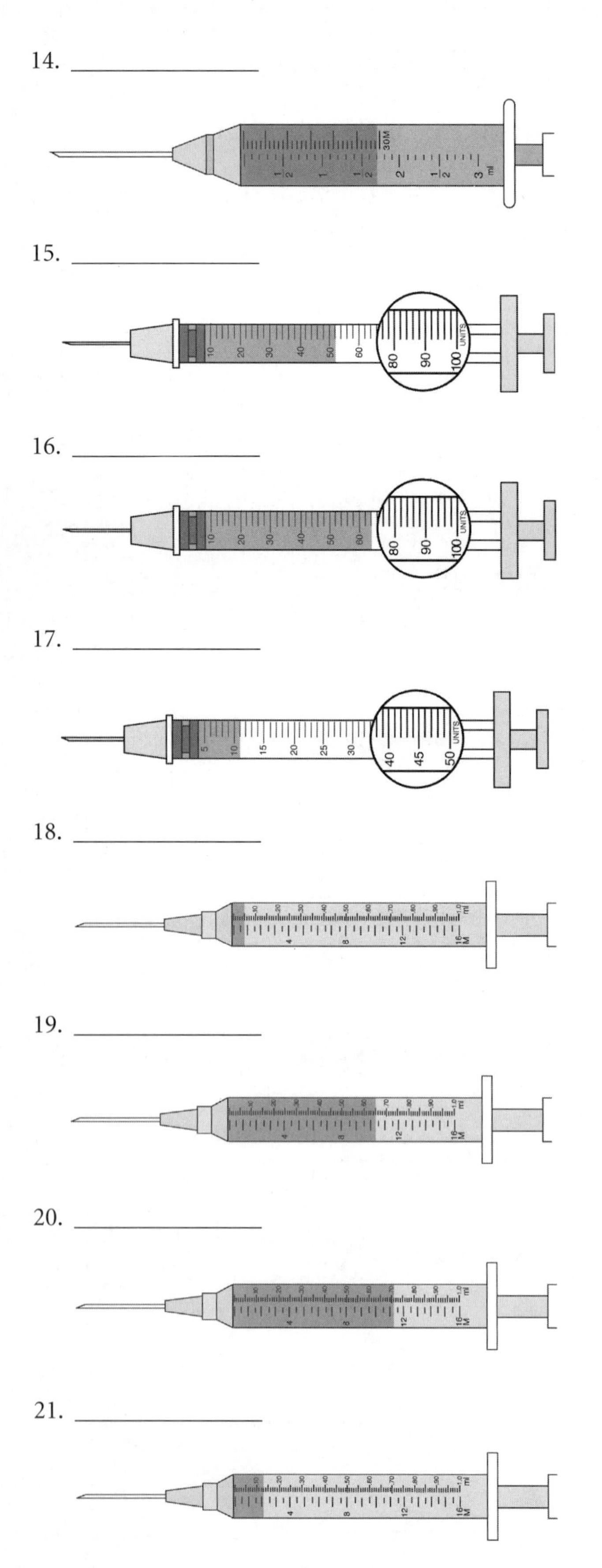

Label the parts of a needle.

22.

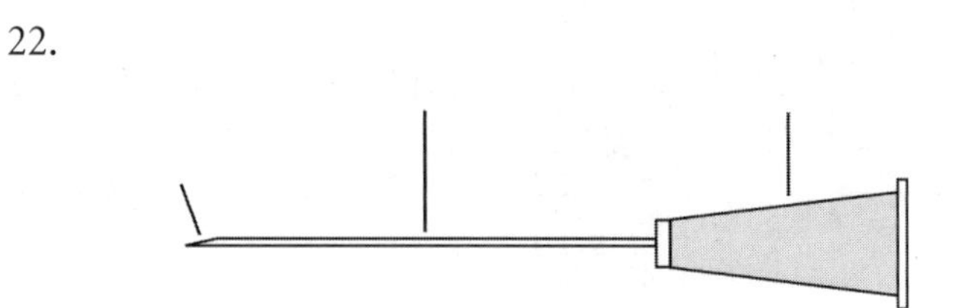

Label the following.

23. This is known as a(n) ____________________.

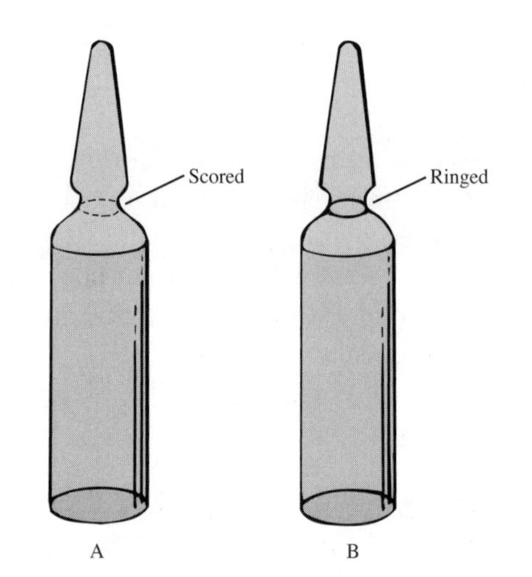

Explain how to withdraw fluid from this receptacle.

24. This is known as a(n) ____________________.

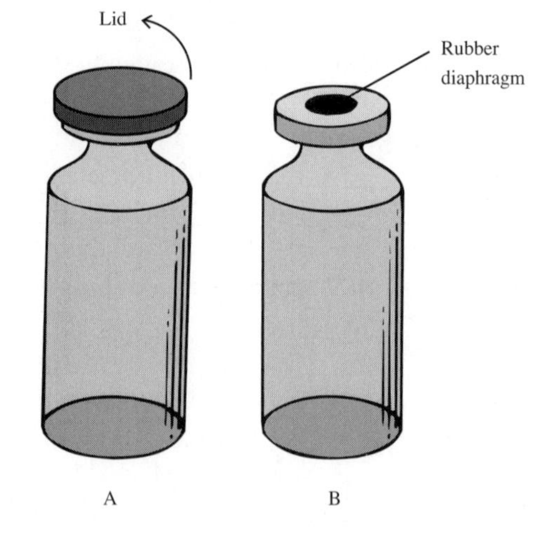

Explain how to withdraw fluid from this receptacle.

25. This is known as a(n) ____________________.

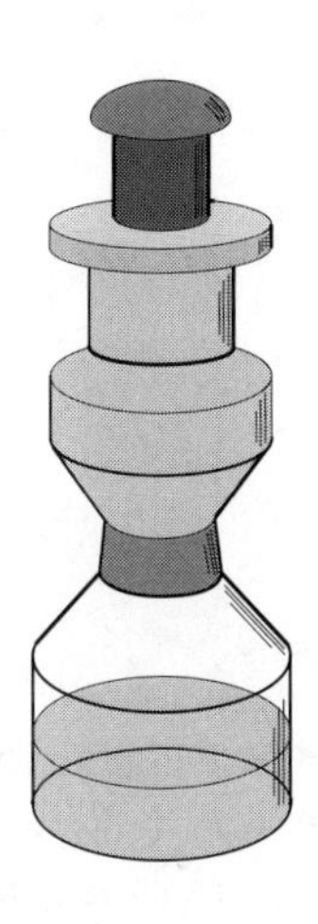

Explain how to withdraw fluid from this receptacle.

TRUE OR FALSE

Mark "T" for true and "F" for false for each statement. Correct all false statements.

_____ 26. When drugs are given parenterally rather than orally, the onset of drug action is generally more rapid but of shorter duration.

_____ 27. Injection of drugs requires skill and special care because of the trauma at the site of needle puncture, possibility of infection, chance of allergic reaction, and that once medication is injected, the drug is irretrievable.

_____ 28. Insulin is now manufactured in U-50 concentration in the United States.

_____ 29. Low-dose insulin syringes are used for patients receiving 80 units or less of U-100 insulin.

_____ 30. Ampules are glass containers that usually contain a single dose of medication.

CHAPTER 10

Student Name____________________

Parenteral Administration: Safe Preparation of Parenteral Medications

Practice Questions for the NCLEX Examination

_____ 1. When preparing to administer a medication from an ampule, the nurse should:
1. move all of the solution to the top of the ampule.
2. cover the ampule neck with a sterile gauze pledget or antiseptic swab while breaking the top off.
3. use a 23-gauge needle to withdraw the medication from the ampule.
4. keep the needle straight and turn the ampule to the side so that all of the medication is removed.

_____ 2. When reconstituting a sterile powder from a vial in preparation for parenteral administration, the nurse should perform which of the following actions? (Select all that apply.)
1. Pull back on the plunger of the syringe to fill with an amount of air equal to the volume of solution to be withdrawn.
2. Withdraw the measured volume of diluent required for reconstitution of the powdered drug.
3. Insert the needle in the diaphragm of the bottle with the powder and inject the diluent into the powder.
4. Withdraw the appropriate amount of reconstituted sterile powder and immediately administer the drug to the patient.

_____ 3. When administering medications in the operating room, the nurse should always follow which of the following actions? (Select all that apply.)
1. Save unused portions of medications for use in other surgical procedures.
2. Tell the surgeon the name and dosage or concentration of the medication or solution handed to him or her.
3. Repeat the entire medication order back to the surgeon at the time the request is made to verify all aspects of the order.
4. Check the accuracy of the drug order against the medication being prepared at least three times during the preparation phase.

_____ 4. Which of the following actions does the nurse identify as appropriate when administering two forms of insulin?
1. Discard NPH insulin if it is cloudy.
2. First, inject the amount of air equal to the amount of insulin to be withdrawn into the regular insulin.
3. First, draw up the NPH insulin to be administered.
4. Be careful not to inject any of the first type of insulin already in the syringe into the vial.

_____ 5. Ms. W. is an overweight adult in need of an intramuscular injection. Which of the following needle lengths would be most effective in ensuring appropriate intramuscular medication administration to Ms. W.?
1. 4 inches
2. 3 inches
3. 2 inches
4. 1 inch

_____ 6. When preparing to administer blood to a patient, the nurse identifies which of the following as an appropriate needle gauge? (Select all that apply.)
1. 18
2. 19
3. 20
4. 22

_____ 7. Which of the following volumes of medication are acceptable for intramuscular administration at one site to an older infant? (Select all that apply.)
1. 0.5 mL
2. 1.0 mL
3. 1.5 mL
4. 2.0 mL

_____ 8. Which of the following statements about insulin syringes are true? (Select all that apply.)
1. If an insulin syringe is not available, a tuberculin syringe may be substituted for insulin administration, as they both hold about 1 mL.
2. The U-100 insulin syringe holds 100 units of insulin per mL.
3. Low-dose insulin syringes may be used for patients receiving 50 units or less of U-100 insulin.
4. The small lines on the insulin syringe represent volume of the insulin as measured in minims.

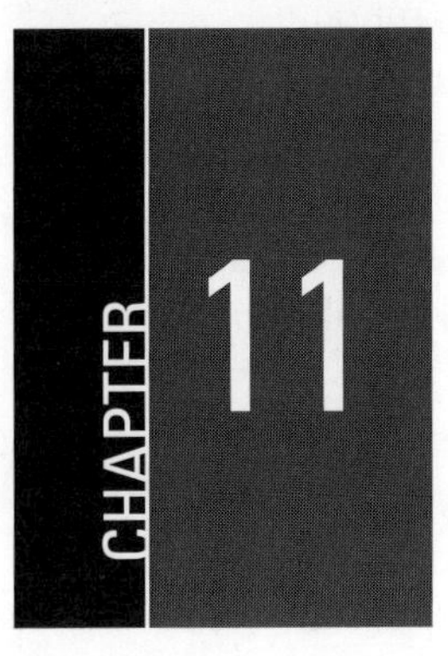

Parenteral Administration: Intradermal, Subcutaneous, and Intramuscular Routes

Review Sheet

The QUESTION column and the ANSWER column have been offset so you can cover the answer while reading the question, allowing you to assess your knowledge.

Question

1. Identify the layer of skin in which an intradermal injection is deposited.
2. Name the common intradermal injection sites.
3. Prior to allergy sensitivity testing, what medications should be stopped for 24 to 48 hours?
4. What volume can safely be injected at one site for intradermal, subcutaneous, IM, and IV medications?
5. What is the angle of the needle inserted for an intradermal injection?
6. How do you "read" a skin test?
7. List the terms associated with intradermal administration and reading of the reactions.
8. Describe patient education that should be done in advance and at the time of performing intradermal testing.
9. What types of subcutaneous injections do NOT require aspiration prior to injection of the medication?
10. List the injection sites used for IM injections.
11. Why is the gluteal area NOT used for IM injections in children under 3 years of age?
12. When is the Z-track method of IM injection used?

Answer

1. Intradermal injections are made into the dermal layer of skin below the epidermis.
2. Upper chest, scapular area of back, inner aspect of forearm.
3. Antihistamines, antiinflammatory agents, certain sleep medications, and immunosuppressants. (Always check with MD before discontinuing medications.)
4. Review Table 10-1 in Chapter 10.
5. A 15-degree angle with the needle bevel upward.
6. Positive reactions are measured, both the wheal and erythema, and by palpation and measurement of the size of any induration present.
7. See textbook, pp. 163-165.
8. See textbook, p. 163.
9. Heparin and insulin do not require aspiration prior to injection.
10. See textbook, pp. 168-171.
11. The gluteal muscle is not adequately developed.

13. What is the purpose of performing a premedication assessment?

12. The Z-track method is used with medications that are particularly irritating or that will stain the skin (e.g., injectable iron).
13. Premedication assessment is performed to prevent the administration of a medication to a patient whose diagnosis, symptoms, or other data indicate the medication should not be administered.

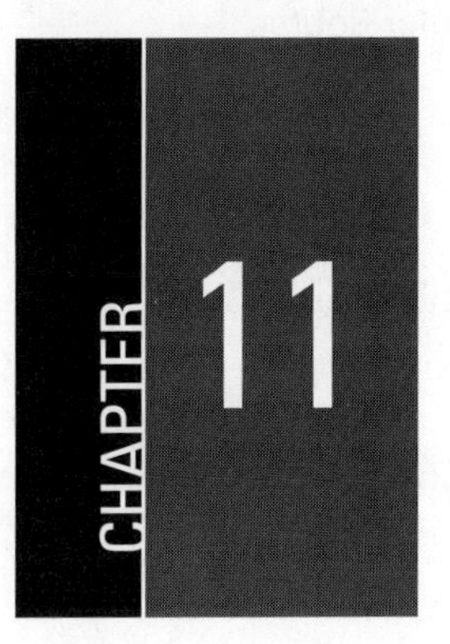

Student Name ____________________

Parenteral Administration: Intradermal, Subcutaneous, and Intramuscular Routes

Learning Activities

FILL-IN-THE-BLANK

Finish each of the following statements using the correct term.

1. ____________________ injections are made by penetrating a needle through the dermis and subcutaneous tissue into the muscle layer.
2. Intramuscular injections should be made at a(n) ________-degree angle.
3. When a drug that is irritating needs to be administered intramuscularly, the ____________________ method is commonly used.
4. To use the ____________________ area for intramuscular injection, the patient should be placed in the prone position on a flat surface.
5. When administering __________________ and __________________ subcutaneously, the nurse should not aspirate after the needle has been inserted.

LABELING

Label the following syringes.

6. ______________

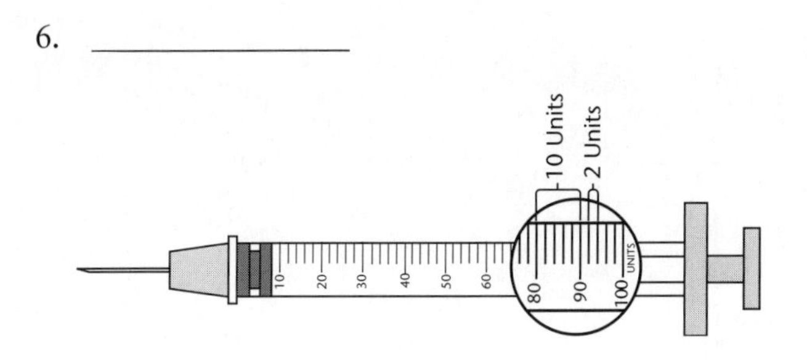

7. ______________

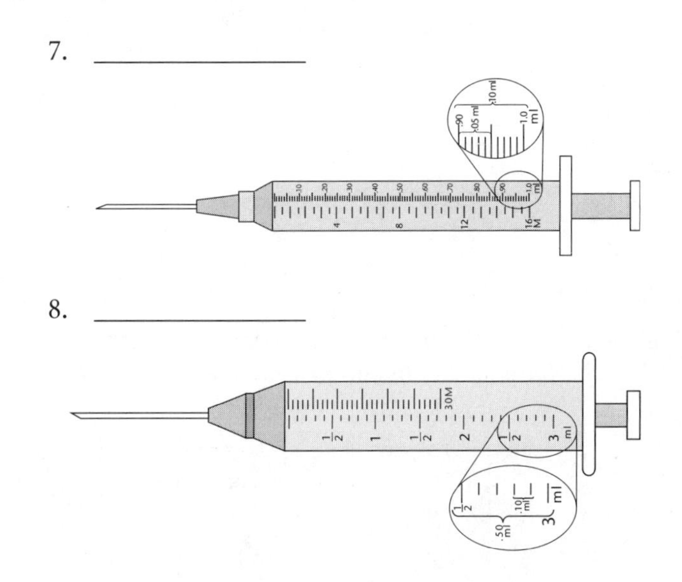

8. ______________

Read the following syringes.

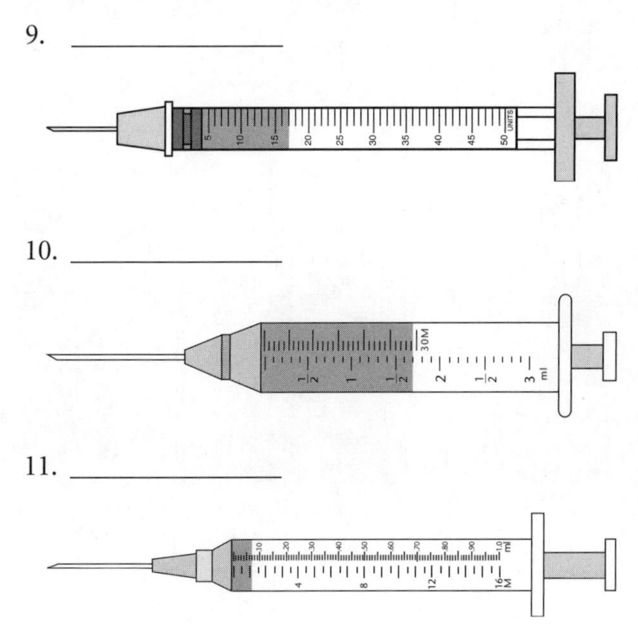

9. ______________

10. ______________

11. ______________

12. ________________

13. ________________

14. ________________

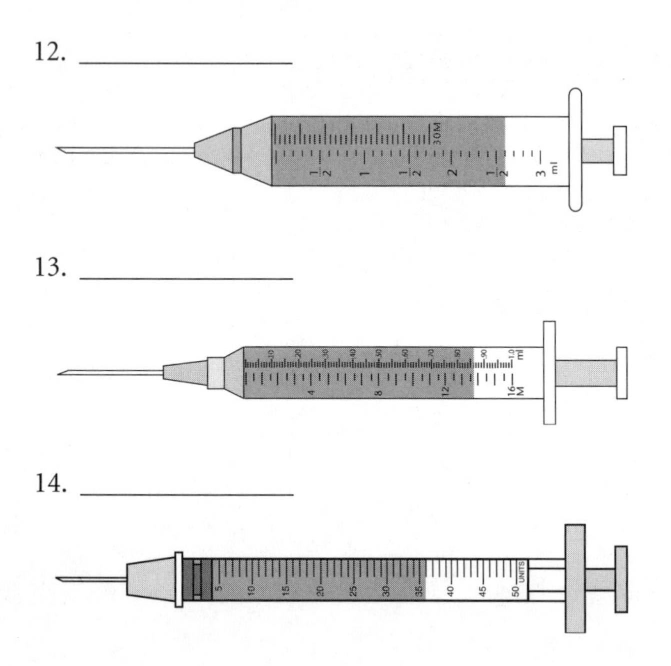

15. Label the figure below with the injection sites used for subcutaneous drug administration.

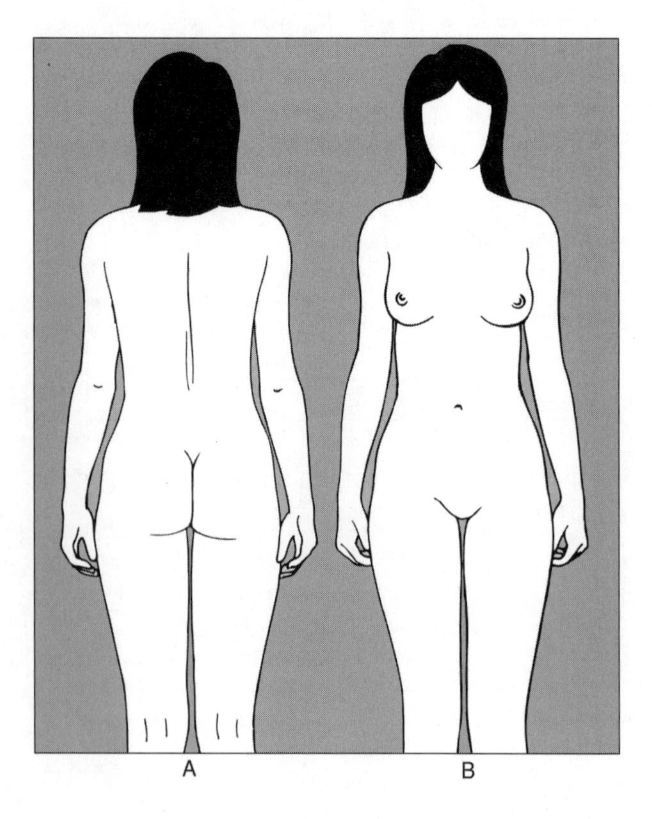

16. Label the pictures below with the sites for intramuscular injection in a child and an adult.

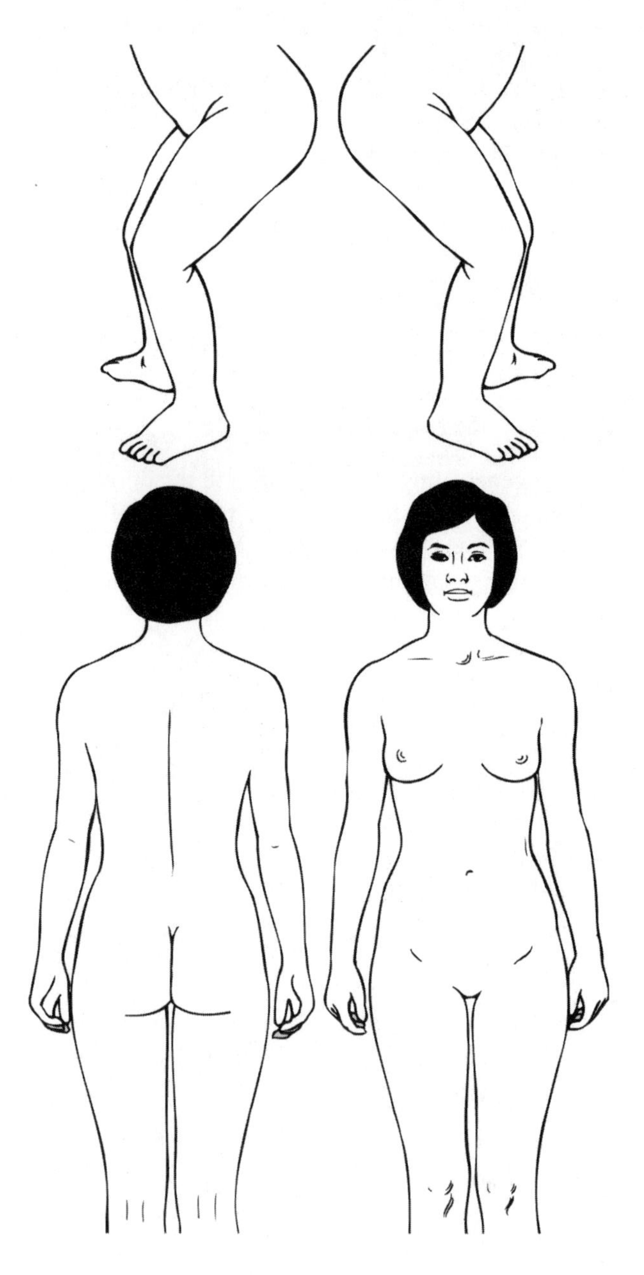

TRUE OR FALSE

Mark "T" for true and "F" for false for each statement. Correct all false statements.

_____ 17. Intradermal injections are made into the dermal layer of skin just below the epidermis.

_____ 18. The usual amount of volume injected subcutaneously is 2 to 5 mL.

_____ 19. When administering heparin subcutaneously, insert the needle quickly at a 45-degree angle, do not aspirate, and slowly inject the medication.

_____ 20. The gluteal area must not be used for intramuscular injection of medication in children under 3 years of age because the muscle is not yet well-developed from walking.

_____ 21. When using the deltoid muscle for intramuscular drug administration in adults, the volume should be limited to 2 mL or less, and the substance must not cause irritation.

CHAPTER 11

Student Name__________

Parenteral Administration: Intradermal, Subcutaneous, and Intramuscular Routes

Practice Questions for the NCLEX Examination

_____ 1. When preparing to provide allergy testing to a patient using the intradermal injection technique, the nurse should:
1. insert the needle at a 90-degree angle with the needle bevel facing down.
2. recap the needle used before disposing of it in a puncture-resistant container.
3. wear gloves.
4. deposit the solution being injected into the subcutaneous tissue under the skin.

_____ 2. The nurse is preparing to administer an intramuscular injection in the dorsogluteal area. Which of the following actions would be most appropriate for the nurse to take?
1. Position the patient in the prone position with the toes pointed inward.
2. Have the patient flex the dorsogluteal muscles to minimize pain from the injection.
3. Identify the site by forming a "V" on the greater trochanter of the femur.
4. Hold the syringe at a 30-degree angle to the surface of the patient's skin.

_____ 3. The usual amount of medication administered via the intramuscular route to adults is:
1. 2 mL.
2. 3 mL.
3. 4 mL.
4. 5 mL.

_____ 4. Which of the following statements by a patient indicates that more teaching is needed about rotating subcutaneous insulin injection sites?
1. "Common sites for subcutaneous administration of insulin include upper arms, anterior thighs, and abdomen."
2. "The fastest site of absorption of insulin is when I inject into the abdomen."
3. "I need to rotate injection sites to prevent lipohypertrophy or lipoatrophy which will slow the absorption of insulin."
4. "Exercise will not affect the rate of insulin absorption."

5. The upper volume of medication that can be delivered to a patient via the subcutaneous route is _____ mL.

6. The upper volume of medication that can be delivered into a muscle is _____ mL.

_____ 7. The most common site for the administration of intradermal medication is the inner aspect of the:
1. thigh.
2. forearm.
3. upper arm.
4. shin.

CHAPTER 12

Parenteral Administration: Intravenous Route

Review Sheet

The QUESTION column and the ANSWER column have been offset so that you can cover the answer while reading the question, allowing you to assess your knowledge.

Question

1. What does the term *intravenous* mean?
2. Nurses having certification for IV therapy can use the initials ____ in their title.
3. Name two agencies that are recommended resources for establishing standards relating to IV therapy.
4. What types of IV administration sets are available?
5. What types of controller clamps are commonly used on IV administration sets?
6. Differentiate between nonvolumetric and volumetric IV infusion controllers.
7. Differentiate among peripheral access devices, midline catheters, central devices, and implantable venous infusion ports. Identify their uses, sites of insertion, and what vessel the catheter tip should be in when placement is complete.
8. How frequently should peripheral catheters be changed?
9. Describe the flushing of Hickman, Broviac, and Groshong catheters.
10. What types of needles are used to access an implanted port and a CathLink 20 port?
11. What does it mean when an IV solution is *isotonic, hypotonic,* or *hypertonic*?
12. What criteria are used to select an isotonic, hypotonic, or hypertonic IV solution for administration to a patient?
13. Compare the preparation for administration of IV solutions delivered in glass bottles with those in plastic bags.

Answer

1. *Intravenous* means "in the vein." In the context of this chapter, it means administration of fluids directly into the bloodstream.
2. CRNI
3. Infusion Nurses Society (INS) and Centers for Disease Control and Prevention (CDC)
4. See textbook, pp. 176-177.
5. Roller and slide clamps. *Note:* A dial-style controller is also available for use.
6. Nonvolumetric infusion devices only monitor the gravity-induced flow by counting drops that pass through the drip chamber; volumetric IV controllers apply external pressure to pump the IV fluid at a specified rate.
7. See textbook, pp. 178-181.
8. 72 to 96 hours (check policy manual where functioning).
9. See textbook, p. 180.
10. All ports except the CathLink 20 are accessed using a Huber needle. The CathLink 20 uses a standard over-the-needle IV catheter (p. 181).
11. See textbook, p. 183.
12. See textbook, p. 183.

14. When setting up an IV fluid or medication for administration as an IV piggyback, how should the piggyback bag be positioned?
15. Compare common peripheral access devices and the intended use of each.
16. Describe vein selection for the initiation of an IV in the hand or forearm.
17. Identify common veins used for initiating IV therapy in infants and children.
18. What are the most common veins used for central venous catheter access?
19. Study and practice IV-related procedures found throughout this chapter in the laboratory setting (e.g., venipuncture, spiking and hanging an IV, adding an IV piggyback to a primary line, giving IV drugs by bolus method, preparing an ADD-Vantage or similar prepackaged system of medication for administration IV, and operating syringe pumps and volumetric and nonvolumetric infusion control devices). Check with the instructor for details.
20. Obtain copies of procedures used at the clinical site where you are assigned for:
    - frequency of changing IV tubing.
    - IV peripheral sites.
    - length of time IV solutions can remain hanging.
    - recording of IV fluids and IV medications on the MAR.
    - procedures for flushing and dressing of heparin, saline, or medlock.
    - central venous catheters and PICC lines.
21. Explain the SASH procedure used for IV therapy.
22. Which type of IV central catheter does not require flushing with heparin?
23. What is a commonly accepted rate for a TKO (to keep open) IV order?
24. What is the purpose of a premedication assessment?

13. See Figure 12-1.
14. See Figure 12-9.
15. See Figures 12-3, 12-4, and textbook, pp. 178-179.
16. See Figures 12-10 and 12-11.
17. See Figure 12-12.
18. The subclavian and jugular veins are most commonly used for central IV access.
19. Consult with your instructor to obtain detailed instructions for practicing and being "checked off" on procedures relating to IV.
20. See general guidelines, textbook pp. 185-187. Guidelines of individual practice settings should always be consulted.
21. **S** = Saline
    A = Administer drug
    S = Saline
    H = Heparin (Not all types of vascular access devices require the use of heparin; check hospital policy.)
22. Groshong
23. A commonly accepted rate for TKO IV is 10 mL/hr.

25. What is the formula used to calculate an IV drip rate?
26. Describe the correct method of monitoring an infusing IV solution and site.
27. Describe how to assess for infiltration at an IV site.
28. If you see air in the tubing of a running IV, what should you do?
29. What are the signs and symptoms of circulatory overload and pulmonary edema?
30. How is a suspected pulmonary embolism verified?
31. Differentiate between the terms *infiltration* and *extravasation.*

24. Premedication assessment is performed to prevent the administration of a medication to a patient whose diagnosis, symptoms, or other data indicate the medication should not be administered.
25. $\frac{\text{mL of solution x number of drops/mL}}{\text{hrs of administration x 60 min/hr}}$ = drops/min
26. Check the ordered IV solution, total amount infused, drip rate, IV tubing for kinks or air in the line, date and time the IV solution was hung, and check for IV site infiltration.
27. Check for limb's color, size, or skin integrity; compare with the opposite limb. See textbook for guidelines to follow and for the infiltration scale, Figure 12-19.
28. Clamp the tubing; use a syringe to withdraw the air bubble.
29. Symptoms of circulatory overload include engorged neck veins; dyspnea; reduced urine output; edema; bounding pulse; and shallow, rapid respirations. Symptoms of pulmonary edema include dyspnea, cough, anxiety, rales, rhonchi, possible cardiac dysrhythmias, thready pulse, frothy sputum, and elevation or drop in blood pressure depending on the severity.
30. A lung scan is done as well as drawing ABGs and baseline prothrombin times.
31. Infiltration is leakage of IV solution into the tissue surrounding the vein; extravasation is leakage of an irritant chemical into the tissue surrounding the vein.

CHAPTER 12

Student Name ______________________________

Parenteral Administration: Intravenous Route

Learning Activities

FILL-IN-THE-BLANK

Finish each of the following statements using the correct term.

1. Macrodrip intravenous chambers provide ____, ____, or ____ drops/mL, whereas microdrip chambers deliver ____ drops/mL.

2. If the IV solution and the blood have approximately the same osmolality, the solution is said to be ____________________; if the solutions has fewer dissolved particles than the blood, they are known as being ____________________, and those with higher concentrations of dissolved particles are considered to be ____________________ solutions.

3. The most commonly used veins for IV administration in infants and children are in the ____________________ region of the scalp, ____________________ of the hand, and ____________________ of the foot.

4. Two types of solutions are used to maintain patency of vascular access devices: ____________________ is used to prevent clot formation and ____________________ is used to clean the interior diameter of the device of blood or particles of medication.

5. Some complications of intravenous therapy include ____________________, which is leakage of an intravenous solution into the tissue surrounding the vein, and ____________________, which is the leakage of an irritant chemical into the tissue surrounding the vein.

6. The usual time interval between tube changes on lipid solutions is _____ hours.

7. Based on drop volume, an IV administration set that delivers 20 gtt/mL is called a(n) ____________________ set.

8. A type of IV device that holds a prefilled syringe is called a(n) ____________________ ____________________.

9. A(n) ____________________-the-needle catheter is commonly inserted peripherally for routine peripheral infusion therapy.

10. This type of IV infusion device is designed for use over a 2- to 4-week period of use. It is known as a(n) ______________ ______________ ______________.

11. A type of central venous catheter that a qualified nurse can insert is known as a(n) ____________________ catheter.

12. A type of tunneled venous catheter that does not require flushing with heparin is known as a(n) ____________________ catheter.

13. Name three types of vessels that comprise the intravascular compartment:
    1) ____________________,
    2) ____________________, and
    3) ____________________.

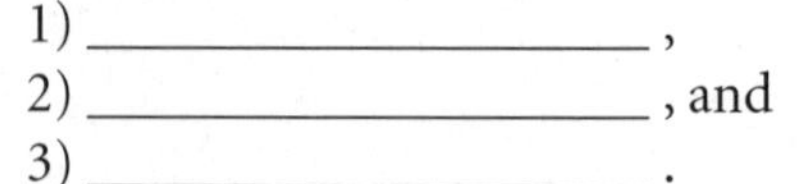

14. Isotonic solutions have an osmolality range of _____ to _____ mOsm/L.

15. Hypertonic solutions (e.g., parenteral nutrition solutions) are administered through central infusion lines directly into the ______________ ______________ ______________.

16. Name the agency that is recognized as a recommended resource to be consulted when establishing guidelines relating to infectious diseases.

____

LABELING

Label the following.

17. What type of drip chamber is this?

____

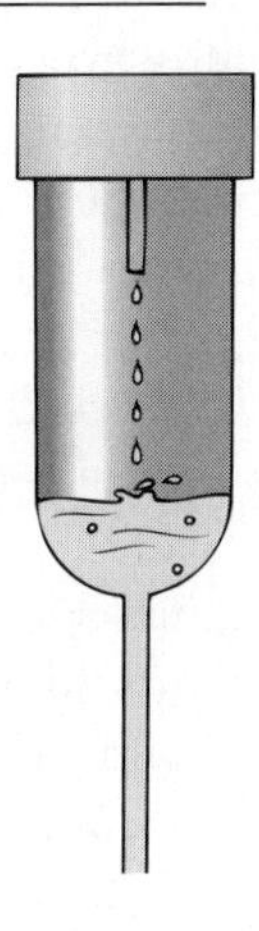

18. Figure A is a(n): ______________

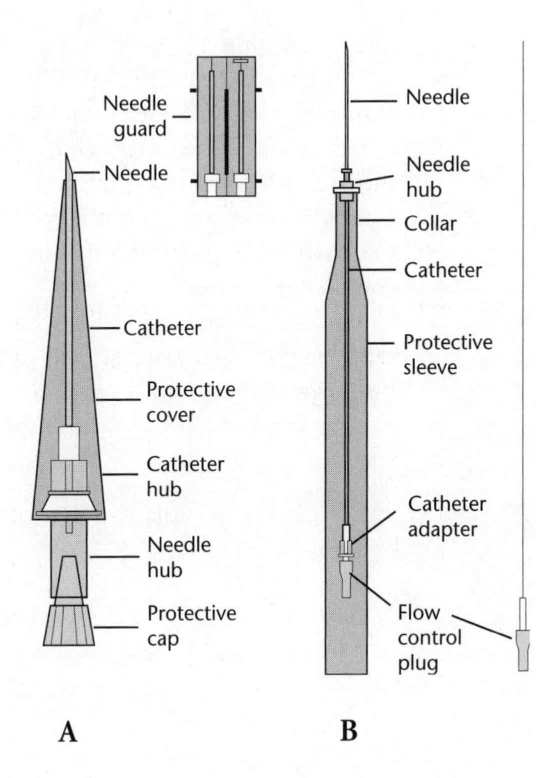

TRUE OR FALSE

Mark "T" for true and "F" for false for each statement. Correct all false statements.

_____ 19. Intravenous administration is the most rapid of all parenteral routes because it bypasses all barriers to drug absorption.

_____ 20. Topical antibiotics or creams should not be used on peripheral intravenous catheters because they have the potential to promote fungal infections and antimicrobial resistance.

_____ 21. Bacteriostatic water or saline containing the benzyl preservative to reconstitute or dilute medications or to flush IV catheters of newborns should not be used because the preservative is toxic to these patients.

_____ 22. Thrombophlebitis is the inflammation of a vein, and phlebitis is inflammation of the vein with the formation of a thrombus in the area of inflammation.

_____ 23. Flushing the IV line by speeding the IV solution is not recommended because the medication still in the line would be administered too rapidly.

CHAPTER 12

Student Name________________________________

Parenteral Administration: Intravenous Route

Practice Questions for the NCLEX Examination

_____ 1. Mr. K. is ordered a peripherally inserted central venous catheter (PICC) for the administration of medications. The nurse has taught Mr. K. about the insertion procedure, use, and care of his PICC line. Which of the following statements by Mr. K. indicates that more teaching is needed?
1. "I will be placed under general anesthesia to have this intravenous line inserted."
2. "I will be able to go home with a PICC."
3. "My PICC line can last up to a year if it is properly cared for."
4. "The PICC line should be flushed with a saline-heparin solution after every use, or daily if not used."

_____ 2. Which of the following statements about implantable infusion ports are correct? (Select all that apply.)
1. Blood products can be administered through an implantable infusion port.
2. One port of a two port system may be reserved for drawing blood samples.
3. An implanted central venous access catheter may remain in place for over a year and only requires a saline-heparin solution flush after every access or once monthly.
4. The CDC recommends that central venous catheters be routinely replaced to prevent catheter-related infection

_____ 3. Mr. R. has been admitted to the health care facility after experiencing a GI bleed at home which has now resolved. Mr. R. has an intravascular fluid volume deficit because he has lost a lot of volume and is in need of fluid replacement. The nurse would anticipate which of the following intravenous fluids to be ordered for Mr. R.?
1. 0.9% sodium chloride
2. 0.2% sodium chloride
3. 0.45% sodium chloride
4. 5% dextrose in water

_____ 4. When providing care to a patient receiving intravenous therapy, the nurse should perform which of the following actions? (Select all that apply.)
1. Wear gloves to inspect the IV site.
2. If it appears that the intravenous access device is clotted, attempt to clear the needle by flushing with fluid.
3. Check the drip chamber; if it is less than half full, squeeze it to fill more completely.
4. Check the temperature of the solution being infused because cold solutions can cause spasms in the vein.

_____ 5. The nurse should follow which of the following practices when administering a medication by a heparin/saline/medlock? (Select all that apply.)
1. Select a syringe several milliliters larger than that required by the volume of the drug.
2. When a blood return is established, inject saline for flush followed by the medication at the rate specified by the manufacturer.
3. After the medication is administered, insert another syringe containing 10 mL of normal saline to flush the remaining drug from the catheter.
4. Maintain constant pressure on the plunger of the syringe used to flush the line after the medication has been administered while simultaneously withdrawing the needle from the diaphragm to prevent backflow of blood.

_____ 6. Which of the following needle gauges does the nurse determine as appropriate for the administration of blood? (Select all that apply.)
1. 26
2. 25
3. 20
4. 16
5. 18

_____ 7. In calculating intravenous fluid rates, microdrip chambers form how many drops per milliliter?
1. 10
2. 15
3. 20
4. 60

_____ 8. Which of the following statements about peripherally inserted central venous catheters (PICC) are correct? (Select all that apply.)
1. They are not available for pediatric use.
2. PICC line insertion is only attempted in the operating room.
3. PICC lines are easier to maintain than short peripheral catheters because there is less frequent infiltration and phlebitis.
4. They should not be used for long-term administration of total parenteral nutrition.

CHAPTER 13

Drugs Affecting the Autonomic Nervous System

Review Sheet

The QUESTION column and the ANSWER column have been offset so that you can cover the answer while reading the question, allowing you to assess your knowledge.

Question

1. The central nervous system is composed of ____________.
2. The autonomic nervous system relays information from the central nervous system to ____________.
3. The autonomic nervous system controls the functions of what types of tissue?
4. What primary function is controlled by the motor nervous system?
5. What neurotransmitter is liberated by cholinergic fibers?
6. What neurotransmitter is liberated by adrenergic fibers?
7. What three major types of receptors are found in the autonomic nervous system?
8. Stimulation of $alpha_1$ receptors causes what action on blood vessels?
9. Stimulation of $beta_1$ receptors produces what type of effect on the heart rate?
10. Stimulation of $beta_2$ receptors produces what effects?
11. Define *adrenergic agent.*

Answer

1. The central nervous system (CNS) is composed of the brain and spinal cord.
2. The autonomic nervous system (ANS) relays information from the CNS to the whole body.
3. The ANS controls the functions of all tissue except striated muscle.
4. Skeletal muscle contractions are controlled by the motor nervous system.
5. The cholinergic fibers secrete acetylcholine.
6. The adrenergic fibers secrete norepinephrine.
7. The three major types of receptors found in the ANS are alpha-, beta-, and dopaminergic receptors.
8. Stimulation of $alpha_1$ receptors causes vasoconstriction. This results in a rise in blood pressure; therefore, before giving $alpha_1$-type medications, the blood pressure should be checked. This action makes these drugs useful in the treatment of hypotension and shock.
9. Stimulation of $beta_1$ receptors increases the heart rate. If excessive doses of a $beta_1$ agonist are administered, the patient may experience tachycardia and dysrhythmias.
10. Stimulation of $beta_2$ receptors relaxes the smooth muscle of the bronchi, uterus, and peripheral blood vessels. These actions make these drugs useful as bronchodilators and inhibitors of preterm labor.

12. When beta-adrenergic agents are administered, what effects will be seen on blood vessels, bronchi, heart rate, blood pressure, respiration, lungs, gastric motility and tone, and blood glucose?
13. What premedication assessments should be completed prior to administering an adrenergic agent?
14. Giving an excessive dose of an adrenergic agent results in what adverse effects?
15. List the primary actions of alpha-adrenergic blocking agents and beta-adrenergic blocking agents.
16. Why/when are alpha- and beta-adrenergic blocking agents prescribed?
17. State the possible effects of administering beta blockers to a patient with a known respiratory disease such as asthma or emphysema.
18. Which portion of the autonomic nervous system do cholinergic agents affect?
19. What effect do beta blockers have on a patient with diabetes mellitus?
20. What pharmacologic effect may be expected when indomethacin and beta blocker therapy are combined?
21. What drug is a specific antidote for cholinergic agents?
22. Under what types of clinical conditions are cholinergic agents used?

11. An adrenergic agent produces or mimics the effects of stimulation of the sympathetic nervous system. Therefore, these drugs are also known as "sympathomimetic" agents.
12. When adrenergic agents are administered, blood vessels dilate, bronchi dilate, heart rate increases, blood pressure may drop, GI peristalsis decreases, relaxation of the gastric smooth muscle occurs, and blood glucose increases.
13. Before administering an adrenergic agent, the following assessments should be completed: baseline vital signs (e.g., heart rate, blood pressure), screen for respiratory tract disease, and ascertain if the patient uses bronchodilators or decongestants.
14. Excessive doses of an adrenergic agent may result in dysrhythmias, hypertension, nervousness, anxiety, and insomnia due to stimulation of the sympathetic nervous system.
15. Alpha-adrenergic blocking agents act by plugging the alpha receptors, preventing vasoconstriction of arterioles. Beta-adrenergic blocking agents act by plugging the beta-adrenergic receptors, preventing beta stimulation, especially from norepinephrine and epinephrine.
16. Alpha-adrenergic blocking agents are used to treat diseases with vasoconstriction (e.g., peripheral vascular disease, Buerger's disease, and Raynaud's disease). Beta blocking agents are used to treat hypertension, angina pectoris, cardiac dysrhythmias, and hyperthyroidism.
17. Administering a beta blocker to a person with a known respiratory disease may cause bronchoconstriction and make the person experience respiratory distress.
18. Cholinergic agents affect the parasympathetic portion of the nervous system.
19. Beta blockers induce hypoglycemia; they decrease the release of insulin in response to hypoglycemia and mask the symptoms normally associated with hypoglycemia.
20. The combination of indomethacin and beta blocker therapy may cause loss of hypertensive control. The dosage of the beta blocker may need to be increased.
21. Atropine sulfate, an anticholinergic agent, is a specific antidote for cholinergic agents.

23. What side effects can be anticipated when an anticholinergic agent is administered?
24. What actions of anticholinergic agents make them useful in the clinical treatment of gastrointestinal disorders?
25. Before administering any anticholinergic agent, the patient's history should be checked for the presence of what type of eye disorder?
26. Atropine is an example of an anticholinergic agent frequently used preoperatively. Which of the drug's anticholinergic properties make this drug useful preoperatively?
27. What premedication assessments should be completed before administering an anticholinergic agent?
28. The postoperative patient who has been given atropine sulfate needs to be monitored for ___________.
29. Describe the action(s) and side effects of the following drug classifications and/or drugs: alpha-adrenergic agents, beta-adrenergic agents, cholinergic agents, anticholinergic agents, beta-adrenergic blocking agents, physostigmine, epinephrine, and atropine.

22. Cholinergic agents can be used to treat glaucoma, urinary retention, myasthenia gravis, as a muscle relaxant to reverse nondepolarizing agents, and for gastrointestinal disorders such as paralytic ileus.
23. Anticholinergic agents produce the following side effects: dryness of mouth and tongue, blurring of vision, mild nausea, and nervousness. Other side effects include constipation, urinary hesitancy or retention, tachycardia, palpitations, mydriasis, muscle cramping, and mild transient postural hypotension.
24. Anticholinergic (also known as *antispasmodic*) agents' actions include decreased secretion of saliva, hydrochloric acid, pepsin, bile, and other enzymatic fluids necessary for digestion, along with relaxation of the sphincter muscles and decreased spasm, which allows peristalsis to move the contents of the stomach and bowel through the gastrointestinal tract.
25. All patients' charts should be screened for the presence of angle-closure glaucoma before any anticholinergic agent is administered.
26. Atropine sulfate is given preoperatively to dry secretions of the mouth, nose, throat, and bronchi, and decrease secretions during surgery. It also prevents vagal stimulation and bradycardia during the placement of the endotracheal tube.
27. Check for a history of angle-closure glaucoma or history of enlarged prostate and urinary hesitancy or retention before administering an anticholinergic agent.
28. The postoperative patient who received atropine sulfate needs to be monitored frequently for urinary retention. There may also be postoperative constipation.
29. See textbook, pp. 212-217. Examine drug monographs and drug classification explanations.

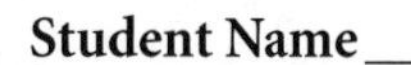

Student Name______________________________

CHAPTER 13

Drugs Affecting the Autonomic Nervous System

Learning Activities

FILL-IN-THE-BLANK

Finish each of the following statements using the correct term.

1. The efferent and afferent nerves are known collectively as the ____________________.

2. The junction between one neuron and the next is called a(n) ____________________.

3. The two major neurotransmitters of the autonomic nervous system are ____________________ and ____________________.

4. The nerve endings that liberate acetylcholine are called ____________________, and those that secrete norepinephrine are called ____________________.

5. Catecholamines that are secreted naturally in the body are ______________, ______________, and ______________.

6. Dopamine is secreted at what three primary sites in the body? ______________, ______________, ______________

7. The three types of sympathetic autonomic nervous system receptors are ______________, ______________, and ______________.

8. Cholinergic agents are also known as ____________________.

9. Stimulation of the adrenergic receptors causes smooth muscle ______________ of the bronchial muscles, which causes ______________ of the airway.

10. Stimulation of the cholinergic receptors causes smooth muscle ____________________ of the bronchial muscles, which causes ____________________ of the airway.

11. The generic names of all $beta_1$ blocking agents end in "-_____."

MATCHING

Match the generic drug name with its corresponding brand name. Each option will be used only once.

_____ 12. propantheline

_____ 13. carvedilol

_____ 14. neostigmine

_____ 15. isoproterenol

_____ 16. terbutaline

a. Isuprel
b. Pro-Banthine
c. Brethine
d. Coreg
e. Prostigmin

TRUE OR FALSE

Mark "T" for true and "F" for false for each statement. Correct all false statements.

_____ 17. The brain and spinal cord make up the central nervous system.

_____ 18. The central nervous system receives signals from afferent nerves throughout the body that are transmitted to the spinal cord and brain.

_____ 19. The transmission of nerve signals or impulses occurs because of the activity of chemical substances called *neurotransmitters.*

_____ 20. Anticholinergic agents are safe to use in patients with closed-angle glaucoma.

_____ 21. Cholinergic drugs are also known as *parasympathetic agents.*

DRUG ACTION/SIDE EFFECTS

22. *State the actions and side effects of the following drug that affects the autonomic nervous system.*

	Actions	Side Effects
CHOLINERGIC AGENTS		

CHAPTER 13

Student Name______________________________

Drugs Affecting the Autonomic Nervous System

Practice Questions for the NCLEX Examination

_____ 1. When administering a drug that stimulates $beta_2$ receptors, the nurse expects the patient to exhibit which one of the following?
1. Bronchoconstriction
2. Uterine relaxation
3. Vasoconstriction
4. Hypertension

_____ 2. Patients with which one of the following conditions would most likely benefit from the dopaminergic effects of adrenergic agents?
1. Parkinson's disease
2. Guillain-Barré syndrome
3. Amyotrophic lateral sclerosis
4. Multiple sclerosis

_____ 3. Ms. U. is taking terbutaline for treatment of chronic obstructive pulmonary disease. When working with Ms. U., the nurse assesses her for which of the following side effects?
1. Hypotension
2. Bradycardia
3. Insomnia and wakefulness
4. Skin rash

_____ 4. Which of the following drugs is the preferred treatment for a patient with asthma in need of treatment with a beta blocker?
1. Propranolol
2. Timolol
3. Nadolol
4. Atenolol

_____ 5. Before administering a beta blocker to a patient, it is most important for the nurse to assess the patient for a history of:
1. hypertension.
2. angina pectoris.
3. diabetes.
4. cardiac dysrhythmias.

_____ 6. Mr. G. experiences orthostatic hypotension as a result of taking an adrenergic agent for treatment of hypertension. Which of the following measures should the nurse incorporate into his care? (Select all that apply.)
1. Monitor the blood pressure in the standing position daily.
2. Monitor the blood pressure daily in the supine position.
3. Teach Mr. G. to rise slowly from a supine or sitting position.
4. Encourage Mr. G. to sit down if feeling faint.

_____ 7. The nurse assessing a patient who is taking a beta-adrenergic blocking agent should report which of the following findings to the primary health care provider? (Select all that apply.)
1. Bradycardia
2. Wheezing
3. Orthopnea
4. Hypoglycemia

_____ 8. Some of the effects of cholinergic agents include which of the following? (Select all that apply.)
1. Increased heartbeat
2. Miosis of the eye
3. Increased contractions of the urinary bladder
4. Sweating

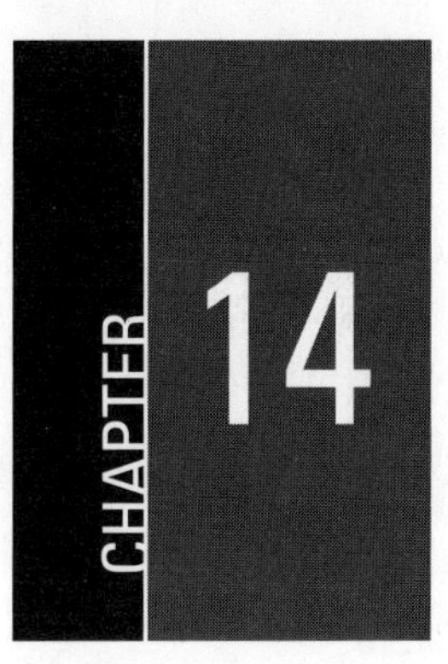

Sedative-Hypnotics

Review Sheet

The QUESTION column and the ANSWER column have been offset so that you can cover the answer while reading the questions, allowing you to assess your knowledge.

Question

1. What are the four stages of sleep?
2. What is another name for paradoxic sleep?
3. What is insomnia?
4. What premedication assessments should be performed prior to administering any sedative-hypnotic agent?
5. Differentiate between the actions of a sedative and a hypnotic.
6. What should a nursing history relating to a patient's complaints of insomnia include?
7. Name two classes of drugs used as sedative-hypnotics. What ending appears on the generic drug names?
8. State the effect of hypnotics on respiratory function.
9. What changes in REM sleep occur with the administration of barbiturates?
10. What is a rebound effect associated with discontinuing barbiturates?
11. What is meant by *morning hangover* associated with barbiturates, benzodiazepines, and miscellaneous agents used as sedative-hypnotics? State the associated health teaching that needs to be initiated.

Answer

1. Sleep stages I-IV are explained in the textbook, p. 218.
2. Rapid eye movement (REM) sleep is also called paradoxic sleep.
3. Insomnia is the inability to sleep.
4. Before administering a sedative-hypnotic agent, assess for level of alertness, orientation, and ability to perform motor functions, as well as current blood pressure, pulse, respirations, sleep pattern, anxiety level, and environmental and nutritional factors that might impede sleep.
5. Hypnotics produce sleep. Sedatives relax the patient.
6. A nursing history related to a patient's complaints of insomnia should include usual pattern of sleep, anxiety level, environmental factors, nutritional habits, and medications or actions tried before seeking current treatment.
7. Two classes of sedative-hypnotics are barbiturates (all end in "-tal") and benzodiazepines (all end in "-am," except chlordiazepoxide [Librium]).
8. Hypnotics produce mild to marked respiratory depression, depending on dosage and pulmonary function.
9. Barbiturates initially decrease REM sleep; however, as tolerance builds, REM sleep returns to normal.
10. A rebound effect associated with discontinuing barbiturates is increase in REM; it may take several weeks following barbiturate therapy for this to resolve.

12. What is a paradoxical response to hypnotics and what nursing actions are required if this response occurs?
13. What laboratory studies are recommended with continued use of barbiturates and benzodiazepines?
14. List the generic and brand names of commonly prescribed barbiturates, benzodiazepines, and miscellaneous sedative-hypnotic agents as assigned by the instructor.
15. In addition to their use as sedative-hypnotics, for what other clinical uses are barbiturates prescribed?
16. What effect can the regular use of barbiturates have on oral contraceptive therapy?
17. What is the blood-brain barrier?
18. What side effects can be expected from the administration of sedative-hypnotics?
19. What are side effects to report when taking sedative-hypnotics?
20. What premedication assessments should be performed before administration of a benzodiazepine?

11. Morning hangover from sedative-hypnotics includes blurred vision, mental dullness, and mild hypotension. Health teaching about this effect should include directions to consult physician if these symptoms become too bothersome; instructions to rise slowly to sitting position, equilibrate, then stand; and a caution regarding use of machinery, etc.
12. Paradoxical response is a period of excitement prior to sedation induced by use of barbiturates and other sedative-hypnotics not usually associated with benzodiazepine therapy. Appropriate nursing actions include protecting the patient from harm providing for channelling of energy.
13. RBC, WBC, and differential count lab studies should be done with continued use of barbiturates and benzodiazepines. Also immediately report sore throat, fever, progressive weakness, purpura, or jaundice.
14. Consult Tables 14-1, 14-2, and 14-3.
15. Specific agents are used as anticonvulsants and induction anesthetics.
16. The client may need to use an alternative form of contraceptive therapy, particularly if spotting or breakthrough bleeding occurs.
17. The blood-brain barrier is a membrane that controls the passage of drugs into the central nervous system to the receptor sites on the cells within the central nervous system.
18. Side effects of sedative-hypnotics include hangover, sedation, lethargy, blurred vision, and transient hypotension.
19. Side effects of sedative-hypnotics to report are excessive use or abuse, paradoxical response, pruritus, rash, high fever, sore throat, purpura, and jaundice.
20. Before administering a benzodiazepine, assess vital signs, including blood pressure in lying and sitting positions. Check whether the client is in the first trimester of pregnancy, breastfeeding, or has a history of a blood dyscrasia or hepatic disease.

Student Name ____________________

Sedative-Hypnotics

Learning Activities

FILL-IN-THE-BLANK

Finish each of the following statements using the correct term.

1. ____________________ is the most common sleep disorder known.
2. A(n) ____________________ is a drug that produces sleep; a(n) __________________ quiets the patient and gives a feeling of relaxation and rest, not necessarily accompanied by sleep.
3. The long-acting barbiturate, phenobarbital, is also used as a(n) ____________________.
4. The ____________________ are the most commonly used sedative-hypnotics.
5. To enhance sleep, patients should be offered foods high in ____________________ and ____________________ products at a specific time before sleep.

Choose from the following vocabulary words to complete the statements: sedative, hypnotic, rebound sleep, paradoxic excitement, initial insomnia, intermittent insomnia, terminal insomnia. Not all words will be used.

Steve has difficulty falling asleep, and the physician he consults tells him this is known as (6.) ____________________. While at the sleep disorder clinic, Steve tells another patient, Walt, about his difficulty sleeping. Walt quickly explains this isn't the same as his problem. He falls asleep, but awakens about 4 AM and can't get back to sleep. Walt's insomnia pattern is called (7.) ____________________.

Prior to surgery, the physician prescribes a(n) (8.) ______________ to help James to sleep. The next morning, a(n) (9.) ___________ is ordered for 8 AM (0800) for the purpose of providing relaxation and rest while awaiting scheduled surgery at 10:30 AM (1030). Two days after surgery, James asks the nurse if it would be OK to ask the doctor for a prescription for the "wonderful medication" he took prior to surgery because he had the best sleep that day. The nurse asks him about his sleep pattern. He describes that he generally has difficulty sleeping all night at home. He sleeps a while, awakens, and sleeps in cycles several times nightly. The nurse tells him this is known as (10.) ____________________.

MATCHING

Match the generic drug name with its corresponding brand name. Each option will be used only once.

_____ 11. triazolam

_____ 12. midazolam

_____ 13. flurazepam

_____ 14. pentobarbital

_____ 15. amobarbital

a. Versed
b. Amytal
c. Dalmane
d. Halcion
e. Nembutal

TRUE OR FALSE

Mark "T" for true and "F" for false for each statement. Correct all false statements.

_____ 16. Insomnia is not a disease but a symptom of physical or mental stress.

_____ 17. A common side effect of barbiturate therapy is daytime sedation.

_____ 18. Most cases of insomnia are short-lived and can be effectively treated by nonpharmacologic methods.

_____ 19. Habitual use of benzodiazepines does not ever result in physical dependence.

_____ 20. Smoking enhances the metabolism of benzodiazepines.

DRUG ACTION/SIDE EFFECTS

21. *State the actions and side effects of the following drug class.*

	Actions	Side Effects
BARBITURATES		

Student Name______________________________

Sedative-Hypnotics

Practice Questions for the NCLEX Examination

_____ 1. When working with patients taking nonbarbiturate, nonbenzodiazepine sedative-hypnotic agents, the nurse knows that:
1. daytime drowsiness is generally not a problem with these agents because of their short half-lives.
2. they do not produce physical dependence with habitual use.
3. these drugs may be abruptly discontinued.
4. if restlessness and/or anxiety develop, the drugs need to be immediately stopped.

_____ 2. Nurses working with pregnant and lactating patients taking benzodiazepines should know that these agents:
1. do not cross the placenta.
2. do not enter the fetal circulation.
3. should not be administered during the first trimester of pregnancy.
4. do not cross into breast milk.

_____ 3. Mr. Q. was taking barbiturates for a sleep disorder for a long period of time. He has been admitted to the hospital because of rapid discontinuation of the barbiturates. The nurse would expect Mr. Q. to exhibit which of the following signs/symptoms of rapid barbiturate discontinuation? (Select all that apply.)
1. Anxiety
2. Delirium
3. Grand mal seizures
4. Hypotension

_____ 4. Mr. I. is ordered a sedative-hypnotic drug PRN. It is 11:00 PM and the nurse is assessing Mr. I.'s status. The most appropriate action the nurse should take with Mr. I. is to:
1. administer the sedative-hypnotic drug to ensure Mr. I. receives a good night's sleep.
2. not offer the sedative-hypnotic unless Mr. I. is having difficulty sleeping, and other measures to meet comfort and psychological needs have failed to produce the desired effect.
3. leave the sedative-hypnotic at Mr. I.'s bedside and instruct him to take it if he has difficulty falling asleep.
4. tell Mr. I. he should not take the sedative-hypnotic under any conditions because he should not risk getting addicted to it.

_____ 5. The nurse would expect to find which of the following signs displayed by a patient who appears to be in REM sleep? (Select all that apply.)
1. Decreased heart rate
2. Irregular breathing
3. Some muscular activity
4. Rapid eye movement

_____ 6. Which of the following pieces of information would the nurse include in patient education about nonpharmacologic methods to enhance sleep? (Select all that apply.)
1. Do not go to bed at the same time each night; go to bed when you feel the most tired.
2. Eat your heaviest meal of the day about 45 minutes before you plan to go to bed.
3. Exercise during the day, not near bedtime.
4. Avoid eating chocolate.

_____ 7. Which of the following side effects would the nurse expect to find when assessing a patient who is taking barbiturate therapy for sleep disturbance? (Select all that apply.)
1. Skin rash
2. Blurred vision
3. Restlessness
4. Transient hypotension on arising

_____ 8. Which of the following medications does the nurse identify as potentially inducing or aggravating insomnia? (Select all that apply.)
1. Corticosteroids
2. SSRI antidepressants
3. Theophylline
4. Levodopa

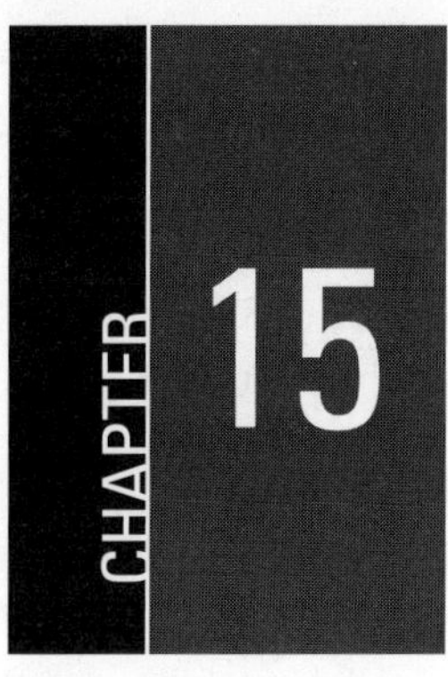

Drugs Used for Parkinson's Disease

Review Sheet

The QUESTION column and the ANSWER column have been offset so that you can cover the answer while reading the question, allowing you to assess your knowledge.

Question

1. Prepare a list of signs and symptoms of parkinsonism.
2. Summarize the purpose of giving medications to treat Parkinson's disease.
3. Identify the basic components of a baseline assessment of a patient's neurologic function.
4. What are the monitoring parameters found on the Unified Parkinson's Disease Rating Scale?
5. What are the meanings of the terms: *dyskinesia; propulsive, uncontrolled movement;* and *akinesia*?
6. Persons taking amantadine hydrochloride may experience confusion, disorientation, and mental depression. What actions should the nurse take if/when this occurs?
7. Because of the many side effects known to occur with medications used to treat parkinsonism, what health teaching should be initiated?
8. Compare the actions of amantadine hydrochloride, bromocriptine mesylate, carbidopa, levodopa, pergolide mesylate, selegiline, and tolcapone.

Answer

1. Signs and symptoms of parkinsonism are expressionlessness; masklike face; tremors of hands, lips, tongue, and jaw; "pill-rolling" movements of fingers; excessive salivation; and dyskinesia.
2. Medications are given to treat Parkinson's disease to provide maximum relief of symptoms and to optimize independence of movement and activity. See also Drug Therapy for Parkinson's Disease, p. 232.
3. Baseline neurologic assessment includes orientation to name, date, time, and place; degree of alertness; ability to comprehend and follow instructions; and degree of involvement in activities of daily life.
4. See textbook, pp. 233-234.
5. Dyskinesia: inability to perform voluntary movements. Propulsive, uncontrolled movement: quick, short steps forward or backward that cannot be controlled. Akinesia: lack of movement.
6. The nurse should provide for patient safety, report alterations for evaluation by the physician, and continue to make regularly scheduled assessments of the individual's neurologic status.
7. Prepare a list of symptoms the patient has before starting therapy and involve the patient in keeping track of alterations (as the individual's abilities permit). Explain the need for continuing therapy for a period sufficient for the effectiveness of medications to be evaluated. Have the patient report effects that are particularly bothersome; work cooperatively to plan approaches to alleviate the problems.

9. Summarize the side effects associated with medication therapy used in the treatment of parkinsonism. State nursing actions that could be used to alleviate and/or prevent the side effects.
10. What type of glaucoma prohibits the use of levodopa?
11. What specific type of vitamin preparation should be used by patients taking levodopa?
12. List three drugs used to treat parkinsonism.
13. What drugs may be combined with levodopa to improve its effectiveness?
14. Persons taking levodopa (Larodopa) for several months may develop what type of central nervous system side effects?
15. Why should a baseline neurologic assessment be done prior to and periodically during the administration of commonly prescribed drugs for treatment of Parkinson's disease?
16. What neurologic side effects are most often seen with pergolide?
17. What is the primary mechanism of action of anticholinergic agents?
18. What are the therapeutic outcomes desired when an anticholinergic agent is prescribed for a Parkinson's patient?
19. When the ability to perform motor functions is impaired, what nursing diagnosis statement could be made?

8. Amantadine hydrochloride slows destruction of dopamine and may aid in release of dopamine from storage sites. Bromocriptine mesylate stimulates dopamine receptors in basal ganglia of the brain. Carbidopa inhibits the metabolism of levodopa. Levodopa replaces dopamine deficiency in the basal ganglia of the brain. Pergolide mesylate stimulates postsynaptic dopamine receptors. Selegiline has an unknown mechanism of action. Tolcapone reduces the destruction of dopamine in peripheral tissue allowing significantly more to reach the brain.
9. See pp. 236, 238 (amantadine), p. 240 (bromocriptine), p. 242 (levodopa), p. 243 (pergolide), p. 246 (entacapone), and pp. 247-248 (anticholinergic agents).
10. Angle-closure glaucoma prohibits the use of levodopa.
11. Pyridoxine-free multiple vitamin (Larobec) should be used by patients taking levodopa.
12. Drugs used to treat parkinsonism include bromocriptine mesylate (Parlodel), levodopa (Larodopa), amantadine (Symmetrel), carbidopa (Sinemet), pergolide mesylate (Permax), and ropinirole (Requip).
13. Carbidopa, an enzyme inhibitor that reduces the metabolism of levodopa, allowing a greater portion of the administered levodopa to reach the receptor sites in the basal ganglia. Entacapone inhibits the metabolism of dopamine, resulting in a more constant dopaminergic stimulation in the brain.
14. Long-term use of levodopa can cause abnormal movements (e.g., rocking, facial grimacing, chewing motions, head and neck bobbing).
15. Several of the drugs used to treat Parkinson's disease can cause adverse effects such as confusion and hallucinations. It is important to know which is a progression of the disease and which is due to an adverse effect of drug therapy.
16. Common neurologic side effects with pergolide include dyskinesia, hallucinations, somnolence, and insomnia.
17. The primary mechanism of action of anticholinergic agents is to reduce overstimulation caused by the excess of acetylcholine, a cholinergic neurotransmitter.
18. The desired effects are reduction in drooling, sweating, tremors, and depression.
19. Risk for injury related to Parkinson's disease; manifested by propulsive gait, unsteadiness, and progressive inability to walk unassisted.

CHAPTER 15

Student Name ____________________

Drugs Used for Parkinson's Disease

Learning Activities

FILL-IN-THE-BLANK

Finish each of the following statements using the correct term.

1. Selegiline may be used to slow the course of Parkinson's disease by possibly slowing the progression of deterioration of ____________________ nerve cells.
2. ____________________ is the impairment of the individual's ability to perform voluntary movements.
3. ____________________ is extremely slow body movement, which may eventually progress to ____________________, or lack of movement.
4. A dermatologic condition known as ____________________ ____________________ is occasionally observed in conjunction with amantadine therapy. It is characterized by diffuse rose-colored mottling of the skin, often accompanied by ankle edema predominantly in the extremities.
5. ____________________ is an antibiotic which inhibits the metabolism of ropinirole.
6. Anticholinergics reduce the severity of the ____________________ and drooling associated with parkinsonism.
7. The goal of treatment of parkinsonism is to restore dopamine neurotransmitter function as close to normal as possible, and relieve symptoms caused by ____________________ acetylcholine.
8. With Parkinson's disease, the neurotransmitter ____________________ is deficient, leaving a relative excess of the neurotransmitter ____________________.
9. To help reduce an excess amount of acetylcholine, ____________________ agents are prescribed.
10. The major action of the drug carbidopa is to reduce metabolism of ____________________.
11. The major action of the drug levodopa is to cross into the brain and be metabolized to ____________________.
12. The major action of the drug entacapone is to reduce destruction of ____________________ in peripheral tissue.
13. The term used for the lack of ability to move is ____________________.

MATCHING

Match the generic drug name with its corresponding brand name. Each option will be used only once.

_____ 14. amantadine hydrochloride

_____ 15. bromocriptine mesylate

_____ 16. carbidopa

_____ 17. benztropine mesylate

_____ 18. trihexyphenidyl hydrochloride

a. Sinemet
b. Symmetrel
c. Cogentin
d. Artane
e. Parlodel

TRUE OR FALSE

Mark "T" for true and "F" for false for each statement. Correct all false statements.

_____ 19. The symptoms associated with parkinsonism are caused by a dopamine deficiency in the extrapyramidal system within the basal ganglia of the brain.

_____ 20. In most cases of drug-induced parkinsonism, there is no recovery if the chemical is discontinued.

_____ 21. There is no cure for parkinsonism.

_____ 22. Orthostatic hypotension is a rare side effect with most of the medicines used to treat Parkinson's disease.

_____ 23. About half of the patients who benefit from amantadine therapy begin to notice a reduction in benefit after 2 or 3 months.

_____ 24. Carbidopa is used to reduce the dose of levodopa required by approximately 75%.

_____ 25. Carbidopa has no effect when used alone; it must be used in combination with levodopa.

_____ 26. Dopamine does not enter the brain when administered orally.

DRUG ACTION/SIDE EFFECTS

27. *State the action and side effects of the following drug classes or drugs used in the treatment of Parkinson's disease.*

	Actions	Side Effects
AMANTADINE HYDROCHLORIDE		

CHAPTER 15

Student Name ____________________

Drugs Used for Parkinson's Disease

Practice Questions for the NCLEX Examination

_____ 1. Constipation resulting from drug therapy for Parkinson's disease is best treated by:
1. limiting fluid intake to four six-ounce glasses of water daily.
2. adding bulk-forming laxatives to the daily regimen.
3. decreasing bulk in the diet.
4. eliminating fruits from the diet.

_____ 2. Tremors associated with Parkinson's disease:
1. are usually a "pill rolling" motion in the fingers and thumbs.
2. are usually increased with voluntary movement.
3. occur primarily with motion.
4. start with rapid movement of the arms and hands.

_____ 3. When performing an admission assessment on a patient with Parkinson's disease, the nurse will most likely find:
1. the spine to be erect and the shoulders to be parallel to the hips.
2. eyes that are bulging.
3. increased salivation.
4. muscle relaxation and weakness.

_____ 4. When teaching a patient about diet therapy and levodopa, which of the following statements should the nurse include?
1. Vitamin C will decrease the effects of levodopa.
2. Pyridoxine (B_6) will reduce the therapeutic effect of levodopa.
3. A low-protein diet is recommended for patients with parkinsonism.
4. Patients taking levodopa therapy should be weighed every other month.

_____ 5. Patients taking which types of drugs for parkinsonism are at risk for the development of sudden sleep events?
1. Amantadine hydrochloride
2. Bromocriptine mesylate
3. Carbidopa
4. Levodopa

_____ 6. Before administering levodopa therapy, it is most important for the nurse to assess the patient for a history of:
1. hypertension.
2. allergy to penicillin.
3. asthma.
4. angle-closure glaucoma.

_____ 7. Which of the following drugs is contraindicated for patients receiving selegiline?
1. Morphine
2. Meperidine
3. Acetaminophen
4. Aspirin

_____ 8. Which of the following foods are high in tyramine content? (Select all that apply.)
1. Chianti wine
2. Chicken
3. Fava beans
4. Cheeses

_____ 9. Which of the following statements would the nurse include when teaching a patient with Parkinson's disease about the drug apomorphine?
1. It is chemically related to morphine, but does not have any opioid activity.
2. It is used to treat hypermobility associated with the "weaning off" of dopamine agonists.
3. It is administered intravenously.
4. It commonly causes hypertension in patients who initially start therapy with this drug.

_____ 10. Which of the following medications used in treating patients with Parkinson's disease slows the course of the disease by possibly slowing the progression of deterioration of dopaminergic nerve cells?
1. Selegiline
2. Symmetrel
3. Parlodel
4. Sinemet

_____ 11. Which of the following signs or symptoms would the nurse most likely find in a patient who has had Parkinson's disease for 12 years? (Select all that apply.)
1. Tremors
2. Dyskinesia
3. Obesity
4. Dry mouth

_____ 12. Which of the following statements about Parkinson's disease and its treatment are true? (Select all that apply.)
1. Parkinson's disease is a progressive neurologic disorder.
2. The symptoms associated with Parkinson's disease develop because of a relative excess of dopamine in the brain.
3. Selegiline therapy is often started first to slow the development of symptoms.
4. Nonpharmacologic treatment of Parkinson's disease is equally important in maintaining the long-term well-being of the patient.

_____ 13. Which of the following statements about the use of apomorphine in the treatment of Parkinson's disease is true? (Select all that apply.)
1. Apomorphine is chemically related to morphine and has twice as much opioid activity as morphine.
2. Apomorphine is used to treat the muscular rigidity associated with Parkinson's disease.
3. Emesis is one of the pharmacologic actions of apomorphine.
4. Apomorphine should not be administered intravenously.

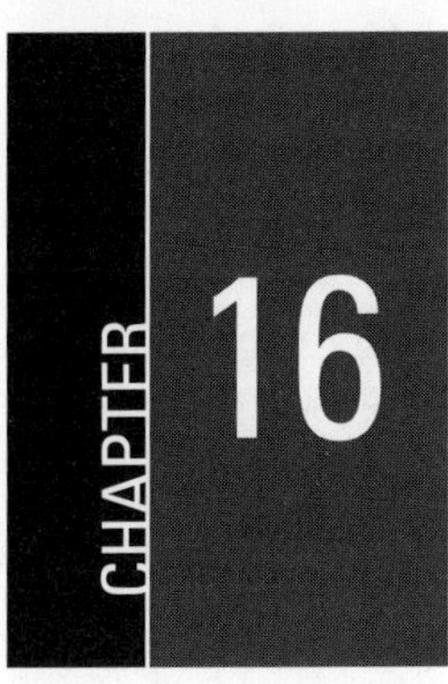

Drugs Used for Anxiety Disorders

Review Sheet

The QUESTION column and the ANSWER column have been offset so that you can cover the answers while reading the questions, allowing you to assess your knowledge.

Question

1. Define *anxiety disorder.*
2. What is a phobia?
3. What is obsessive-compulsive disorder?
4. What is a panic disorder?
5. State another common name for tranquilizers.
6. Summarize nursing assessments and interventions that are used for the patient displaying anxiety.
7. State the action of benzodiazepines.
8. What is the ending spelling of all generic drug names of benzodiazepines except chlordiazepoxide?
9. Name three benzodiazepines that are relatively short-acting and therefore most appropriate for an older adult or an individual with reduced hepatic function.
10. What premedication assessments should be performed prior to administering a benzodiazepine?

Answer

1. Patients are said to suffer from an anxiety disorder when their responses to stressful situations are abnormal, irrational, and impair normal daily functioning.
2. Phobias are irrational fears of a specific object, activity, or situation. The patient recognizes the fear as exaggerated or unrealistic. The fear persists, however, and the patient seeks to avoid the situation.
3. An obsession is an unwanted thought, idea, image, or urge that a patient recognizes as time-consuming and senseless but that repeatedly intrudes into the consciousness despite attempts to ignore, prevent, or counteract it. A compulsion is a repetitive, intentional, purposeful behavior performed to decrease the anxiety associated with an obsession.
4. See textbook, p. 251.
5. Tranquilizers are also called *anxiolytic agents* or *antianxiety* medications.
6. See textbook, pp. 253-254.
7. Benzodiazepines stimulate an inhibitory neurotransmitter gamma-aminobutyric acid (GABA).
8. All generic drug names of benzodiazepines end in "-am."
9. Alprazolam, lorazepam, oxazepam are appropriate benzodiazepines for older adults or individuals with reduced hepatic function.

11. State the desired therapeutic outcome for any drug prescribed for an anxiety disorder.
12. Why is the use of benzodiazepines avoided during the first trimester of pregnancy?
13. Describe side effects to expect with buspirone (BuSpar), hydroxyzine (Vistaril), and meprobamate (Equanil).
14. Based on the side effects of the drugs listed in question 13, what nursing diagnosis could be developed?
15. When you read a drug monograph that lists possible orthostatic hypotension as a side effect, what nursing actions would be appropriate, in addition to teaching the patient to rise slowly from a supine to sitting position?
16. What are additive effects associated with concurrent CNS system depressants?
17. What are symptoms of hepatotoxicity?
18. What are the side effects to expect with hydroxyzine?
19. What is the major advantage of buspirone, an azaspirone agent, over other antianxiety agents?
20. What is the action of fluvoxamine (Luvox), an SSRI agent?
21. When used as a preoperative medication, what are the desired actions of hydroxyzine (Vistaril, Atarax)?

10. Before administering a benzodiazepine, assess for level of anxiety present; vital signs, especially blood pressure in sitting and supine positions; blood dyscrasias; hepatic disease; and whether the patient is in the first trimester of pregnancy or breastfeeding.
11. The desired outcome of drug therapy for anxiety disorders is a decreased level of anxiety so that the individual can function normally in life's daily activities.
12. Use of benzodiazepines in the first trimester of pregnancy is associated with increased incidence of birth defects.
13. Side effects to expect include sedation and lethargy with buspirone; blurred vision, constipation, dryness of mucous membranes, and sedation with hydroxyzine; and sedation, slurred speech, and dizziness with meprobamate.
14. A possible nursing diagnosis is: Injury, high risk for, related to antianxiety drug therapy (meprobamate, buspirone, hydroxyzine) manifested by lethargy, sedation, blurred vision, dizziness.
15. Monitor blood pressure in supine and standing positions every shift and provide for patient safety.
16. Combining more than one drug that depresses the CNS will cause exaggeration of the depressant effects and could reach potentially fatal levels.
17. Symptoms of hepatotoxicity include anorexia, jaundice, nausea, vomiting, hepatomegaly, splenomegaly, and abnormal liver function tests (elevated bilirubin, AST, ALT, GGT, alkaline phosphatase, and prothrombin time).
18. Side effects to expect with hydroxyzine include blurred vision, constipation, dry mucosa (thirst), and sedation.
19. There is lower incidence of sedation with buspirone.
20. Luvox inhibits serotonin reuptake at the nerve endings, prolonging the serotonin activity. It is used to assist patients with obsessive-compulsive disorder to gain better control over obsessive actions.
21. Used preoperatively, hydroxyzine causes sedation, acts as an antiemetic, and reduces the narcotic dose needed for analgesia.

Student Name______________________________

Drugs Used for Anxiety Disorders

Learning Activities

FILL-IN-THE-BLANK

Finish each of the following statements using the correct term.

1. ____________________ is an unpleasant feeling of apprehension or nervousness caused by the perception of potential or actual danger that threatens a person's security.

2. A(n) ____________________ is an unwanted thought, idea, image, or urge that the patient recognizes as time-consuming and senseless but repeatedly intrudes into the consciousness, despite attempts to ignore, prevent, or counteract it.

3. The most common drug class used for the treatment of anxiety disorders are the ____________________.

4. A patient is admitted to the emergency department from his place of employment after he started to breathe fast and feel anxious when a butterfly entered his office space. The patient states, "I am so afraid of butterflies. I know they will kill me, and I can't stop thinking that that butterfly was in my office. I am terrified of them." The nurse understands that the patient most likely is exhibiting evidence of a(n) ____________________ .

5. The ____________________ are the most commonly used drugs for the treatment of anxiety disorders because they are more consistently effective, less likely to interact with other drugs, less likely to cause overdose, and have less potential for abuse than other antianxiety agents.

MATCHING

Match the generic drug name with its corresponding brand name. Each option will be used only once.

_____ 6. alprazolam

_____ 7. diazepam

_____ 8. lorazepam

_____ 9. oxazepam

a. Serax
b. Ativan
c. Valium
d. Xanax

TRUE OR FALSE

Mark "T" for true and "F" for false for each statement. Correct all false statements.

_____ 10. Anxiety disorders are the most commonly encountered mental disorder in clinical practice.

_____ 11. Panic attacks occur on exposure to an anxiety-causing situation.

_____ 12. Patients generally respond to benzodiazepine therapy in one week.

_____ 13. It is recommended that benzodiazepines not be administered during at least the first trimester of pregnancy.

_____ 14. Larger doses of benzodiazepines may be necessary to maintain anxiolytic effects in patients who smoke.

DRUG ACTION/SIDE EFFECTS

15. *State the actions and side effects of the following drug classes or drugs used in the treatment of anxiety disorders.*

	Actions	Side Effects
BENZODIAZEPINES		

CHAPTER 16

Student Name______________________________

Drugs Used for Anxiety Disorders

Practice Questions for the NCLEX Examination

_____ 1. Which of the following statements about buspirone is true?
1. It is a controlled substance.
2. It has a high potential for abuse.
3. It is sometimes called a *midbrain modulator*.
4. It requires 2 to 3 days of treatment before initial signs of improvement are evident.

_____ 2. Which of the following drugs used for anxiety disorders is also used routinely as a preoperative or postoperative sedative to control vomiting, diminish anxiety, and reduce the amount of narcotics needed for anesthesia?
1. Meprobamate
2. Hydroxyzine
3. Buspirone
4. Fluvoxamine

_____ 3. Which of the following interventions by the nurse would be most effective in dealing with a patient who has orthostatic hypotension caused by meprobamate therapy?
1. Tell the patient to rise from a sitting position rapidly.
2. Encourage the patient to sit down if feeling faint.
3. Encourage the patient to sleep in a chair at night; do not lie down.
4. Tell the patient to reduce the dose of meprobamate by half.

_____ 4. Which of the following is the most effective treatment for patients with anxiety disorders?
1. Combination of pharmacologic and nonpharmacologic therapies
2. Stress management
3. Biofeedback
4. Benzodiazepines

_____ 5. The most common adverse effect of buspirone therapy is:
1. constipation.
2. dry mouth.
3. CNS disturbances.
4. hepatotoxicity.

_____ 6. Anxiety is a component of many medical illnesses involving which of the following systems? (Select all that apply.)
1. Cardiovascular
2. Pulmonary
3. Digestive
4. Endocrine

_____ 7. Common withdrawal symptoms the nurse should look for in patients discontinuing long-term treatment with benzodiazepines include: (Select all that apply.)
1. restlessness.
2. worsening of anxiety.
3. tremor.
4. muscle tension.

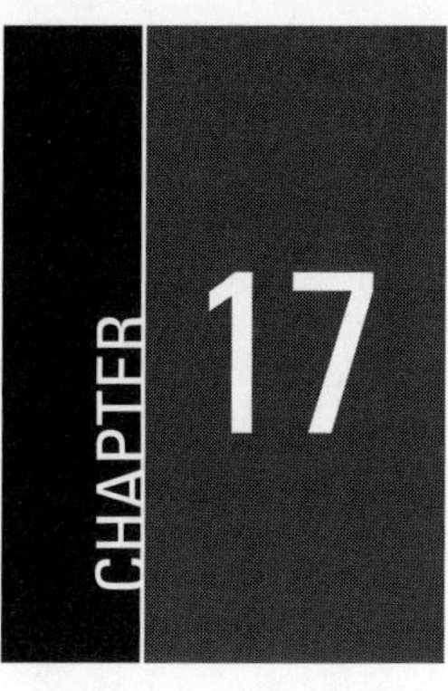

Drugs Used for Mood Disorders

Review Sheet

The QUESTION column and the ANSWER column have been offset so that you can cover the answers while reading the questions, allowing you to assess your knowledge.

Question

1. Define *mood disorders.*
2. Which neurotransmitters are affected by depression?
3. What are characteristic symptoms found in a person experiencing depression?
4. Define *bipolar disorder.*
5. Define *flight of ideas.*
6. Cite the incidence of attempted suicide in individuals with mood disorders.
7. Cite the three stages that patients with mood disorders experience as they strive for achievement of full functioning status.
8. Give two examples of cognitive symptoms and psychomotor symptoms.
9. Define *labile moods.*
10. Define *grandiose thinking.*
11. List the drug classifications used in the treatment of depression.

Answer

1. Mood disorders are also known as *affective disorders*. The person's ability to function is impaired for a prolonged period of time going beyond brief periods of emotional upset from negative life experiences. Mood disorders are characterized by abnormal feelings of euphoria and/or depression.
2. Norepinephrine, serotonin, and dopamine are the neurotransmitters affected by depression.
3. Characteristic symptoms of depression are persistent, reduced ability to experience pleasure in life's usual activities, sometimes accompanied by personality change and sadness.
4. Bipolar disorder is characterized by distinct episodes of mania (euphoria) and depression separated by intervals without mood disturbances.
5. Quick thoughts that rapidly change from one topic to another are called *flight of ideas.*
6. The frequency of suicide attempts in individuals with mood disorders is 15%, 30 times higher than general population.
7. The stages one goes through during treatment of a mood disorder are: acute, continuation, and maintenance. See textbook, p. 264, for definitions of each.
8. Cognitive symptoms involve the ability to concentrate, altered clarity of thought (e.g., confusion, poor short-term memory). Psychomotor symptoms include slowed or retarded movements, pacing, and outbursts of shouting.
9. Labile moods are rapid shifts in mood. A person may be happy, then rapidly switch to anger and irritability.
10. Grandiose thinking is overestimation of oneself and one's abilities or importance.

12. Describe basic components of assessment for an individual with a mood disorder.
13. In general, what is the decision-making capacity of an individual with a mood disorder?
14. What are the basic actions of medicines used to treat depression?
15. Why is it necessary to closely monitor patients taking antidepressants?
16. What is the anticipated therapeutic outcome for antidepressant therapy?
17. Discuss premedication assessments needed for an individual who is to receive 1) MAOIs; 2) SSRIs; 3) tricyclic antidepressants; or 4) miscellaneous agents, including bupropion, maprotiline, mirtazapine, nefazodone, trazodone, and venlafaxine.
18. State appropriate nursing diagnoses as indicators of antidepressant therapy.
19. Name the drug used to treat manic episodes. List the important premedication assessments as well as assessments needed for long-term therapy.
20. List the normal serum level for lithium.
21. Describe teaching that should be completed about sodium intake while receiving lithium therapy.

11. Drugs used in the treatment of depression include MAOIs, tricyclic antidepressants, SSRIs, and a miscellaneous group of monocyclic and tetracyclic agents.
12. Basic components of assessment for mood disorders include history of mood disorders, basic mental status, interpersonal relationships, mood/affect, clarity of thought, thoughts of death, psychomotor function, sleep pattern, and dietary history.
13. The decision-making capacity of an individual with a mood disorder is highly variable. The nurse must evaluate the individual's abilities and need to be protected from self-harm.
14. All antidepressants block the uptake and destruction of the neurotransmitters serotonin, norepinephrine, and/or dopamine.
15. Patients taking antidepressants may be suicidal. When drug therapy is initiated, it may take 1–4 weeks before a therapeutic response is evident. An early improvement in mood or other symptoms should not be used as an indicator that the depression is no longer present. Individuals may require 4–6 weeks to reach a full therapeutic level of the medicine.
16. The anticipated therapeutic outcome for individuals taking antidepressants is improvement of mood with a concurrent reduction in the feelings of depression.
17. MAOIs, textbook pp. 270-271; SSRIs, textbook pp. 272-273; tricyclic antidepressants, textbook p. 274; miscellaneous agents, textbook pp. 276-280.
18. Risk for violence: self-inflicted—hopelessness—dysfunctional grieving—ineffective individual coping—social isolation, and disturbed perception.
19. Lithium carbonate (Eskalith, Lithane) is used to treat manic episodes. Before beginning lithium therapy, stress importance of the need for adequate hydration and sodium intake. Teach the patient the signs of lithium toxicity (e.g., nausea, vomiting, abdominal pain, diarrhea, lethargy, speech difficulty, mild dizziness, muscle twitching, and tremors).
20. Normal serum lithium range is 0.4–1.5 mEq/L.

22. Why is behavioral monitoring during antidepressant therapy done?

21. During lithium therapy, normal daily intake of sodium is essential, as is adequate hydration. Stress using salt in cooking and at the table. The person should also drink 10 to 12 8-oz glasses of water daily.
22. Behavioral monitoring during antidepressant therapy is done to detect development of extrapyramidal symptoms and to monitor for degree of therapeutic response to therapy.

Student Name____________________

Drugs Used for Mood Disorders

Learning Activities

FILL-IN-THE-BLANK

Finish each of the following statements using the correct term.

1. Bipolar disorder was formerly known as ____________________ ____________________.

2. The most common gastrointestinal side effect when taking tricyclic antidepressants is ____________________.

3. St. John's wort may ____________________ toxic effects of antidepressant medicines.

4. ____________________ is used to treat acute mania and for the prophylaxis of recurrent manic and depressive episodes in bipolar disorder.

5. Periods of elation or euphoria are known as ____________________.

6. People taking MAOIs must omit foods containing ____________________.

MATCHING

Match the generic drug name with its corresponding brand name. Each option will be used only once.

_____ 7. sertraline

_____ 8. paroxetine

_____ 9. fluvoxamine

_____ 10. fluoxetine

_____ 11. citalopram

_____ 12. imipramine

_____ 13. clomipramine

_____ 14. amitriptyline

a. Elavil
b. Anafranil
c. Tofranil
d. Celexa
e. Luvox
f. Paxil
g. Zoloft
h. Prozac

TRUE OR FALSE

Mark "T" for true and "F" for false for each statement. Correct all false statements.

_____ 15. Major depression currently ranks as the second leading cause of disease burden in the United States.

_____ 16. Anxiety symptoms are present in almost 90% of depressed patients.

_____ 17. All patients with depression should be assessed for suicidal thoughts.

_____ 18. For most antidepressants, the lag time between initiation of therapy and therapeutic response is one week.

_____ 19. Electroconvulsive therapy is contraindicated in the treatment of patients with cardiovascular disease.

_____ 20. Dosages of fluvoxamine may need to be decreased for full therapeutic response in patients who smoke.

DRUG ACTION/SIDE EFFECTS

21. *State the action and side effects of the following drug classes or drugs used in the treatment of mood disorders.*

	Actions	Side Effects
MONOAMINE OXIDASE INHIBITORS		

CHAPTER 17

Student Name ______________________________

Drugs Used for Mood Disorders

Practice Questions for the NCLEX Examination

_____ 1. The highest priority of care for a patient with severe mood disorders is:
1. monitoring serum drug levels.
2. the provision of patient safety and supervision at intervals consistent with severity of the suicidal threat.
3. maintaining a calm environment.
4. maintenance of physical restraints.

_____ 2. Patients with severe mood disorders would most likely benefit from which type of diet?
1. High protein
2. High sodium
3. High fat
4. Low calorie

_____ 3. When foods with high tyramine content are ingested by a patient taking monoamine oxidase inhibitors, the most common adverse effect is:
1. allergic reaction.
2. renal failure.
3. hypertensive crisis.
4. respiratory depression.

_____ 4. Which of the following drugs for pain is contraindicated for use in a patient who is receiving monoamine oxidase inhibitor therapy?
1. Meperidine
2. Morphine
3. Acetaminophen
4. Codeine

_____ 5. For a patient on bupropion hydrochloride therapy, the concurrent use of nicotine patches may cause:
1. the development of a rash.
2. low heart rate.
3. chronic cough.
4. high blood pressure.

_____ 6. The fluid and electrolyte status of patients taking lithium carbonate need to be closely monitored by the nurse, because lithium may:
1. deplete potassium stores.
2. enhance sodium depletion.
3. cause calcium toxicity.
4. result in acidosis.

_____ 7. Which of the following should be included when teaching patients about lithium therapy?
1. If nausea should occur, discontinue therapy immediately.
2. Continue with the usual dose of lithium if weakness should develop.
3. Maintain a normal dietary intake of sodium with adequate maintenance fluids.
4. Lithium will cause a metallic taste in your mouth that you will get used to.

_____ 8. When interacting with patients who are in the manic phase, the nurse should:
1. allow the patient to make decisions if capable.
2. maintain flexibility with unit rules.
3. isolate patients who are highly agitated.
4. medicate the patient immediately.

_____ 9. The nurse who is teaching a patient taking an MAOI for the treatment of depression should teach the patient to avoid which of the following foods? (Select all that apply.)
1. Red wine
2. Pickles
3. Cheddar cheese
4. Avocados
5. Yogurt

_____ 10. Which of the following medications for pain is appropriate for use in the patient who is taking MAOIs for the treatment of depression? (Select all that apply.)
1. Morphine
2. Meperidine
3. Ibuprofen
4. Acetaminophen

_____ 11. The most widely used drug class of antidepressant medications are the:
1. SSRIs.
2. MAOIs.
3. tricyclic antidepressants.
4. miscellaneous agents.

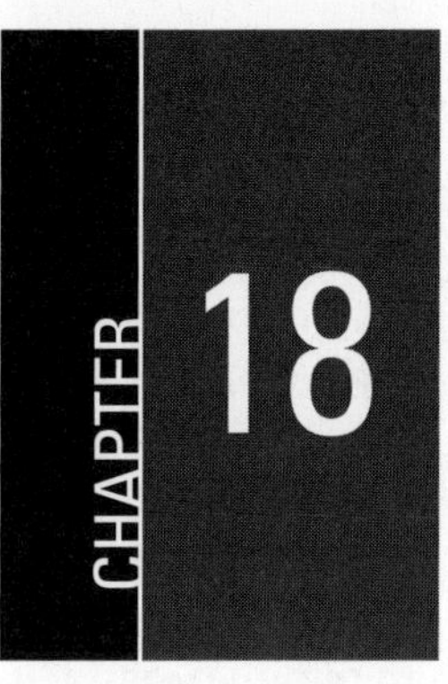

Drugs Used for Psychoses

Review Sheet

The QUESTION column and the ANSWER column have been offset so that you can cover the answer while reading the questions, allowing you to assess your knowledge.

Question

1. Define *psychosis.*
2. Differentiate among delusions, hallucinations, and disorganized thinking.
3. What is change in affect?
4. What is meant by *target symptoms*?
5. What rating scales have been developed for objective measurement of target symptoms due to psychotherapy and pharmacology?
6. What is another name for an antipsychotic agent?
7. Differentiate between the terms *low-potency* and *high-potency* antipsychotic agents.
8. What are typical and atypical antipsychotic agents?

Answer

1. Psychosis does not have a single definition, but is a clinical descriptor that means that a person is out of touch with reality.
2. Delusions are false, irrational beliefs unchanged in the presence of data to the contrary. Hallucinations are false sensory perceptions experienced by an individual without external stimulus. Disorganized thinking is recognized when an individual switches rapidly from one idea or thought to another unrelated topic.
3. Change in affect is characterized by diminished emotional expression, reduced spontaneous movement, and poor eye contact. The individual withdraws from effective functioning in interpersonal relations, work, education, and self-care.
4. Target symptoms are those symptoms to be assessed to evaluate therapeutic response to drug therapy and nonpharmacologic interventions.
5. Brief Psychiatric Rating Scale (BPRS), the Positive and Negative Scale for Schizophrenia (PANSS), the Clinical Global Impression (CGI) scale, and the Rating of Aggression Against People and/or Property (RAAPP) Scale are recently developed scales in use for objective measurement of target symptoms. (Note: Students could benefit from further online research of the scales listed.)
6. Neuroleptic agent—usually reserved for the typical antipsychotic agents.
7. These terms refer ONLY to the milligram doses and not to the difference in effectiveness of antipsychotic agents.

9. Cite the desired therapeutic outcome(s) from antipsychotic therapy.

10. Define *extrapyramidal symptoms*, including dystonia, pseudoparkinsonian symptoms, akathisia, and tardive dyskinesia.

11. What causes pseudoparkinsonian symptoms?

12. What monitoring scales are used to rate dystonia?

13. What are the DISCUS or AIMS scales?

14. Describe common adverse effects associated with antipsychotic therapy.

15. What is neuroleptic malignant syndrome? What are the symptoms, and how is it treated?

16. Summarize nursing implementations and patient education used for patients being treated for psychoses.

17. Memorize the generic and brand names of these commonly prescribed antipsychotic agents: Thorazine, Trilafon, Compazine, Mellaril, Clozaril, Haldol, and Risperdal.

8. Typical agents are listed in Table 18-1. Atypical antipsychotic agents include clozapine, olanzapine, quetiapine, risperidone, and ziprasidone. These classifications are based on the drugs' mechanisms of action.
9. Calmed the individual, reduced psychomotor agitation and insomnia, reduced thought disorders so the individual is able to function with minimal exacerbation of psychotic symptoms.
10. Dystonia is spasmodic movements of muscle groups (e.g., tongue protrusion, rolling back of the eyes). Pseudoparkinsonian symptoms are tremors, muscular rigidity, masklike expression, shuffling gait, and loss or weakness of motor function. Akathisia is a feeling of anxiety, restlessness, pacing, rocking, and inability to sit still. Tardive dyskinesia is progressive symptoms of involuntary, hyperkinetic, abnormal movements.
11. Pseudoparkinsonian symptoms are caused by a relative deficiency of dopamine and an excess of acetylcholine, caused by antipsychotic agents.
12. Toronto Western Spasmodic Torticollis Rating Scale (TWSTRS), Global Dystonia Scale (GDS), Unified Dystonia Scale (UDRS), and the Fahn-Marsden Scale. (See also related websites on documentation of dystonia.)
13. Both the DISCUS and AIMS scales are involuntary movement scales for rating dyskinetic movements. (See textbook Appendix G for the DISCUS scale.)
14. Adverse effects of antipsychotic therapy include sedation, drowsiness, appetite stimulation, postural hypotension, reflex tachycardia, lowering of seizure threshold, and development of symptoms of tardive dyskinesia.
15. See textbook, p. 289. Symptoms of neuroleptic malignant syndrome include fever, extrapyramidal symptoms, and lead-pipe rigidity, probably due to excessive dopamine depletion. It is treated with bromocriptine or amantadine as dopamine agonists and dantrolene, a muscle relaxant. Fever is treated with cooling blankets, adequate hydration, and antipyretics.
16. See textbook, pp. 290-292.
17. The generic and brand names of commonly prescribed antipsychotic agents are: chlorpromazine (Thorazine); perphenazine (Trilafon); prochlorperazine (Compazine); thioridazine (Mellaril); clozapine (Clozaril); haloperidol (Haldol); and risperidone (Risperdal).

Student Name______________________________

Drugs Used for Psychoses

Learning Activities

FILL-IN-THE-BLANK

Finish each of the following statements using the correct term.

1. ____________________ does not have a single definition but is a clinical descriptor that means being out of touch with reality.

2. A(n) ____________________ is a false or irrational belief that is firmly held despite obvious evidence to the contrary.

3. The typical antipsychotic agents antagonize the neurotransmitter ____________________ in the central nervous system.

4. With the use of antipsychotic therapy, reduction in hallucinations, delusions, and thought disorder often requires _____ to _____ weeks of therapy for full therapeutic effect.

5. ________________ ________________ syndrome is a potentially fatal adverse effect of antipsychotic therapy in which the patient displays extrapyramidal manifestations as part of the symptoms of the disorder.

6. ____________________ is a syndrome consisting of subjective feelings of anxiety and restlessness and objective signs of pacing, rocking, and inability to sit or stand in one place for extended periods.

7. A(n) ____________________ is a false sensory perception that is experienced without an external stimulus but that nevertheless seems real to the patient.

8. Persistent and involuntary hyperkinetic abnormal movements in a patient taking antipsychotic drugs is called ____________________ ____________________.

MATCHING

Match the generic drug name with its corresponding brand name. Each option will be used only once.

_____ 9. risperidone

_____ 10. haloperidol

_____ 11. chlorpromazine

_____ 12. prochlorperazine

_____ 13. olanzepine

a. Haldol
b. Risperdal
c. Thorazine
d. Zyprexa
e. Compazine

Select the definition that best describes the term(s) listed. Not all definitions will be used.

_____ 14. hallucinations

_____ 15. delusions

_____ 16. akathisia

_____ 17. tardive dyskinesia

_____ 18. dystonia

a. Syndrome demonstrated by anxiety, restlessness, pacing, and rocking
b. Alternating feelings of danger and elation
c. Involuntary hyperkinetic abnormal movements
d. False sensory perceptions experienced without external stimulus
e. Prolonged spasmodic movements of muscle groups
f. A false, irrational belief that a patient embraces despite evidence to the contrary

TRUE OR FALSE

Mark "T" for true and "F" for false for each statement. Correct all false statements.

_____ 19. In some instances, it is necessary to use injection of long-acting medicines to overcome the non-adherence problem in selected patients with psychotic symptoms.

_____ 20. Rapid increases in dosages of antipsychotic medication will reduce the antipsychotic response time and decrease the frequency of adverse effects.

_____ 21. Extrapyramidal effects are the most troublesome side effects and the most common cause of nonadherence associated with antipsychotic therapy.

_____ 22. Acute dystonia has the latest onset of all the extrapyramidal symptoms.

_____ 23. With the possible exception of clozapine, all antipsychotic agents have the potential to produce tardive dyskinesia.

_____ 24. It is hypothesized that the cause of the symptoms seen in neuroleptic malignant syndrome is excessive dopamine depletion.

_____ 25. Patients taking clozapine are particularly susceptible to developing agranulocytosis.

DRUG ACTION/SIDE EFFECTS

26. *State the action and side effects of the following drug classes or drugs used in the treatment of psychoses.*

	Actions	Side Effects
ANTIPSYCHOTIC AGENTS		

CHAPTER 18

Student Name________________________________

Drugs Used for Psychoses

Practice Questions for the NCLEX Examination

_____ 1. Which of the following statements should the nurse include when teaching patients taking antipsychotic agents about acute dystonia?
1. Acute dystonia reactions occur most often in the first 72 hours of therapy.
2. Dystonic reactions occur most often in females.
3. There are no treatments for dystonic reactions.
4. Dystonic reactions usually last for 1 week.

_____ 2. When working with diabetic or prediabetic patients who are taking antipsychotic drugs, it is most important for the nurse to:
1. monitor the patient for the development of hyperglycemia, particularly during the early weeks of therapy.
2. reduce the amount of oral hypoglycemic agents by one-half.
3. increase the amount of insulin by one unit per milligram of antipsychotic agent taken.
4. discontinue blood glucose monitoring.

_____ 3. Which of the following statements should the nurse include when teaching patients about drug therapy for psychoses?
1. Expect a rash to develop and continue taking the medication.
2. If fine tremors of the tongue or lip smacking develops, discontinue use of the antipsychotic drug immediately.
3. Avoid prolonged exposure to sunlight and ultraviolet light.
4. Hypertension is a common side effect from the use of these drugs.

_____ 4. Patients experiencing neuroleptic malignant syndrome usually manifest which of the following signs and symptoms? (Select all that apply.)
1. Lead-pipe rigidity
2. Tachycardia
3. Labile hypertension
4. Hypothermia

_____ 5. The best treatment approach to tardive dyskinesia for patients receiving antipsychotic therapy is:
1. reduction of antipsychotic drug dose.
2. discontinuation of the antipsychotic drug.
3. dopamine agonists.
4. assessment for early signs of tardive dyskinesia, at least semiannually and preferably quarterly.

_____ 6. Which of the following statements about tardive dyskinesia is true?
1. Symptoms improve when the antipsychotic dosage is decreased.
2. It typically appears after antipsychotic disease reduction or discontinuation takes place.
3. It improves with administration of anticholinergic agents.
4. It rapidly goes away after antipsychotic medications are discontinued.

_____ 7. A patient receiving antipsychotic therapy develops pseudoparkinsonian symptoms. His wife wants to know what to expect now that these symptoms have developed. The nurse should include which of the following statements in speaking to the patient's wife?
1. "The antipsychotic medication will need to be discontinued due to this complication."
2. "These symptoms are a side effect of the antipsychotic drug therapy and no treatment is effective."
3. "Your husband has now developed Parkinsonism and there is no treatment."
4. "These symptoms are well-controlled by anticholinergic antiparkinsonian agents."

_____ 8. The most common cause of nonadherence associated with antipsychotic therapy is:
1. the high cost of these medications.
2. extrapyramidal effects.
3. drowsiness.
4. hypertension.

_____ 9. A patient in the emergency department tells the nurse that he is the creator of the universe. The nurse identifies the patient as experiencing:
1. disorganized thinking.
2. change of affect.
3. hallucinations.
4. delusions.

_____ 10. Patients taking antipsychotic drug therapy are most likely to experience which of the following adverse effects? (Select all that apply.)
1. Pseudoparkinsonism
2. Weight loss
3. Hypoglycemia
4. Akathisia

_____ 11. Patients taking antipsychotic medications may experience which of the following side effects as a result of the anticholinergic effects produced by these agents? (Select all that apply.)
1. Diarrhea
2. Chronic fatigue
3. Dry mouth
4. Blurred vision

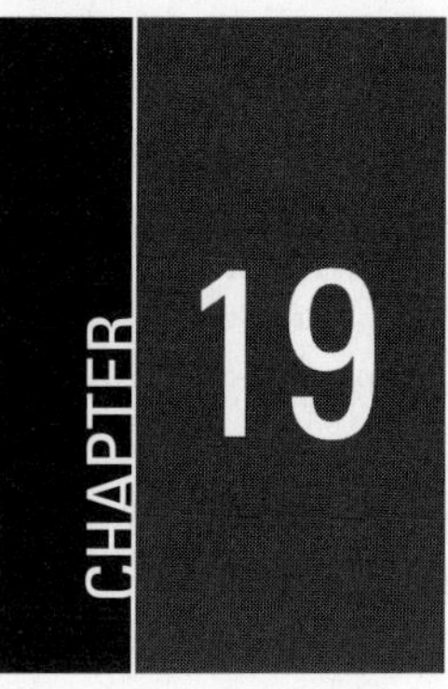

Drugs Used for Seizure Disorders

Review Sheet

The QUESTION column and the ANSWER column have been offset so that you can cover the answer while reading the question, allowing you to assess your knowledge.

Question

1. Define *seizures.*
2. Define *epilepsy.*
3. What are the most common types of generalized convulsive seizures?
4. Differentiate among the symptoms of each type of generalized convulsive seizure.
5. Define the types of partial seizures and differentiate among the symptoms of each.
6. Differentiate among tonic phase, clonic phase, and postictal state.
7. What is status epilepticus?
8. What is an atonic seizure or "drop attack"?
9. Define an *absence* or *petit mal seizure.*

Answer

1. Seizures are brief periods of abnormal electrical activity in the brain that may or may not produce violent, involuntary muscle activity.
2. Epilepsy is diagnosed when a patient has chronic, recurrent seizures.
3. Tonic-clonic, atonic, and myoclonic seizures are the types of generalized seizures.
4. See textbook, p. 297.
5. See textbook, p. 297.
6. Tonic phase is when the patient has intense muscle contractions, loss of consciousness, and rigidity of the body. The clonic phase is characterized by alternating jerking and relaxation of the muscles of the extremities. The patient may defecate or urinate during this phase. The postictal period is the period immediately following a seizure, during which the patient rests. The patient has no recollection of the attack after awakening.
7. Status epilepticus is a rapidly recurring generalized seizure that does not allow the individual to regain normal function between seizures.
8. Atonic seizures are characterized by a sudden loss of muscle tone, causing the head or limb to suddenly "drop." There is also loss of consciousness.

10. What are first-line agents and how are they selected?
11. What is the general action of all anticonvulsants?
12. What assessments should the nurse make during seizure activity?
13. What is meant by *postictal* behavior?
14. What are the treatments used for status epilepticus?
15. What action should a patient requiring seizure medications take upon learning she is pregnant?
16. What actions do benzodiazepines have on seizure activity?
17. What symptoms would be seen if benzodiazepines are suddenly stopped?
18. What time period should be used for the gradual withdrawal of benzodiazepines?
19. What precaution should be used when preparing diazepam or phenytoin for administration?
20. What precautions are required when giving IV diazepam or phenytoin?

9. Petit mal seizures occur primarily in children. These seizures are characterized by a 5–20 second period of altered consciousness accompanied by a few rhythmic movements with no frank convulsive movements and no memory of events during the seizure. Partial seizures are localized convulsions of voluntary muscles. The person does not lose consciousness unless the partial seizure progresses into generalized seizure.
10. See textbook, pp. 297-298.
11. Anticonvulsants increase the seizure threshold and regulate neuronal firing with inhibiting excitatory processes or enhancing inhibitory processes. Medications can also prevent seizures from spreading to adjacent neurons.
12. During seizure activity, the nurse should note a description of the seizure, including onset, duration, body parts involved, any progression of symptoms, state of consciousness, respiratory pattern, salivation, pupil size and eye movement, and incontinence.
13. Postictal behavior is the person's state following a seizure. See textbook, p. 299.
14. Status epilepticus treatment is found on p. 300.
15. Do not discontinue medications; contact the health care provider immediately to discuss the medications being taken and appropriate actions for the well-being of the child and the mother.
16. The mechanism of action for benzodiazepines is not fully understood, but it is thought that the benzodiazepines inhibit neurotransmission by enhancing the effects of GABA in postsynaptic clefts between nerve cells.
17. Rapid withdrawal of benzodiazepines can result in symptoms similar to those seen with alcohol withdrawal. These may vary from weakness and anxiety to delirium and generalized tonic-clonic seizures.
18. Benzodiazepines require a 2- to 4-week period of gradual withdrawal.
19. Never mix diazepam or phenytoin in a syringe with another medication; either drug will form a precipitate in the syringe when combined with a second drug.

21. Name the drugs known as hydantoins.
22. What nursing action should be taken when a patient with diabetes is receiving phenytoin?
23. Explain health teaching that should be performed to reduce the severity of gingival hyperplasia.
24. What is the therapeutic range of a blood serum level for phenytoin?
25. List the signs and symptoms of phenytoin toxicity.
26. What is a brand name of phenytoin?
27. What over-the-counter drug decreases the therapeutic effects of hydantoins?
28. If a female patient receiving seizure medications tells the nurse that she has started spotting or bleeding between her regular menstrual cycles, what should the nurse advise?
29. In what way is the spelling of all succinimide anticonvulsants similar?
30. What are the uses of carbamazepine (Tegretol)? What laboratory studies are recommended with its use?
31. What is the action of lamotrigine (Lamictal)?
32. Why is it necessary to check on whether a patient is already taking valproic acid before initiating therapy with lamotrigine?

20. Do not administer diazepam IV at a rate of more than 5 mg per minute. Do not administer IV phenytoin at a rate over 25–50 mg per minute. Take the pulse before and periodically during IV administration of either drug—check for bradycardia. If this occurs, the rate of administration should be slowed until the pulse returns to normal. If possible, have an ECG in use when administering IV diazepam or IV phenytoin.
21. Hydantoins include phenytoin, ethotoin, and fosphenytoin (Note that these drug names all end in "-toin.")
22. Monitor the patient's blood sugar levels periodically because hyperglycemia may be caused by hydantoin therapy.
23. Provide for good oral hygiene that includes gum massage, proper brushing, and frequent dental care to prevent gum overgrowth (gingival hyperplasia).
24. Look up the therapeutic range of phenytoin in Appendix D.
25. Signs and symptoms of phenytoin toxicity include nystagmus, sedation, and lethargy.
26. Dilantin is the brand name of phenytoin.
27. Antacids decrease the therapeutic effects of hydantoins by interfering with their absorption.
28. The nurse should first check a drug reference to see if the seizure medication can reduce the effectiveness of an oral contraceptive; advise the patient appropriately to use an alternate form of contraceptive. This should also be documented in the chart and reported to the physician.
29. All succinimide medications end in "-suximide;" (e.g., ethosuximide, methsuximide, and phensuximide).
30. Carbamazepine (Tegretol) may be used to treat seizures in combination with other anticonvulsant agents and to treat pain associated with trigeminal neuralgia. Blood studies to detect hepatotoxicity, nephrotoxicity, and/or blood dyscrasias should be performed.
31. Lamotrigine blocks voltage-sensitive sodium channels in neuronal membranes.

33. Summarize the premedication assessments for each class of antiepileptics.

34. Review side effects to expect and report for seizure drugs.

32. Approximately 10% of patients receiving lamotrigine develop a skin rash and urticaria in the first 46 weeks of therapy. Combination therapy with valproic acid appears more likely to precipitate a serious rash. (See textbook, p. 307.)

33. Summary of premedication assessments for antiepileptics:
    - For the drug classes benzodiazepines, hydantoins, succinimides, and miscellaneous agents:
        - Baseline assessment of speech pattern, alertness, orientation, and behavioral response to therapy.
    - For the drug classes hydantoins, succinimides, and for miscellaneous agent valproic acid:
        - Review blood reports to detect blood dyscrasias and hepatotoxicity.
    - Hydantoins:
        - Check blood sugar for diabetics (hyperglycemia with hydantoins).
    - Miscellaneous agents:
        - Carbamazepine (Tegretol)—CBC, liver and renal function tests, and ophthalmologic exam
        - Oxcarbazepine (Trileptal)—requires electrolyte studies periodically during this drug's use
        - Valproic acid (Depakene)—liver function tests, bleeding time, and platelet counts
        - Zonisamide (Zonegran)—check for allergy to sulfonamide medicines (do not administer drug until health care provider has approved its use). Check for history of skin rashes; if rash occurs, notify health care provider immediately. Review baseline CBC, liver function, renal lab studies.

34. See individual monographs throughout chapter.

CHAPTER 19

Student Name ______________________________

Drugs Used for Seizure Disorders

Learning Activities

FILL-IN-THE-BLANK

Finish each of the following statements using the correct term.

1. A patient having seizures that are chronic and recurrent is diagnosed as having ____________________.

2. ______________ ______________ is a rapidly recurring generalized seizure that does not allow the individual to regain normal function between seizures.

3. The period of time immediately after the seizure is complete is referred to as the ____________________ period.

4. In describing seizures, a sudden loss of muscle tone is known as a(n) ____________________ seizure or drop attack.

5. ____________________ is by far the most commonly used anticonvulsant of the hydantoins.

6. Zonisamide acts by blocking ____________________ and ____________________ channels to stabilize the neuronal membranes.

7. Diazepam, clonazepam, and clorazepate are anticonvulsants classified as ____________________.

8. Phenytoin can cause ____________________ in a diabetic patient.

9. A decrease in therapeutic effectiveness of phenytoin can occur when an OTC ____________________ is taken concurrently.

MATCHING

Match the generic drug name with its corresponding brand name. Each option will be used only once.

_____ 10. phenytoin

_____ 11. lorazepam

_____ 12. diazepam

_____ 13. clonazepam

a. Klonopin
b. Valium
c. Dilantin
d. Ativan

TRUE OR FALSE

Mark "T" for true and "F" for false for each statement. Correct all false statements.

_____ 14. *Generalized seizures* refer to those that affect both hemispheres of the brain, are accompanied by loss of consciousness, and may be subdivided into convulsive and nonconvulsive types.

_____ 15. Epilepsy is treated almost exclusively with medications known as *anticonvulsants*.

_____ 16. In children, anticonvulsant therapy may cause a change in personality and possible indifference to school and family activities.

_____ 17. Individuals who are having a seizure should be restrained to protect them from further injury.

_____ 18. Smaller doses of benzodiazepines may be necessary to maintain effects in patients who smoke.

_____ 19. The mechanism of action of the hydantoins is unknown.

_____ 20. Hypoglycemia may be caused by hydantoin therapy in patients with diabetes.

_____ 21. Carbamazepine is not effective in controlling myoclonic or absence seizures.

DRUG ACTION/SIDE EFFECTS

22. *State the action and side effects of the following drug classes or drugs used in the treatment of seizure disorders.*

	Actions	Side Effects
BENZODIAZEPINES		

CHAPTER 19

Student Name______________________________

Drugs Used for Seizure Disorders

Practice Questions for the NCLEX Examination

_____ 1. When administering diazepam intravenously, the nurse should: (Select all that apply.)
1. administer slowly at a rate of 5 mg over at least one minute.
2. administer diazepam via continuous infusion.
3. not administer diazepam with any other drugs.
4. assess the injection site for venous irritation.

_____ 2. Patients taking which group of anticonvulsants are most at risk for the development of gingival hyperplasia?
1. Barbiturates
2. Benzodiazepines
3. Hydantoins
4. Succinimides

_____ 3. Patients receiving zonisamide for the treatment of seizure disorder should be assessed for an allergy to:
1. penicillin.
2. furosemide.
3. sulfonamides.
4. digitalis.

_____ 4. A patient who has been taking lamotrigine for treatment of a seizure disorder develops a skin rash in the second week of therapy. The nurse should:
1. discontinue the lamotrigine.
2. promptly notify the health care provider of development of the rash.
3. administer Benadryl to the patient.
4. pack the area of the skin rash in ice.

_____ 5. Before starting treatment with valproic acid, which of the following baseline studies should be completed? (Select all that apply.)
1. Electrocardiogram
2. Liver function tests
3. Bleeding time determination
4. Platelet count

_____ 6. A female patient taking topiramate for seizure control who also is taking oral contraceptives should be informed that:
1. she will not be able to become pregnant because of the topiramate therapy.
2. topiramate therapy should be stopped if she experiences spotting or bleeding.
3. an alternative form of birth control should be used when taking topiramate with oral contraceptives.
4. there are no contraindications of using these two drugs together.

_____ 7. A patient taking oxcarbazepine therapy for the treatment of a seizure disorder develops nausea, malaise, headache, lethargy, and is confused. The patient is experiencing symptoms of:
1. hyponatremia.
2. hypokalemia.
3. hypocalcemia.
4. hypomagnesemia.

_____ 8. If sedation, drowsiness, dizziness, or blurred vision should develop in a patient taking gabapentin for treatment of a seizure disorder, the patient should:
1. discontinue use of the gabapentin.
2. reduce the dose of the gabapentin by half.
3. not discontinue use of the gabapentin without first consulting the health care provider.
4. take the gabapentin before going to sleep.

_____ 9. Which of the following actions should the nurse take when working with a patient experiencing a seizure?
1. Restrain the patient
2. Place a tongue blade in the patient's mouth
3. Once the patient enters into the relaxation stage, turn him or her slightly onto the side to allow secretions to drain from the mouth.
4. Medicate the patient immediately.

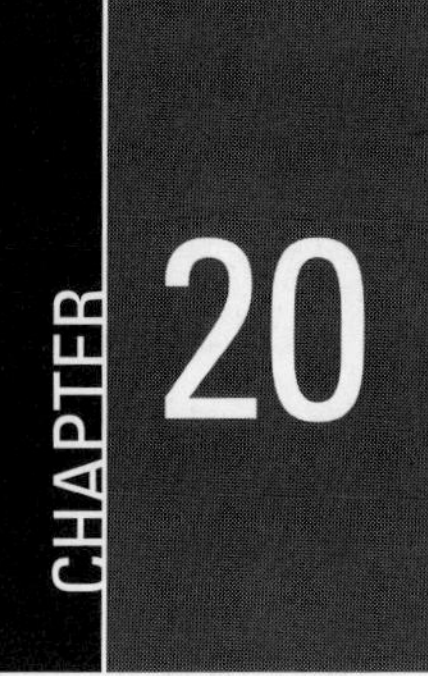

Drugs Used for Pain Management

Review Sheet

The QUESTION column and the ANSWER column have been offset so that you can cover the answer while reading the questions, allowing you to assess your knowledge.

Question

1. Define *pain perception*, *pain threshold*, and *pain tolerance*.
2. Compare nociceptive pain, somatic pain, visceral pain, neuropathic pain, and idiopathic pain.
3. Define *analgesic*.
4. Name the classes of analgesics.
5. What neurotransmitters are known to stimulate nociceptors?
6. What are the four types of opiate receptors?
7. What drug is usually prescribed for severe, chronic pain?
8. Summarize the nursing process for pain management.
9. Discuss the World Health Organization's stepwise approach to pain management.
10. What are the primary therapeutic outcomes appropriate for pain management therapy?
11. Read the Pain Care Bill of Rights.
12. Obtain a copy of the pain assessment tools used in local clinical sites and discuss the appropriate assessments and recording of pain events using the tools assembled.

Answer

1. Pain perception is awareness of the pain sensation. Pain threshold is the point at which pain is felt. Pain tolerance is an individual's ability to withstand the pain experience.
2. Nociceptive pain is a result of stimulus to pain receptors (dull, aching); somatic pain originates in the skin, bone, or muscle; visceral pain originates in the organs of the thorax or abdomen; neuropathic pain results from injury to the peripheral or central nervous systems; and idiopathic pain is of unknown origin.
3. Analgesics are drugs that relieve pain.
4. Opiate agonists, opiate partial agonists, opiate antagonists, antiinflammatory, nonsteroidal antiinflammatory, and miscellaneous agents
5. The neurotransmitters bradykinin, prostaglandins, leukotrienes, histamines, and serotonin sensitize nociceptors.
6. The four types of opiate receptors are mu, delta, kappa, and sigma receptors.
7. Morphine sulfate is usually prescribed for severe, chronic pain. It may also be combined with other drugs such as antidepressants.
8. See textbook, pp. 319-328.
9. See textbook, p. 318.
10. See textbook, p. 319.
11. See Table 20-1, p. 320.

13. What is the most effective route for administering an analgesic when immediate relief is needed?
14. Explain the benefits of patient-controlled analgesia (PCA).
15. What is meant by "on demand" in relation to the use of a PCA pump?
16. Differentiate among addiction, physical dependence, and tolerance.
17. Define *agonists, antagonists,* and *partial agonists.*
18. Opiate agonists are subdivided into what four groups?
19. Identify pain assessment data needed to establish a baseline for monitoring therapy before initiating treatment for pain.
20. For what type(s) of pain are opiate agonists used?
21. What premedication assessments should be performed before administering an opiate agonist?
22. Will naloxone reverse CNS depression caused by sedative/hypnotics or tranquilizers?
23. When is naloxone effective?
24. What three drugs are antidotes for opiate agonists and opiate partial agonists?
25. Do opiate partial agonists relieve pain effectively in people who have recently taken opiate agonists?

12. Individualize to local clinical facilities.
13. The intravenous route gives the most immediate pain relief.
14. With PCA, the patient can initiate the administration of analgesics, allowing pain relief to be obtained rapidly. Most important is the sense of control a patient feels toward the pain and scheduling daily activities. The PCA system monitors the total dose(s) administered and limits can be set on the total amount that can be self-administered during a specified period.
15. "On demand" means the patient can self-administer a dosage of pain medication when needed. There is a "lock-out" safety device that limits the number of administrations over a specific period of time.
16. Research on the Internet definitions of *addiction, physical dependence,* and *tolerance.*
17. Agonists interact with receptors to stimulate response. Antagonists attach to a receptor but do not stimulate a response or block a response. Partial agonists are drugs that interact with a receptor to stimulate a response, but may inhibit other responses.
18. Opiate agonists are divided into four groups: morphinelike derivatives, meperidinelike derivatives, methadonelike derivatives, and other opiate agonists.
19. Baseline vital signs, neurologic exam, prior analgesics administered, and degree of pain control; voiding and bowel pattern.
20. Opiate agonists are used for moderate to severe pain.
21. Baseline vital signs, neurologic exam, prior analgesics administered, degree of pain control; voiding and bowel pattern.
22. Naloxone will not reverse CNS depression caused by sedative/hypnotics or tranquilizers.
23. Naloxone reverses the CNS depressant effects of the opiate agonists.
24. Nalmefene, naloxone, and naltrexone are antidotes for opiate agonists and opiate partial agonists.

26. Give an example of an opiate partial agonist.
27. What is the most common drug used as an analgesic for relief of mild to moderate pain?
28. What three pharmacologic effects are associated with the salicylates?
29. When is ASA (aspirin) indicated?
30. What is salicylism?
31. What is the antidote for salicylism?
32. What are premedication assessments to perform before administering nonsteroidal antiinflammatory drugs (NSAIDs)?
33. What are NSAIDs?
34. How do NSAIDs act?
35. What are the primary therapeutic outcomes expected from the NSAIDs?
36. What is the major adverse effect of NSAIDs?
37. Name five commonly used NSAIDs.
38. Name the synthetic nonopiate analgesic used frequently for mild to moderate pain.
39. Compare the action of the drug in question 34 with the action of acetaminophen (Tylenol).
40. What are early indications of acetaminophen toxicity?

25. Opiate partial agonists usually do not alleviate pain in people who have recently taken opiate agonists.
26. See Table 20-3, p. 332.
27. Aspirin is the most common drug used to relieve mild to moderate pain.
28. Three pharmacologic effects of salicylates are analgesic, antipyretic, and antiinflammatory.
29. ASA is indicated for analgesic effect, fever reduction, and antiinflammatory effects. Do not give aspirin to children who may be developing a viral infection. Salicylates have been associated with Reye's syndrome.
30. Salicylism is seen with high doses of salicylates. Symptoms include tinnitus, impaired hearing, sweating, dizziness, mental confusion, and nausea and vomiting.
31. There is no antidote for salicylism. Use gastric lavage, force IV fluids, and alkalization of urine with IV sodium bicarbonate; stop salicylates.
32. See textbook, p. 341.
33. NSAIDs are also known as "aspirinlike" drugs. They are chemically unrelated to the salicylates but are prostaglandin inhibitors and share many of the same therapeutic actions and side effects.
34. NSAIDs act by blocking cyclooxygenase (COX-1 and COX-2).
35. The primary therapeutic outcomes expected from the NSAIDs are reduced pain, reduced inflammation, and elimination of fever.
36. The major adverse effect of NSAID therapy is increased risk of potentially fatal cardiovascular adverse effects including heart attack and stroke, gastric irritation, gastric bleeding, constipation, dizziness, drowsiness, confusion, hives, pruritus, rash, nephrotoxicity, hepatotoxicity, and blood dyscrasias.
37. See Table 20-4, pp. 337-339.
38. Acetaminophen (Tylenol, Datril, Tempra) is a synthetic nonopiate analgesic used frequently for mild to moderate pain.
39. Acetaminophen has no antiinflammatory effect. However, it is a very good antipyretic and analgesic.

41. What premedication assessments are required for each classification of drug used to treat pain?
42. What effect does aspirin have on phenytoin, valproic acid, and oral hypoglycemic agents?

40. Early indications of acetaminophen toxicity include nausea, anorexia, vomiting, and jaundice accompanied by an elevation in liver function tests.
41. This information can be found in sections listed as premedication assessments in the drug monographs throughout Chapter 20.
42. When taken with aspirin, phenytoin levels are increased, causing toxicity: nystagmus, lethargy, sedation. Dosage adjustment may be required. Valproic acid levels are increased when taken with aspirin; dose adjustment may be needed. With oral hypoglycemics, aspirin increases potential for hypoglycemia.

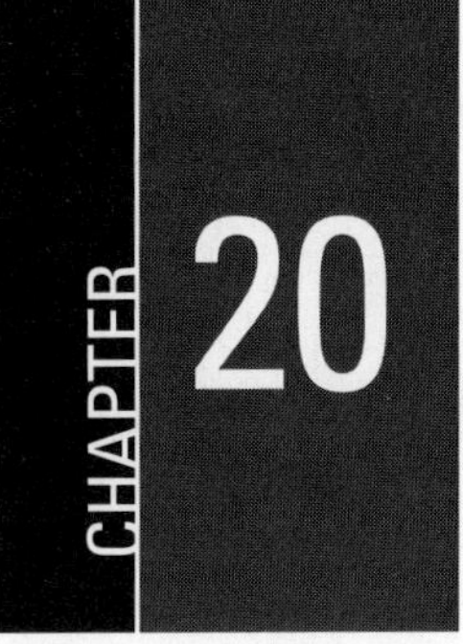

Student Name____

Drugs Used for Pain Management

Learning Activities

FILL-IN-THE-BLANK

Finish each of the following statements using the correct term.

1. The three terms used in relationship to the pain experience are pain ____________________, pain ____________________, and pain ____________________.

2. ____________________ pain is a nonspecific pain of unknown origin.

3. ____________________ are drugs that relieve pain without producing loss of consciousness or reflex activity.

4. Antidotes for opiate antagonists include ____________________, ____________________, and naltrexone.

5. Opiate partial agonist drugs should be held and the health care provider notified if the patient's respirations are below ____________________.

6. NSAID is an abbreviation for ____.

7. The primary therapeutic outcomes expected from acetaminophen are _______________ and _______________.

MATCHING

Match the generic drug name with its corresponding brand name. Each option will be used only once.

_____ 8. butorphanol

_____ 9. buprenorphine

_____ 10. nalbuphine

_____ 11. oxaprozin

_____ 12. naproxen

_____ 13. meloxicam

a. Daypro
b. Aleve
c. Mobic
d. Stadol
e. Buprenex
f. Nubain

TRUE OR FALSE

Mark "T" for true and "F" for false for each statement. Correct all false statements.

_____ 14. The sympathetic nervous system is activated when a person experiences acute pain.

_____ 15. Chronic pain has a slower onset and lasts longer than 6 months beyond the healing process.

_____ 16. The first step leading to the sensation of pain is the stimulation of receptors known as *nociceptors*.

_____ 17. Pain is expected with aging.

_____ 18. Patients should be taught to request pain medication before the pain escalates and becomes severe for optimal effectiveness.

_____ 19. The word *narcotic* should be abandoned in exchange for *opiate agonists* and *opiate partial agonists.*

_____ 20. Symptoms of withdrawal from opiate agonists reach a peak at 12 hours after discontinuation of the medication and disappear over the next 24 hours.

_____ 21. Tramadol is a new synthetic opiate agonist that is anticipated to have the same physical addiction that occurs with morphine.

_____ 22. Urinary retention can occur with the use of opiate agonists.

_____ 23. A unique property of aspirin when compared with other salicylates is inhibition of platelet aggregation and enhancement of bleeding time.

_____ 24. Although considered acceptable at one time, placebo therapy should never be used with pain management.

_____ 25. The rating of pain has been designated "the fifth vital sign."

DRUG ACTION/SIDE EFFECTS

26. *State the action and side effects of the following drug classes or drugs used for pain management.*

	Actions	Side Effects
OPIATE AGONISTS		

CHAPTER 20

Student Name______________________________

Drugs Used for Pain Management

Practice Questions for the NCLEX Examination

_____ 1. Patients experiencing acute pain would be most likely to exhibit:
1. bradypnea.
2. bradycardia.
3. constricted pupils.
4. hypertension.

_____ 2. Which type of pain originates from the abdominal and thoracic organs?
1. Nociceptive pain
2. Somatic pain
3. Visceral pain
4. Neuropathic pain

_____ 3. Which of the following statements about the use of the transdermal opioid analgesic Duragesic is true?
1. Duragesic is commonly used for acute pain.
2. It takes approximately 2 hours for the initial patch of medication to reach a steady blood level.
3. The patch provides relief for up to 72 hours.
4. No other analgesics may be used with Duragesic.

_____ 4. When working with a patient who is receiving drugs for pain, which statement about nutritional aspects of care is correct?
1. Constipation is a common effect from opiate use.
2. Caffeine should be encouraged to counteract the sedating effects of other medications.
3. Limit fluid intake to four 8-ounce glasses daily.
4. Stool softeners are contraindicated in patients using pain medications.

_____ 5. When working with a patient suspected of being addicted to opiate agonists, the nurse knows that:
1. patients need to undergo the symptoms of withdrawal to be treated for addiction.
2. patients are treated with an abrupt reduction of daily opiate doses.
3. if withdrawal symptoms become severe, the patient may receive methadone.
4. tranquilizers and sedatives are contraindicated in the treatment of patients withdrawing from opiate agonist addiction.

_____ 6. If an opiate partial agonist is administered to a patient addicted to a opiate agonist, the nurse must assess for:
1. withdrawal symptoms from the opiate agonist.
2. constipation.
3. hypotension.
4. hypothermia.

_____ 7. Ms. L. has been taking an oral hypoglycemic agent to control her diabetes mellitus. She is now ordered salicylate drug therapy for pain management. The nurse recognizes that when these two types of drugs are taken together:
1. Ms. L. will need to switch to subcutaneous insulin therapy for the duration of time she is taking the salicylates.
2. urine glucose determinations with Clinitest will be the most accurate method of blood glucose measurements for Ms. L. at this time.
3. the dose of the oral hypoglycemic agent should be doubled while Ms. L. is on salicylate drug therapy.
4. salicylates may enhance the hypoglycemic effects of oral hypoglycemic agents; therefore Ms. L. should be monitored for hypoglycemia.

_____ 8. Which of the following statements about opiate partial agonists is true?
1. Constipation does not occur with use of these drugs.
2. These drugs have no effect on the respiratory center of the brain.
3. Addiction is not an issue with use of these drugs.
4. The potency with the first few weeks of therapy is similar to that of morphine; however, after prolonged use, tolerance may develop.

_____ 9. Visceral pain usually originates from: (Select all that apply.)
1. skin.
2. bones.
3. abdominal organs.
4. joints.
5. thoracic organs.

_____ 10. Comfort measures the nurse may provide for the patient with pain may include: (Select all that apply.)
1. backrubs.
2. cold applications.
3. exercise.
4. transcutaneous electrical nerve stimulation (TENS).

_____ 11. A patient is receiving opiate agonists for pain control. Which of the following side effects (if any) should the nurse report to the primary care provider? (Select all that apply.)
1. Patient complaint of feeling lightheaded
2. Respiratory rate of 7
3. Orthostatic hypotension
4. Urinary retention
5. Constipation

_____ 12. The drug of choice for treating respiratory depression when excessive doses of opiate agonists, opiate partial agonists, or propoxyphene have been administered, or when the causative agent is unknown, is:
1. naloxone.
2. nalbuphine.
3. meperidine.
4. tramadol.

_____ 13. Patients who overdose on acetaminophen most likely sustain damage to the ____________________ system.
1. cardiovascular
2. hepatic
3. central nervous
4. reproductive

CHAPTER 21

Introduction to Cardiovascular Disease and Metabolic Syndrome

Review Sheet

The QUESTION column and the ANSWER column have been offset so that you can cover the answer while reading the question, allowing you to assess you knowledge.

Question

1. Define *cardiovascular disease.*
2. What are the characteristics of metabolic syndrome?
3. What are the risk factors for the development of metabolic syndrome?
4. In addition to type 2 diabetes and heart disease, what other consequences are associated with metabolic syndrome?
5. Summarize the overall treatment goals for metabolic syndrome.
6. What is the drug therapy for hypertension associated with metabolic syndrome?
7. What is the treatment for dyslipidemia associated with metabolic syndrome?
8. What is the mechanism of action of the thiazolidinediones in the treatment of type 2 diabetes mellitus in metabolic syndrome?
9. What is the mechanism of action of metformin in the treatment of type 2 diabetes mellitus in metabolic syndrome?
10. What is mechanism of action of the alpha-glycosidase inhibitors in the treatment of type 2 diabetes mellitus in metabolic syndrome?

Answer

1. *Cardiovascular disease* is a collective term used to refer to disorders of the circulatory system.
2. The presence of type 2 diabetes mellitus, abdominal obesity, hypertriglyceridemia, low high-density lipoproteins (HDL), and hypertension.
3. Poor diet, sedentary lifestyle, and genetic predisposition.
4. Renal disease, obstructive sleep apnea, polycystic ovary syndrome, cognitive decline in older adults, and dementia in older adults.
5. Refer to Box 21-2, p. 350.
6. A combination of a thiazide diuretic plus an angiotensin-converting enzyme inhibitor or a beta blocker.
7. Treatment of dyslipidemia is generally to lower the triglycerides and LDL-cholesterol and raise the HDL-cholesterol. After lifestyle changes, medicines most commonly used are the 3-hydroxy-methylglutaryl coenzyme A reductase inhibitors, fibrinic acid derivatives, and niacin.
8. The thiazolidinediones reduce insulin resistance in peripheral tissues.
9. Metformin decreases production of glucose by the liver and to a lesser extent, reduces insulin resistance in peripheral tissues.

11. What is the mechanism of action of the sulfonylureas and meglitinides in the treatment of type 2 diabetes mellitus in metabolic syndrome?

10. The alpha-glycosidase inhibitors reduce the absorption of glucose from the intestine, reducing postprandial hyperglycemia.

11. The sulfonylureas and meglitinides stimulate the beta cells of the pancreas to release more insulin.

CHAPTER 21

Student Name______________________________

Introduction to Cardiovascular Disease and Metabolic Syndrome

Learning Activities

FILL-IN-THE-BLANK

Finish each of the following statements using the correct term.

1. ______________ ______________ ______________ is the term pertaining to narrowing or obstruction of the arteries of the heart which leads to angina pectoris and myocardial infarction.

2. __________________ has been recognized as the greatest contributor to the development of cardiovascular disease.

3. Weight in proportion to height is referred to as ______________ ______________ ______________.

4. __________________ diseases are a major cause of premature death in the United States.

TRUE OR FALSE

Mark "T" for true and "F" for false for each statement. Correct all false statements.

_____ 5. The treatment of dyslipidemia is generally to lower the triglycerides and HDL-cholesterol and raise the LDL-cholesterol.

_____ 6. Insulin injections are used in the treatment of patients with metabolic syndrome who do not secrete adequate amounts of insulin.

_____ 7. The reductase inhibitors used to treat dyslipidemias are also known as "statins."

_____ 8. A weight loss of 10 to 15 pounds can improve hypertension and hyperglycemia associated with metabolic syndrome.

_____ 9. A hemoglobin A1c of 10% is considered as meeting the general treatment goals for patients with metabolic syndrome.

CHAPTER 21

Student Name________________________________

Introduction to Cardiovascular Disease and Metabolic Syndrome

Practice Questions for the NCLEX Examination

_____ 1. When teaching a group of patients about metabolic syndrome, the nurse should include which of the following statements? (Select all that apply.)
1. Type 1 diabetes mellitus is a common characteristic of metabolic syndrome.
2. Mexican-American women have the highest rate of metabolic syndrome in the United States within ethnic groups.
3. Patients with metabolic syndrome commonly have low high-density lipoproteins.
4. Hypertension is commonly found in patients with metabolic syndrome.
5. Hypertriglyceridemia is commonly found in patients with metabolic syndrome.

_____ 2. Which of the following lab values indicate that the general treatment goals for patients with metabolic syndrome are being met? (Select all that apply.)
1. Blood pressure 128/78
2. High-density lipoproteins 45 mg/dL
3. Triglycerides 140 mg/dL
4. Hemoglobin A1c of 5%
5. Fasting plasma glucose 118 mg/dL

_____ 3. Which of the following drugs used in the treatment of type 2 diabetes mellitus reduces insulin resistance in peripheral tissues?
1. Meglitinides
2. Alpha-glycosidase inhibitors
3. Sulfonylureas
4. Thiazolidinediones

_____ 4. When teaching a group of patients with metabolic syndrome the importance of weight loss and healthy diet, which of the following statements should the nurse include?
1. "Restrict the total amount of fat you consume each day to approximately 45% of your total calories."
2. "You must limit the amount of protein you eat to 2 ounces once a day."
3. "Most of the dietary fat you consume should be saturated."
4. "Olive oil is an example of the type of 'good' fat you may eat."

_____ 5. Which of the following drugs used to treat type 2 diabetes mellitus associated with metabolic syndrome stimulates the beta cells of the pancreas to release more insulin? (Select all that apply.)
1. Sulfonylureas
2. Metformin
3. Alpha-glycosidase
4. Meglitinides
5. Thiazolidinediones

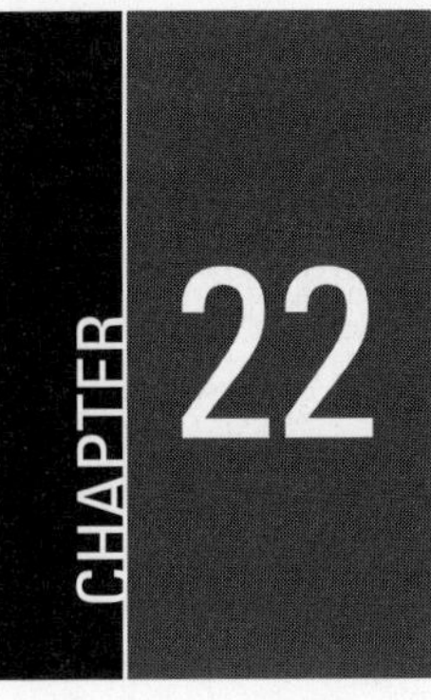

Drugs Used to Treat Dyslipidemias

Review Sheet

The QUESTION column and the ANSWER column have been offset so that you can cover the answer while reading the questions, allowing you to assess your knowledge.

Question

1. Define *atherosclerosis, hyperlipidemia, dyslipidemia, chylomicrons, triglycerides,* and *lipoproteins.*
2. List the key characteristics of metabolic syndrome.
3. What lifestyle changes should be used to treat hyperlipidemia prior to starting drug therapy?
4. What are the primary drugs for lowering serum cholesterol levels?
5. Why aren't fibric acid agents used as first-line drugs for the treatment of hyperlipidemias?
6. Which class of drugs used to treat hyperlipidemia is the most expensive?
7. Summarize nursing assessments needed for a patient with hyperlipidemia.
8. Why are supplemental vitamins required with bile acid-binding resins?
9. What are the signs and symptoms of a vitamin K deficiency?
10. Describe the proper preparation of cholestyramine for administration.

Answer

1. See textbook, p. 352.
2. Metabolic syndrome, also known as *syndrome X*, includes type II diabetes mellitus, abdominal obesity, hypertriglyceridemia, low HDL cholesterol, and hypertension.
3. Lifestyle changes should be attempted for treatment of hyperlipidemia before starting drug therapy, including dietary changes (e.g., fat intake less than 30% of calories, decreased cholesterol and saturated fat intake, increased polyunsaturated and monounsaturated fats), weight reduction, and regular exercise.
4. Bile acid resins, niacin, and HMG-CoA are the primary classes of lipid-lowering drugs. Ezetimibe (Zetia) represents a new class of drugs whose clinical role is yet to be determined.
5. Fibric acid agents do not result in substantial reduction of LDL-C, but are effective in lowering triglycerides.
6. HMG-CoA drugs, known as *statins*, are the most expensive.
7. Nursing assessments needed for patients with hyperlipidemia include risk factors (e.g., family history of increased cholesterol and lipids), smoking, dietary habits, glucose intolerance, elevated serum lipids, obesity, and sedentary lifestyle.
8. Bile acid-binding resins may deplete the body of its needed supply of fat-soluble vitamins (DEAK).
9. Bruising; bleeding gums; dark, tarry stools; and "coffee ground" emesis are signs and symptoms of a vitamin K deficiency.

11. What drug interactions can occur with the use of bile acid-binding resins?
12. Discuss patient teaching needed to minimize the common side effects to expect with bile acid-binding resins therapy such as constipation, bloating, fullness, nausea, and flatulence.
13. What is the primary desired therapeutic outcome from niacin?
14. What premedication assessments should be performed before administration of niacin?
15. Why is niacin not used with diabetic patients?
16. What suggestions can be given to patients taking niacin to minimize the side effects of flushing, itching, rash, tingling, and headache?
17. Cite the premedication assessments that should be done prior to niacin therapy.
18. Name three statin drugs.
19. How long is the trial period used to evaluate the use of statins for hyperlipidemias?
20. What are common side effects to expect from antilipemic therapy?
21. What is the effect on triglycerides of fibric acid agents?
22. What anticipated alterations may occur in the blood glucose level with gemfibrozil?
23. What is the mechanism of action of ezetimibe (Zetia)?

10. To prepare cholestyramine for administration, mix powdered resin with 2–6 oz water, soup, juice, or crushed pineapple; allow to stand until drug is absorbed and dispersed. Follow with an additional glass of water.
11. Bile acid-binding resins bind to drugs such as warfarin, thyroxine, thiazide diuretics, NSAIDs, and beta blockers, and therefore reduce absorption of these drugs. Minimize this effect by administering 1 hour before or 4 hours after giving a resin. (See also textbook p. 356.)
12. See drug monograph, textbook p. 356.
13. The primary desired therapeutic outcome of niacin is decreased LDL and total cholesterol, decreased triglycerides, and increased HDL levels.
14. Before administering niacin, assess serum triglyceride and cholesterol levels, liver function, baseline uric acid and blood glucose levels, and vital signs. Document existing gastrointestinal symptoms.
15. Niacin is not recommended for diabetics because of glucose intolerance.
16. Take niacin with food, take aspirin 30 minutes before each dose of niacin (unless contraindicated). Tell the patient that tolerance develops quickly.
17. See textbook, p. 357.
18. The statin drugs include atorvastatin, fluvastatin, lovastatin, pravastatin, and simvastatin.
19. The trial period used to evaluate the therapeutic success of statins for hyperlipidemias is a period of up to 3 months.
20. Nausea, diarrhea, flatulence, bloating, and abdominal distress are side effects to expect with antilipemic therapy.
21. Fibrates are the most effective triglyceride-lowering agents.
22. Gemfibrozil may cause moderate hyperglycemia.
23. Ezetimibe (Zetia) acts by blocking the absorption of cholesterol by the small intestines. Note that it also does not elevate triglycerides.

CHAPTER 22

Student Name___________________________

Drugs Used to Treat Dyslipidemias

Learning Activities

FILL-IN-THE-BLANK

Finish each of the following statements using the correct term.

1. ____________________ is characterized by the accumulation of fatty deposits on the inner walls of arteries and arterioles throughout the body that reduces the blood supply to vital organs resulting in strokes, angina pectoris, myocardial infarction, and peripheral vascular disease.

2. ____________________ is sometimes referred to as "good" lipoproteins since high levels indicate that cholesterol is being removed from vascular tissue where it may participate in the development of CAD.

3. It is becoming recognized that our ____________________ may be the greatest contributor to causing hyperlipidemia.

4. Pharmacologic antilipemic therapy is often started with the ______________ ______________ ______________ because of their safety record and success in lowering cholesterol levels.

5. The primary medicines used to lower elevated cholesterol levels are the bile acid-binding resins, ____________________, and ____________________.

6. ____________________ is the first of a new class of agents used to reduce atherosclerosis by blocking the absorption of cholesterol by the small intestine.

7. ____________________ is the first of a new class of drugs used to decrease atherosclerosis by combining two omega-3 fatty acids which act to decrease the synthesis of triglycerides in the liver.

8. ____________________ is the only form of vitamin B_3 that is approved by the FDA for the treatment of dyslipidemias.

MATCHING

Match the generic drug name with its corresponding brand name. Each option will be used only once.

_____ 9. simvastatin

_____ 10. lovastatin

_____ 11. fluvastatin

_____ 12. atorvastatin

a. Lipitor
b. Zocor
c. Lescol
d. Mevacor

TRUE OR FALSE

Mark "T" for true and "F" for false for each statement. Correct all false statements.

_____ 13. Coronary artery disease is a major cause of premature death in the United States.

_____ 14. Drug therapy for the treatment of hyperlipidemias usually lasts for a few weeks and is then discontinued.

_____ 15. The most cost-effective and successful forms of treatment for hyperlipidemias are smoking cessation, weight reduction, exercise, and dietary modifications.

_____ 16. The primary therapeutic outcome expected from bile acid-binding resin therapy is reduction of LDL and total cholesterol levels.

_____ 17. Antilipemic agents may be used to treat hyperlipidemias only if diet, exercise, and weight reduction are not successful in adequately lowering LDL-C levels.

_____ 18. The statins are the most potent antilipemic agents available with the added benefits of decreasing inflammation, decreasing platelet aggregation, decreasing thrombin formation, and decreasing platelet viscosity resulting in decreased heart attacks and stroke.

_____ 19. HDLs (high-density lipoproteins) are also referred to as "good cholesterol" because they are beneficial in preventing coronary heart disease.

_____ 20. Niacin is effective in lowering triglycerides and cholesterol and raises LDL cholesterol levels.

_____ 21. Smoking contributes to the development and progression of coronary heart disease.

_____ 22. The use of bile acid-binding resins could potentially result in the development of a bleeding disorder if vitamins or a balanced diet are not taken regularly.

_____ 23. Bile acid-binding resins may bind with warfarin, NSAIDs, tetracycline, and beta blockers, thereby enhancing the drugs' effectiveness.

_____ 24. Common side effects of niacin use are headache and flushing.

_____ 25. Gemfibrozil may cause hypoglycemia.

_____ 26. Vitamins A, C, and B are significantly affected by bile acid-binding resin drugs.

DRUG ACTION/SIDE EFFECTS

27. *State the action and side effects of the following drug classes or drugs used in the treatment of hyperlipidemias.*

	Actions	Side Effects
FIBRIC ACIDS		

CHAPTER 22

Student Name______________________________

Drugs Used to Treat Dyslipidemias

Practice Questions for the NCLEX Examination

_____ 1. Which of the following statements should be included in the teaching for patients receiving bile acid-sequestering resins?
1. "You should limit your water intake to 4 glasses a day."
2. "Eat foods that are low in bulk to avoid diarrhea."
3. "You may need to take supplemental vitamins"
4. "Now that you are on a medication to lower your lipids, there is no need to monitor your cholesterol intake."

_____ 2. Patients taking bile acid-sequestering resins are most at risk for the development of:
1. hypertension.
2. tachycardia.
3. nephrotoxicity.
4. vitamin K deficiency.

_____ 3. Mr. X. has been prescribed the following medications: digoxin, Lasix, and cholestyramine, which is a bile acid-binding resin. Which action should the nurse take?
1. Administer all of the medications together to avoid unnecessary interruption of the patient's rest.
2. Mix the cholestyramine with soda pop and have Mr. X. immediately consume it.
3. Administer the Lasix and digoxin 1 hour before or 4 hours after administration of cholestyramine to avoid interference with their absorption.
4. Limit water intake with the administration of cholestyramine to 2 ounces.

_____ 4. A patient taking HMG-CoA reductase inhibitors for the treatment of hyperlipidemia should be instructed to:
1. avoid grapefruit juice.
2. increase any anticoagulants taken by twice as much.
3. expect muscle weakness as a common expected effect.
4. take these medications on an empty stomach to increase absorption.

_____ 5. Patients with a deficiency of which vitamin are most at risk for the development of bleeding disorders?
1. Vitamin A
2. Vitamin D
3. Vitamin E
4. Vitamin K

_____ 6. Which of the following drugs used to treat hyperlipidemias has an expected side effect of flushing, itching, rash, tingling, and headache associated with its use?
1. Niacin
2. HMG-CoA reductase inhibitors
3. Fibric acids
4. Bile acid-binding resins

_____ 7. The most common expected side effect of drugs used to treat hyperlipidemias includes:
1. abdominal discomfort and gas.
2. myopathy.
3. jaundice.
4. sweating.

_____ 8. When assessing a patient with signs and symptoms of vitamin K deficiency, the nurse would expect to find which of the following? (Select all that apply.)
1. Bleeding gums
2. Bruising
3. Dark tarry stools
4. "Coffee-ground" emesis

_____ 9. A patient taking a bile acid-binding resin for the treatment of dyslipidemia tells the nurse that ever since he began taking the medication, he experiences bloating and fullness. The nurse should instruct the patient to: (Select all that apply.)
1. swallow the medication without gulping air.
2. maintain adequate fiber in his diet.
3. limit his fluid intake.
4. take the medication with carbonated beverages.

_____ 10. When teaching a patient about niacin therapy, the nurse should tell the patient to report which of the following side effects to the primary care provider? (Select all that apply.)
1. Flushing
2. Tingling
3. Fatigue
4. Muscle aches

_____ 11. Which of the following statements is true about the HMG-CoA reductase inhibitors? (Select all that apply.)
1. They are the most potent antilipemic agents available.
2. They reduce inflammation, platelet aggregation, thrombin formation, and plasma viscosity.
3. Rhabdomyolysis and myoglobinuria have been reported as side effects of these drugs.
4. Patients who are pregnant should not take these medications.

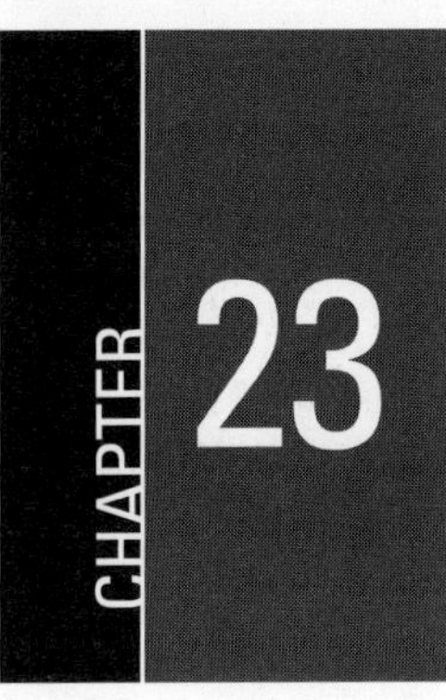

Drugs Used to Treat Hypertension

Review Sheet

The QUESTION column and the ANSWER column have been offset so that you can cover the answer while reading the questions, allowing you to assess your knowledge.

Question

1. What are systolic and diastolic blood pressure?
2. How is the mean arterial pressure or average pressure calculated?
3. What are the primary determinants of systolic and diastolic blood pressure?
4. What is the definition of *hypertension*?
5. Differentiate among prehypertension, primary hypertension, and secondary hypertension.
6. State the procedure for measuring blood pressure as recommended by JNC 7 guidelines.
7. Identify the goals of blood pressure therapy.

Answer

1. Systolic blood pressure is pressure exerted as blood is pumped from the heart; diastolic blood pressure is the pressure present during the resting phase of the heartbeat.
2. See textbook, p. 363.
3. The primary determinant of systolic blood pressure is cardiac output, and the determinant for diastolic blood pressure is peripheral vascular resistance.
4. Hypertension is an elevation in either the systolic or diastolic blood pressure or both. See textbook, pp. 364-365, for discussion of recommended screening in adults.
5. Prehypertension is a range of blood pressure readings that indicates a high probability of developing a heart attack, heart failure, stroke, or renal disease. Primary hypertension is a controllable but not curable form of hypertension of unknown etiology. There are known risk factors that contribute to the development of primary hypertension. Secondary hypertension occurs following the development of another disorder in the body (e.g., renal disease, head trauma).
6. Sit the patient in a chair with feet on the floor and the arm supported at heart level for at least 5 minutes. Use an appropriate size cuff (cuff bladder encircles at least 80 percent of the arm).
   Verify readings in the opposite arm. The person needs two or more readings on separate occasions to be classified as having hypertension.
   When readings of the systolic and diastolic fall into two different stages, the higher of the two stages is used to classify the degree of hypertension present.

8. List the drug classifications used in the treatment of hypertension.
9. What is therapeutic outcome for antihypertensive therapy?
10. Describe significant nursing processes for people with hypertension.
11. How does JNC 7 classify antihypertensive agents in current use?
12. What class of drugs is used initially in the treatment of uncomplicated hypertension when lifestyle changes are not effective?
13. What is the treatment algorithm used for hypertension?
14. What are the nutritional goals for the treatment of hypertension?
15. Summarize the premedication assessments used prior to administration of antihypertensive drugs. (Examine differences among the various types of agents usually prescribed.)
16. What are the four classes of diuretic agents used to treat hypertension?
17. What laboratory test is used as a guide to indicate when a patient needs to switch from a thiazide-type to a loop diuretic?
18. What are the major side effects to expect and report with beta-adrenergic blocking agents?
19. What types of patients should avoid the use of beta blocking agents?

7. Reduction and maintenance of BP below 140/90 mm Hg. Patients with concurrent conditions—e.g., diabetes mellitus, heart failure, and renal disease—less than 130/80. Weight reduction, DASH diet, dietary sodium reduction, physical activity, and moderation of alcohol consumption are recommended. Smoking cessation and stress reduction are also recommended.
8. Hypertension is treated primarily with preferred agents: diuretics and beta-adrenergic blockers; alternative agents: angiotensin-converting enzyme (ACE) inhibitors, angiotensin II receptor antagonists, calcium ion antagonists, $alpha_1$-adrenergic blockers; and adjunctive agents: centrally acting $alpha_2$ agonists, peripheral-acting adrenergic antagonists, and direct vasodilators.
9. The therapeutic outcome for antihypertensive therapy is to lower blood pressure by reducing peripheral resistance.
10. See textbook, pp. 367-372.
11. See Table 23-1.
12. If lifestyle changes do not sufficiently reduce blood pressure, a diuretic or a beta blocker are generally the initial treatment of choice.
13. See Figure 23-2.
14. See textbook, p. 365.
15. See sections labeled "premedication assessments" in the drug monographs throughout Chapter 23.
16. The four classes of diuretic agents used to treat hypertension are carbonic anhydrase inhibitors, thiazide and thiazide-like agents, loop diuretics, and potassium-sparing diuretics. Thiazide diuretics are most often used. Carbonic anhydrase inhibitors are rarely used to treat hypertension.
17. The creatinine clearance test is used when a patient needs to switch from a thiazide-like to a loop diuretic.
18. The major side effects to expect and report with beta-adrenergic agents include bradycardia, peripheral vasoconstriction, bronchospasm, wheezing, hypoglycemia in diabetic patients, and heart failure.

20. What precautions should be instituted when beta blocker therapy is to be discontinued?
21. What effect does angiotensin II have on blood vessels?
22. What effect does an increase in aldosterone secretion have on blood pressure?
23. Summarize the side effects to expect and to report with the use of ACE inhibitors.
24. What is the action of angiotensin II receptor antagonists?
25. What is the action of eplerenone, the aldosterone receptor blocking agent?
26. What are contraindications to the administration of the aldosterone receptor blocking agent eplerenone (Inspira)?
27. Review the side effects to report with use of eplerenone (Inspira), the aldosterone receptor blocking agent.
28. Which herbal product and fruit juice slows the absorption of eplerenone?
29. What is the action of calcium ion antagonists on the blood pressure?
30. What are side effects to expect with $alpha_1$-adrenergic blockers?
31. Why should centrally acting $alpha_2$ agonists (e.g., clonidine, guanabenz, guanfacine, methyldopa) be discontinued gradually?

19. Beta blocking agents are not as effective in African-American patients and should be avoided in patients with asthma, type 1 diabetes mellitus, heart failure with an etiology of systolic dysfunction, and in patients with peripheral vascular disease.
20. After long-term treatment with beta blockers, discontinue gradually over 1–2 weeks and monitor for anginal symptoms.
21. Angiotensin II produces vasoconstriction, which results in an increase in blood pressure.
22. Aldosterone results in sodium retention, which causes water retention and increased cardiac output, thereby increasing blood pressure.
23. Side effects to expect with ACE inhibitors include nausea, fatigue, headache, diarrhea, and orthostatic hypotension. Side effects to report include swelling face, eyes, lips; dyspnea; neutropenia; nephrotoxicity; hyperkalemia; chronic cough; and can cause fetal and neonatal harm during pregnancy.
24. Angiotensin II receptor inhibitors block the angiotensin II from binding to receptor sites in vascular smooth muscle and the adrenal glands. This prevents elevation of pressure and sodium-retaining properties of angiotensin II.
25. Eplerenone (Inspira), an aldosterone receptor blocking agent, blocks the stimulation of the mineralocorticoid receptors by aldosterone, thereby preventing sodium reabsorption.
26. Eplerenone (Inspira) is contraindicated in patients with serum potassium greater than 5.5 mEq/L, type 2 diabetes with microalbuminuria, serum creatinine greater than 2.0 mg/dL in males or 1.8 mg/dL in females; creatinine clearance less than 50 mL/min, patients taking potassium-sparing diuretics (e.g., amiloride, triamterene), and patients taking strong metabolic enzyme inhibitors (e.g., ketoconazole, cimetidine, others).
27. See textbook, p. 379.
28. Grapefruit juice and St. John's wort.
29. Calcium ion antagonists inhibit the movement of calcium ions across cell membranes. This causes slower rate of heart contraction and relaxation of smooth muscles of blood vessels, resulting in vasodilation and reduction of the blood pressure.
30. Side effects to expect with $alpha_1$-adrenergic blockers include drowsiness, headache, dizziness, weakness, tachycardia, and fainting.

32. What is an anticipated side effect seen with minoxidil (Loniten, Minodyl)?
33. To what drug class does guanadrel (Hylorel) belong?
34. What is the ending of generic drug names belonging to the class of ACE inhibitors?
35. What is the ending of generic drug names belonging to the class of angiotensin II receptor antagonists?
36. What is the ending of generic drug names belonging to the class of calcium ion antagonists?
37. What is the ending of generic drug names belonging to the class of $alpha_1$-adrenergic blocking agents?

31. Sudden discontinuation of centrally acting $alpha_2$ agonists can produce a rebound effect with sudden increase in blood pressure.
32. The anticipated side effect seen with minoxidil is hair growth on the body.
33. Guanadrel is a peripheral-acting adrenergic antagonist.
34. Generic drug names of ACE inhibitors end in "-pril" (enalapril, captopril, etc.).
35. Generic drug names of angiotensin II receptor antagonists end in "-sartan" (e.g., candesartan, losartan).
36. Generic drug names of calcium ion antagonists end in "-pine," with the exceptions of diltiazem and verapamil.
37. Generic drug names of $alpha_1$-adrenergic blocking agents end in "-azosin."

CHAPTER 23

Student Name ____________________

Drugs Used to Treat Hypertension

Learning Activities

FILL-IN-THE-BLANK

Finish each of the following statements using the correct term.

1. The difference between the systolic and diastolic pressure is called the ____________________ pressure.

2. To reduce the frequency of cardiovascular disease in patients with conditions such as diabetes mellitus, heart failure or renal disease, a goal blood pressure of __________ mm Hg is suggested.

3. The Dietary Approaches to Stop Hypertension (DASH) diet includes dietary ____________________ reduction, physical activity, and moderation of ____________________ consumption.

4. The ____________________ act as antihypertensive agents by causing volume depletion, sodium excretion, and vasodilatation of peripheral arterioles.

5. After a first dose of an ACE inhibitor, a patient develops swelling of the face, eyes, lips, tongue, and difficulty breathing. This is referred to as ____________________.

6. Patients should be cautioned against the sudden discontinuation of beta-adrenergic blocking agents for the treatment of hypertension because exacerbation of ____________________ symptoms may occur, followed in some cases by myocardial infarction.

7. The physiologic goal of antihypertensive therapy is a decrease in blood pressure through reduction in ____________________ ____________________.

8. Smoking causes ____________________ of blood vessels and results in increased peripheral resistance.

MATCHING

Match the generic drug name with its corresponding brand name. Each option will be used only once.

_____ 9. enalapril

_____ 10. losartan

_____ 11. nifedipine

_____ 12. doxazosin

a. Cardura
b. Procardia
c. Cozaar
d. Vasotec

Select the correct statement associated with the terms.

_____ 13. diuretics

_____ 14. beta-adrenergic blockers

_____ 15. angiotensin-converting enzyme (ACE) inhibitors

_____ 16. calcium antagonists

a. block beta receptors to inhibit cardiac response to sympathetic nerve stimulation
b. block flow of calcium ions across cell membranes
c. may produce swelling lips and tongue, dyspnea, neutropenia, nephrotoxicity, and/or chronic cough
d. depletes norepinephrine from adrenergic nerve endings
e. enhances fluid volume excretion, sodium excretion, and vasodilation of peripheral arterioles

Select the correct drug class associated with the drug names.

_____ 17. thiazide diuretic

_____ 18. beta-adrenergic blocker

_____ 19. angiotensin-converting enzyme (ACE) inhibitor

_____ 20. angiotensin II receptor antagonist

_____ 21. calcium ion antagonist

a. Atenolol
b. Hydrochlorothiazide
c. Nifedipine
d. Doxazosin
e. Clonidine
f. Captopril
g. Losartan

TRUE OR FALSE

Mark "T" for true and "F" for false for each statement. Correct all false statements.

_____ 22. Peripheral vascular resistance is regulated primarily by contraction and dilation of arterioles.

_____ 23. The cause of most cases of hypertension is unknown.

_____ 24. The most accurate method of obtaining a blood pressure is to have the patient sit on an examination table with the legs dangling over the side.

_____ 25. Recent evidence indicates that systolic hypertension is the least common form of hypertension, and is present in about 2% of individuals older than 60 years of age.

_____ 26. Patients taking beta-adrenergic blocking agents are most at risk for the development of tachycardia.

_____ 27. The ACE inhibitors reduce blood pressure, preserve cardiac output, and increase renal blood flow.

_____ 28. The chronic, dry, nonproductive, persistent cough associated with ACE inhibitor therapy is thought to be due to an accumulation of bradykinin.

_____ 29. The angiotensin-converting enzyme inhibitors are safe to use for the treatment of hypertension in pregnancy.

_____ 30. Orthostatic hypotension is a possible side effect seen with most antihypertensive drugs.

_____ 31. Primary hypertension is caused by such disorders as renal disease or head trauma.

_____ 32. The primary goal of antihypertensive therapy is to reduce morbidity and mortality.

_____ 33. Angiotensin-converting enzyme (ACE) inhibitors and diuretics are the preferred agents for initiating treatment of hypertension.

_____ 34. The lifestyle changes required to reduce blood pressure are increased exercise, diet, and weight reduction.

_____ 35. The action of smoking on the blood vessels is vasodilation.

_____ 36. An order stating "take orthostatic blood pressure readings" means to take blood pressure every shift without fail.

_____ 37. An important nursing diagnosis when initiating antihypertensive therapy would be *Injury, risk for, r/t antihypertensive therapy.*

_____ 38. Drowsiness and fatigue are common during the first 2 weeks of antihypertensive therapy.

_____ 39. Potassium-sparing and loop diuretics are commonly used for initiating the step approach to antihypertensive therapy.

_____ 40. Blood pressure readings in supine and standing positions are all the data needed to initiate antihypertensive therapy with a diuretic.

DRUG ACTION/SIDE EFFECTS

41. *State the action and side effects of the following drug classes or drugs used in the treatment of hypertension.*

	Actions	Side Effects
ANGIOTENSIN-CONVERTING ENZYME INHIBITORS		

CHAPTER 23

Student Name______________________________

Drugs Used to Treat Hypertension

Practice Questions for the NCLEX Examination

_____ 1. A patient has a blood pressure reading of 170/102. The nurse would identify this patient as having which classification of hypertension?
1. Normal
2. Prehypertension
3. Stage 1 hypertension
4. Stage 2 hypertension

_____ 2. The nurse obtains a blood pressure of 182/112 on an individual at a community health fair. The nurse should inform the patient to:
1. have their blood pressure rechecked in 2 years.
2. have their blood pressure rechecked in 1 year.
3. evaluate or refer to their source of care within 1 month.
4. evaluate or refer to their source of care immediately or within 1 week, depending on the clinical situation.

_____ 3. Which of the following statements should the nurse include when providing patient teaching on the use of beta-adrenergic blockers for the treatment of hypertension?
1. "Do not suddenly discontinue beta-adrenergic therapy, because increased angina and myocardial infarction can develop."
2. "Beta-adrenergic blockers are the antihypertensive drug of choice for patients with diabetes mellitus because they help to lower blood sugar."
3. "Wheezing is a normal response to this drug. If wheezing occurs, continue taking the medication and see your primary health care provider at the next scheduled visit."
4. "If you are taking NSAIDs and beta-adrenergic blockers for the treatment of hypertension, the dose of NSAID will need to be increased because beta-adrenergic blockers decrease the effectiveness of NSAIDs."

_____ 4. Patients on angiotensin-converting enzyme inhibitor therapy for the treatment of hypertension should be monitored for the development of which common electrolyte imbalance?
1. Hyperkalemia
2. Hypocalcemia
3. Hypernatremia
4. Hypomagnesemia

_____ 5. Mr. G. has been ordered to receive an angiotensin II receptor blocker for the treatment of hypertension. Which of the following medications should not be administered without specific approval from the health care provider?
1. Digoxin
2. Spironolactone
3. Lasix
4. Vitamin D

_____ 6. The action of hydralazine to lower blood pressure is:
1. inhibition of the release of norepinephrine.
2. blockage of aldosterone receptors.
3. direct arteriolar smooth muscle relaxation.
4. volume depletion.

_____ 7. Patients taking which one of the following medications for the treatment of hypertension should be assessed for the development of severe depression?
1. Nitroprusside sodium
2. Clonidine
3. Reserpine
4. Diltiazem

_____ 8. Which statement by a patient identifies the need for further teaching regarding use of minoxidil for the treatment of hypertension?
1. "I can expect to have an increase in fine body hair due to this drug."
2. "My salt intake will not need to be monitored."
3. "I should take my pulse every day."
4. "I should report weight gain to my primary care provider."

_____ 9. Which of the following statements should the nurse incorporate into the teaching plan for a patient who is starting on a beta-adrenergic blocking agent for the treatment of hypertension? (The nurse should also take into consideration that the patient is diabetic and has asthma.) (Select all that apply.)
1. "Monitor for hyperglycemia, as beta-adrenergic blocking agents often cause this."
2. "You should notice an improvement in your asthma symptoms because these drugs will help your airways to dilate."
3. "Call your primary care provider if you experience any swelling in your feet."
4. "Do not suddenly discontinue use of this medication."

_____ 10. Patients taking angiotensin-converting enzyme inhibitors should be taught to report which of the following side effects to their primary health care provider? (Select all that apply.)
1. Swelling of the face
2. Chronic cough
3. Muscle cramps
4. Tremor

_____ 11. Which of the following are identifiable causes of hypertension? (Select all that apply.)
1. Sleep apnea
2. Chronic kidney disease
3. Primary aldosteronism
4. Pheochromocytoma
5. Thyroid disease

_____ 12. Which of the following drugs are direct vasodilators? (Select all that apply.)
1. Reserpine
2. Minoxidil
3. Guanadrel
4. Hydralazine

_____ 13. Which of the following statements should the nurse include when teaching a patient about aldosterone receptor antagonist therapy for the treatment of hypertension? (Select all that apply.)
1. "Do not take this drug with grapefruit juice."
2. "Do not take this medication with St. John's wort."
3. "Avoid the use of salt substitutes in seasoning your food."
4. "Avoid foods that are marketed as low sodium."

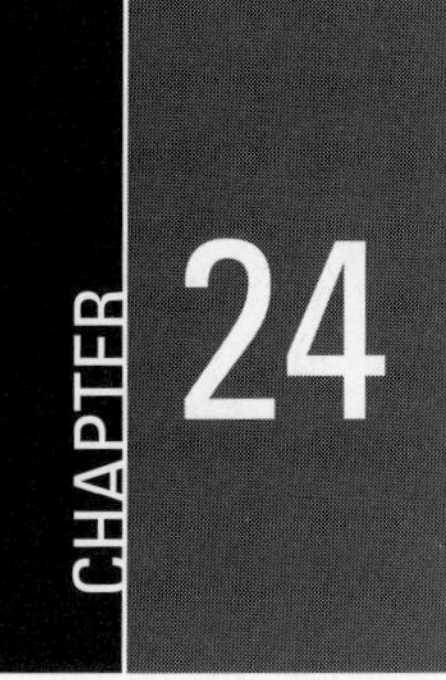

Drugs Used to Treat Dysrhythmias

Review Sheet

The QUESTION column and the ANSWER column have been offset so that you can cover the answer while reading the question, allowing you to assess your knowledge.

Question

1. Define *dysrhythmia.*
2. What function does the electrical system of the heart have on heart action?
3. Review the sequence of the heart's conduction system.
4. How are dysrhythmias produced?
5. Define *sinus dysrhythmia, sinus tachycardia, sinus bradycardia*, and *premature ventricular contraction.*
6. What is a "pulse deficit"?
7. What electrolyte is responsible for electrical system conduction for the SA and AV nodes?
8. What electrolyte is responsible for electrical system conduction for the atrial muscle, the His-Purkinje system, and the ventricular muscle?

Answer

1. Any heart rate or rhythm other than normal sinus rhythm is a dysrhythmia.
2. The electrical system of the heart sequences the muscle contractions of the heart to provide an optimal volume of blood per beat of the heart.
3. The heart's conduction system goes from SA node to AV node to bundle of His to Purkinje fibers to ventricular muscle tissue.
4. Dysrhythmias are produced by the abnormal firing of the pacemaker cells and/or the blockage of the normal electrical system pathway.
5. Sinus dysrhythmia is a variable increase in heart rate originating from the SA node. The increase in rate may parallel the inspiratory phase of respirations. Sinus tachycardia is a regular rhythm of the heartbeat with a rate greater than 100 beats per minute. Sinus bradycardia is a regular rhythm of the heartbeat, but the rate is slower than 60 beats per minute. In premature ventricular contractions, the contraction occurs before the regular ventricular contraction as a result of an electrical impulse arising in the ventricular muscle outside the normal conduction pathway.
6. "Pulse deficit" is the difference between the apical and radial pulse rates; radial is generally lower than apical. For example: apical pulse = 74, radial pulse = 64, pulse deficit = 10.
7. Calcium ions are responsible for electrical system conduction for the SA and AV nodes.

9. What is the goal of treatment for dysrhythmias?
10. What effect do Class I, Ia, Ib, and Ic agents have on the electrical conduction system of the heart?
11. What methods are used to assess dysrhythmias?
12. Review the six cardinal signs of cardiovascular disease.
13. Why can mental status/level of consciousness (LOC) be important when assessing a cardiac patient?
14. What type of changes in the vital signs should be reported to the health care provider?
15. Why is it important to monitor hourly urine output in a patient with dysrhythmias?
16. When is the use of adenosine (Adenocard) indicated?
17. Review the drug monograph for amiodarone hydrochloride (Cordarone) in the text and identify uses, actions, side effects, and premedication assessments for this drug.
18. When beta-adrenergic blocking agents are administered, what cardiac response can be anticipated?
19. Bretylium tosylate (Bretylol) belongs to which class of antidysrhythmic agents?
20. When lidocaine (Xylocaine) is ordered for a dysrhythmia, what should the nurse check on the bottle BEFORE using the medication for IV administration?
21. In general, what agent is the drug of choice for treatment of ventricular dysrhythmias associated with acute myocardial infarction and ventricular tachycardia?

8. Sodium is responsible for electrical system conduction for the atrial muscle, the His-Purkinje system, and the ventricular muscle.
9. The goal of treatment for dysrhythmias is to restore normal sinus rhythm and maintain adequate cardiac output to maintain tissue perfusion.
10. The effects of Class I, Ia, Ib, and Ic agents are as follows: I is a myocardial depressant (inhibits sodium ion movement); Ia causes prolonged duration of electrical stimulation on cells and refractory time between electrical impulses; Ib shortens duration of electrical stimulation and time interval between electrical impulses; Ic is the most potent antidysrhythmic, causing myocardial depression and slowing conduction rate through the atria and the ventricles.
11. ECG monitoring, EPS (electrophysiologic studies), exercise electrocardiography, and laboratory values are used to assess for cardiac dysrhythmias.
12. The six cardinal signs of cardiac disease are dyspnea, chest pain, fatigue, edema, syncope, and palpitations.
13. Mental status/LOC indicates whether there is adequate cerebral tissue perfusion.
14. See textbook, p. 394.
15. Hourly outputs reflect whether the kidney tissues are being adequately perfused.
16. Adenosine is indicated in treatment of paroxysmal supraventricular tachycardia that involves conduction in the SA node, atrium, or AV node.
17. See textbook, pp. 396-398.
18. Reduction in heart rate, systolic blood pressure, and cardiac output result from use of beta-adrenergic blocking agents.
19. Bretylium tosylate is an adrenergic blocking agent, class III antidysrhythmic agent.
20. The bottle must be labeled "Xylocaine for Dysrhythmia" or "Lidocaine Without Preservatives."

22. Describe the initial manifestations of mexiletine neurotoxicity.
23. What drug, also used for seizure disorders, may be used to treat paroxysmal atrial tachycardia and ventricular dysrhythmias, particularly those induced by digoxin toxicity?
24. What action does quinidine have on the heart?
25. When should blood samples for quinidine sulfate levels be drawn in relationship to doses being administered?
26. What is cinchonism?
27. What initial assessments of the heart disorder should be performed when a dysrhythmia is suspected?
28. Review assessments performed for an individual with a heart disorder and compare these with premedication assessments listed throughout this chapter.
29. Why is physical activity curtailed in a patient having dysrhythmias?
30. Why is O_2 administration required PRN when a dysrhythmia occurs?
31. What are the drawbacks of using amiodarone hydrochloride (Cordarone)?

21. Lidocaine (Xylocaine) is generally the drug of choice.
22. Mexiletine has dose-related effects on the CNS. Serum levels greater than 2.0 mcg/mL may precipitate neurologic toxicity and occasionally paradoxic seizure activity. Fine hand tremor is often the first indication, but ataxia, dizziness, light-headedness, nystagmus, paresthesia, blurred vision, diplopia, dysarthria, confusion, and drowsiness are also signs of impending toxicity.
23. Phenytoin may be used to treat some cardiac dysrhythmias, as well as seizure disorders.
24. Quinidine stabilizes the rate of conduction resulting in a slow, regular pulse rate.
25. Blood samples for quinidine sulfate levels should be drawn before the daily dose or at least 6 hours after administration.
26. The signs and symptoms associated with quinidine toxicity (known as cinchonism) include rash, chills, fever, tinnitus, headache, and mental confusion.
27. Electrocardiogram should be performed when a dysrhythmia is suspected.
28. Refer to the textbook for individual monographs throughout the chapter.
29. To conserve oxygen so that the available oxygen can be used to meet the body's basic needs, physical activity is curtailed in patients with dysrhythmias. Reduced oxygen levels (hypoxia) induce dysrhythmias.
30. To prevent hypoxia and the development of dysrhythmias, O_2 is administered PRN.
31. Amiodarone hydrochloride requires hospitalization during loading dose and the maintenance dose is difficult to establish. Life-threatening dysrhythmias may recur at unpredictable intervals. Once the drug is used, switching to a different antidysrhythmic is difficult because the body may store the drug; therefore, a drug interaction with the newly prescribed antidysrhythmic may occur.

CHAPTER 24

Student Name ____________________

Drugs Used to Treat Dysrhythmias

Learning Activities

FILL-IN-THE-BLANK

Finish each of the following statements using the correct term.

1. Adenosine is recommended for the treatment of paroxysmal supraventricular tachycardia because of its strong depressant effects on the ____________________ and ____________________ nodes of the heart.

2. The therapeutic blood level of procainamide is _____ to _____ mg/L.

3. ____________________ was introduced about 50 years ago for the treatment of epilepsy, but it is also effective in controlling dysrhythmias.

4. Rash, chills, fever, and tinnitus caused by the use of quinidine are known as ____________________.

MATCHING

Match the generic drug name with its corresponding brand name. Each option will be used only once.

_____ 5. verapamil

_____ 6. phenytoin

_____ 7. propranolol

_____ 8. amiodarone

_____ 9. procainamide

a. Pronestyl
b. Inderal
c. Cordarone
d. Calan
e. Dilantin

TRUE OR FALSE

Mark "T" for true and "F" for false for each statement. Correct all false statements.

_____ 10. Antidysrhythmic agents are classified according to their effects on the electrical conduction system of the heart.

_____ 11. Currently there are two classifications of antidysrhythmic agents used in clinical practice.

_____ 12. Adenosine is a naturally occurring chemical found only in cardiac cells.

_____ 13. Patients must be hospitalized while the loading dose of amiodarone is administered.

_____ 14. Bretylium, an adrenergic-blocking agent, inhibits the release of norepinephrine.

_____ 15. Bretylium is the treatment of choice for digitalis-induced dysrhythmias.

_____ 16. With amiodarone hydrochloride therapy, it is difficult to predict the degree and duration of antidysrhythmic response.

_____ 17. When beta-adrenergic blockers are being taken, the diabetic patient must be monitored for hyperglycemia due to masking of the symptoms by the drug.

_____ 18. The basic causes of dysrhythmias are the abnormal firing of pacemaker cells, blockage of normal electrical pathways, or a combination of the two.

_____ 19. The most potent antidysrhythmic agents that act as myocardial depressants and slow conduction rate through the atria and ventricles are Class Ia antidysrhythmic agents.

_____ 20. The nursing assessment of a patient should cite specifically whether dyspnea is present with or without exertion.

_____ 21. A narrowing pulse pressure is the difference between the apical and radial pulse rates.

_____ 22. The most frequently used drug for treatment of ventricular dysrhythmias associated with an acute myocardial infarction is digitalis.

DRUG ACTION/SIDE EFFECTS

23. *State the action and side effects of the following drug that is used to treat dysrhythmias.*

	Actions	Side Effects
LIDOCAINE		

CHAPTER 24

Student Name______________________________

Drugs Used to Treat Dysrhythmias

Practice Questions for the NCLEX Examination

_____ 1. A patient starting amiodarone therapy for treatment of a dysrhythmia asks the nurse how long it will take before it is known if this drug will work for him. The best response is:
1. "In 24 hours, we will know if the drug is working for you."
2. "It takes at least 3 days for the full therapeutic effect of the drug to be known."
3. "The response to this drug requires 2 weeks or more."
4. "A blood test has already been completed for you and we are certain this drug will be effective for you."

_____ 2. When caring for a patient taking warfarin as well as amiodarone, the nurse should be particularly aware of the status and results of which laboratory test?
1. PT
2. APTT
3. AST
4. BUN

_____ 3. Which of the following is an expected side effect of quinidine that usually subsides?
1. Diarrhea
2. Headache
3. Blurred vision
4. Urine discoloration

_____ 4. Patients on procainamide therapy are at risk for the development of neuromuscular blockade and respiratory depression when taking which types of antibiotics?
1. Penicillins
2. Tetracyclines
3. Macrolides
4. Aminoglycosides

_____ 5. Before administering disopyramide therapy, it is most important for the nurse to ask the patient about a history of:
1. atrial fibrillation.
2. digitalis use.
3. diabetes mellitus.
4. urinary obstruction.

_____ 6. Patients taking flecainide acetate should report which of the following side effects to the primary care provider immediately?
1. Nausea
2. Dizziness
3. Increasing dyspnea
4. Headache

_____ 7. Which of the following is the drug of choice for the treatment of ventricular dysrhythmias associated with acute myocardial infarction and ventricular tachycardia?
1. Moricizine
2. Mexilentine
3. Lidocaine
4. Procainamide hydrochloride

_____ 8. What information should the nurse provide a patient who is taking phenytoin and oral contraceptives?
1. "Stop taking the oral contraceptives and restart them when the phenytoin therapy is complete."
2. "You can expect to have no bleeding with use of these two medications."
3. "Tell your cardiologist that you cannot take the pronestyl because the oral contraceptives will cause it not to work."
4. "Use of an alternative form of birth control is recommended when phenytoin and oral contraceptives are administered together."

_____ 9. Nurses administering antidysrhythmic agents to patients should take an apical pulse before PO administration and notify the primary care provider if the patient's heart rate is less than:
1. 45.
2. 50.
3. 55.
4. 60.

_____ 10. Which of the following statements is true about amiodarone therapy for the treatment of dysrhythmias? (Select all that apply.)
1. Patients must be hospitalized while the loading dose is given.
2. Amiodarone therapy is contraindicated in the treatment of patients who have pacemakers.
3. Response from amiodarone therapy often requires 2 weeks or more of treatment.
4. Amiodarone should be administered with food or milk if gastric irritation develops.

CHAPTER 25

Drugs Used to Treat Angina Pectoris

Review Sheet

The QUESTION column and the ANSWER column have been offset so that you can cover the answer while reading the questions, allowing you to assess your knowledge.

Question

1. Explain the underlying cause of anginal pain.
2. Review the various presenting symptoms of angina.
3. Compare the precipitating factors associated with chronic stable angina, unstable angina, and variant angina.
4. What are the desired therapeutic outcomes during treatment of angina?
5. What questions should be asked during a nursing assessment related to an angina attack?

Answer

1. The pain and discomfort of angina is caused by the lack of an adequate oxygen supply to the cells in the heart (ischemic heart disease). The underlying etiology is vasospasm of a coronary artery that reduces blood flow through the coronary arteries to the heart tissue.
2. See textbook, p. 408.
3. Chronic stable angina is precipitated by physical exertion or stress. Unstable angina is precipitated by unpredictable factors such as atherosclerotic narrowing, vasospasm, or thrombus formation. Variant angina occurs at rest. The underlying etiology is vasospasm of a coronary artery that reduces blood flow through the coronary arteries to the heart tissue.
4. The goals in treatment of angina pectoris are to prevent myocardial infarction and death, thereby prolonging life, and to relieve anginal pain symptoms, thereby improving the quality of life. The pharmacologic treatment of angina is aimed at decreasing oxygen demand by decreasing heart rate, myocardial contractility, and ventricular volume without inducing heart failure. Because platelet aggregation, blood flow turbulence, and blood viscosity also play a role, especially in unstable angina, platelet-active agents are also prescribed to prevent anginal attacks (see Chapter 27). Since atherosclerosis causes narrowing and closure of coronary arteries inducing angina and myocardial infarction, the use of the HMG-CoA reductase inhibitors (statins) has also become standard therapy in the treatment of angina pectoris when the LDL cholesterol is elevated (see Chapter 22).

6. What are the actions of nitrates, beta-adrenergic blockers, calcium channel blockers, and angiotensin-converting enzyme inhibitors on the myocardial tissue of the heart? Name two examples of each drug class used to treat angina pectoris.
7. Compare the premedication assessments required for nitrates, beta-adrenergic blockers, calcium channel blockers, and angiotensin-converting enzyme inhibitors.
8. What is the drug of choice for acute attacks of angina pectoris?
9. Why is it important to teach patients taking nitroglycerin not to use alcohol?
10. What dose forms are available for nitroglycerin?
11. What side effects can be expected when rapid-acting nitrates (e.g., nitroglycerin, amyl nitrite) are used?

5. See textbook, pp. 409-410.
6. Nitrates do not increase total coronary artery blood flow. They cause relaxation of peripheral vascular smooth muscle that results in dilation of arteries and veins, reducing preload and leading to decreased oxygen demands on the heart. They dilate large coronary arteries and redistribute blood flow within the heart. Examples: isosorbide mononitrate (Imdur), nitroglycerin (Nitro-Bid).

   Beta-adrenergic blocking agents decrease myocardial oxygen demands by blocking beta-adrenergic receptors in the heart, reducing stimulation by norepinephrine and epinephrine, which normally increases heart rate. Beta blockers also reduce blood pressure. Examples: atenolol (Tenormin), metoprolol (Lopressor).

   Calcium channel blockers decrease myocardial oxygen demands and increase myocardial blood supply by coronary artery dilation. These agents block movement of calcium ions across the cell membrane, resulting in 1) inhibition of smooth muscle contraction; 2) dilation of blood vessels, including coronary arteries; and 3) decreased resistance to blood flow as a result of dilation of peripheral vessels. Examples: amlodipine (Norvase), nifedipine (Procardia).

   The angiotensin-converting enzymes inhibit the enzyme's action on the endothelial wall of coronary arteries promoting vasodilation and minimizing cellular aggregation, preventing further thrombus formation. Examples: captopril (Capoten), lisinopril (Zestril).
7. See textbook, pp. 412-416.
8. Nitroglycerin, administered sublingually, is the drug of choice for acute attacks of angina pectoris.
9. Alcohol use results in vasodilation and may lead to postural hypotension.
10. Sublingual tablets, transmucosal tablets, translingual spray, topical disks, sustained-release capsules, topical ointment, and intravenous forms of nitroglycerin are available.

12. What premedication assessments should be performed prior to therapy with nitrates?
13. Describe the procedure for administering nitroglycerin sublingually, via translingual spray, topical ointment, transmucosal tablets, and topical disk.
14. How does one evaluate anginal attacks and what health teaching is needed for an individual who has anginal attacks?
15. What are some guidelines used during the preparation and administration of IV nitroglycerin?
16. What are the desired therapeutic outcomes for the use of beta blocker therapy in the treatment of anginal pain?
17. What is the desired result of the use of calcium ion antagonists to treat angina?
18. What are common side effects associated with angiotensin-converting enzyme inhibitors?

11. Headache and hypotension caused by the vasodilation of blood vessels are side effects of nitroglycerin and amyl nitrite treatment.
12. Assess for pain level, location, duration, intensity, and pattern, and obtain a history of most recent nitrate use before beginning amyl nitrate therapy.
13. Procedure for administration of the various forms of nitroglycerin can be found in the textbook in Chapter 8 and pp. 411-414.
14. See textbook, pp. 409-411.
15. See textbook, p. 414.
16. The desired therapeutic outcomes of beta blocker therapy are decreased frequency and severity of anginal attacks, increased tolerance of activities, and decreased use of nitroglycerin for acute anginal attacks. Before administering beta blockers, take BP in supine and standing position, check for history of respiratory disorders such as COPD, and check for history of diabetes. If patient is a diabetic, determine whether the physician wants baseline blood glucose studies before initiating the medication.
17. The desired action of calcium ion antagonists in the treatment of angina is to decrease myocardial oxygen demands by increasing myocardial blood supply via coronary arteries and decrease resistance to blood flow and dilate peripheral vessels, resulting in decreased workload of the heart.
18. ACE inhibitors cause hypotension with dizziness, tachycardia, fainting, and nonproductive cough.

Student Name ____________________

CHAPTER 25 Drugs Used to Treat Angina Pectoris

Learning Activities

FILL-IN-THE-BLANK

Finish each of the following statements using the correct term.

1. ____________________, clopidogrel, or ____________________ are platelet-active agents that may also slow platelet aggregation.
2. Patients taking nitroglycerin should be instructed to not ingest alcohol, because alcohol consumed in combination with nitroglycerin causes ____________________, potentially resulting in postural ____________________.
3. ____________________ is currently the drug of choice for treatment of angina pectoris.
4. The initial dose of angiotensin-converting inhibitors may cause hypotension with dizziness, ____________________, and fainting.

MATCHING

Match the generic drug name with its corresponding brand name. Each option will be used only once.

_____ 5. verapamil

_____ 6. nifedipine

_____ 7. diltiazem

_____ 8. amlodipine

a. Procardia, Adalat
b. Calan, Isoptin
c. Norvasc
d. Cardizem

TRUE OR FALSE

Mark "T" for true and "F" for false for each statement. Correct all false statements.

_____ 9. Cancer is the leading cause of disability, socioeconomic loss, and death in the United States.

_____ 10. Calcium ion antagonists decrease myocardial oxygen demand, and increase myocardial blood supply by coronary artery dilation.

_____ 11. Isosorbide dinitrate is available for inhalation administration.

_____ 12. Transdermal disk administration of nitrates provides controlled release of nitroglycerin for a 48-hour period when applied to intact skin.

_____ 13. Sildenafil is commonly administered with nitrates to provide optimal therapeutic effects.

_____ 14. Statins are used to lower LDL cholesterol levels.

_____ 15. If more than three nitroglycerin tablets within 15 minutes are required to control pain, the patient should seek medical attention.

_____ 16. Patients should be taught that nitroglycerin tablets must be replaced every month.

DRUG ACTION/SIDE EFFECTS

17. *State the action and side effects of the following drug classes or drugs used in the treatment of angina pectoris.*

	Actions	Side Effects
NITRATES		

CHAPTER 25

Student Name______________________________

Drugs Used to Treat Angina Pectoris

Practice Questions for the NCLEX Examination

_____ 1. Which of the following statements should the nurse include when teaching patients about the use of nitrates?
1. "Store nitroglycerin in the original, dark-colored glass container with a tight lid."
2. "Four tablets may be taken prophylactically a few minutes before engaging in activities that may trigger an anginal attack."
3. "If a slight stinging or burning sensation occurs when you take the medication, report this to your primary care provider at once."
4. "If you develop a headache from taking this medication, take aspirin as indicated."

_____ 2. When administering angiotensin-converting enzyme inhibitors, the nurse is aware that the action of these drugs includes: (Select all that apply.)
1. prevention of thrombus formation.
2. minimization of cellular aggregation.
3. dissolving clots.
4. promotion of coronary artery dilatation.

_____ 3. Patients prescribed beta-adrenergic blocking agents should be assessed for a history of:
1. high blood pressure.
2. gastric ulcer.
3. anemia.
4. respiratory disorders.

_____ 4. The nurse teaches the patient that at the first sign of an anginal attack, she should:
1. call 911.
2. sit or lie down.
3. take two nitroglycerin tablets.
4. take an extra dose of transdermal nitroglycerin.

_____ 5. Which of the following actions by the nurse is appropriate when administering intravenous nitroglycerin?
1. Administer the nitroglycerin with another intravenous medication to avoid fluid overload.
2. Use standard plastic administration sets when infusing this medication.
3. Follow the practice of gradual weaning under controlled conditions.
4. Administer the intravenous nitroglycerin via gravity drip.

_____ 6. When applying transdermal nitroglycerin via disk, the nurse would use which of the following sites? (Select all that apply.)
1. Newly shaved area of the chest
2. Pelvis
3. Inner arm
4. Side

_____ 7. A nurse teaching a patient appropriate use of translingual nitroglycerin spray should include which of the following statements? (Select all that apply.)
1. "Do not shake the container before administration."
2. "Hold the canister vertically when administering the medication."
3. "Spray the dose onto the roof of your mouth."
4. "Do not inhale the spray."

_____ 8. Which of the following is the most common side effect of nitrate therapy?
1. Excessive hypotension
2. Tolerance
3. Nausea
4. Prolonged headache

_____ 9. Nitroglycerin may be administered to the patient by which of the following routes? (Select all that apply.)
1. Transmucosal tablets
2. Transdermal patches
3. Translingual spray
4. Inhalation

_____ 10. Which of the following statements should the nurse include when teaching a patient about nitroglycerin tablets for the treatment of angina? (Select all that apply.)
1. "Every 3 months, the nitroglycerin prescription should be refilled and the old tablets safely discarded."
2. "Nitroglycerin should be stored in the original, dark-colored glass c ontainer with a tight lid."
3. "When taking the drug, you should feel a slight stinging or burning sensation, which usually indicates that it is still potent."
4. "Carry the nitroglycerin with you at all times, but not in a pocket directly next to your body because heat hastens the deterioration of the medication."

_____ 11. The most common side effect of nitrate therapy is:
1. syncope.
2. hypertension.
3. vomiting.
4. headache.

_____ 12. A patient who has been admitted to the hospital with angina has been ordered to receive a nonselective beta blocker along with other therapies. It is most important for the nurse to assess for which of the following? (Select all that apply.)
1. Emphysema
2. Asthma
3. Diabetes mellitus
4. Chronic bronchitis

_____ 13. Mr. Y. has been ordered transdermal nitrate therapy for the treatment of angina as well as nitroglycerin sublingual tablets for acute anginal attacks. When providing teaching, the nurse should include which of the following statements? (Select all that apply.)
1. "Take your pulse in the morning, at lunch, and before bed to be sure the medication is working."
2. "If you need to take more than 3 tablets within 15 minutes to control pain, you should seek medical attention."
3. "When using the ointment, be aware that the medication may discolor clothing."
4. "Always place the nitroglycerin ointment on the area of the chest on top of the heart so it is able to work fast."

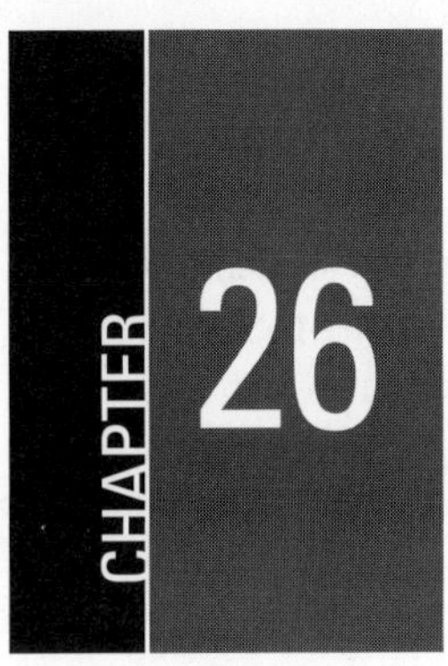

Drugs Used to Treat Peripheral Vascular Disease

Review Sheet

The QUESTION column and the ANSWER column have been offset so that you can cover the answer before reading the questions, thus allowing you to assess your knowledge.

Question

1. Explain the pathophysiology of intermittent claudication, vasospasm, paresthesia, arteriosclerosis obliterans, and Raynaud's disease.
2. What are the goals of treatment of arteriosclerosis obliterans?
3. List the agents specifically approved by the FDA to treat chronic occlusive arterial disease.
4. Name the three calcium ion antagonists used in the treatment of Raynaud's disease.
5. What is the action of an ACE inhibitor in the treatment of peripheral vascular disease (PVD)?
6. What preventive actions can be taken by a patient with Raynaud's disease to reduce or stop vasospastic attacks?
7. What nursing assessments should be made on a regular basis when peripheral vasodilators are prescribed?
8. Describe the health teaching needed when PVD is diagnosed that would promote improved tissue perfusion.
9. What is the action of pentoxifylline (Trental) and cilostazol (Pletal)?
10. What type of vascular conditions may be treated using peripheral vasodilating agents?

Answer

1. See textbook, pp. 419-420.
2. Improve blood flow, relieve pain, and prevent skin ulcerations and/or gangrene.
3. Pentoxifylline and cilostazol
4. Diltiazem, verapamil, and nifedipine
5. Vasodilation
6. Avoid cold temperature, emotional stress, tobacco, and drugs known to induce attacks.
7. Assess for color and temperature of the hands, fingers, legs, and feet. Check for signs and symptoms of skin breakdown, presence of limb pain, or a reduction in sensation in the extremities. Pedal pulses and radial pulse rates should be taken and recorded every 4 hours during hospitalization and twice a day upon discharge.
8. See textbook, pp. 422-423.
9. Trental increases RBC (red blood cell) flexibility, decreases concentration of fibrinogen in the blood, and prevents aggregation of RBCs and platelets, thus preventing blood clotting. Cilostazol inhibits platelet aggregation and promotes vasodilation.

11. What is the mechanism of action of vasodilators used to treat PVD?

12. What are the side effects to expect with the administration of vasodilating agents?
13. List the premedication assessments required for all prescribed medications for PVD.

10. Intermittent claudication, arteriosclerosis obliterans, vasospasms associated with thrombophlebitis, nocturnal leg cramps, and Raynaud's disease.
11. Relaxation of peripheral arterial blood vessels, thereby increasing blood flow to the extremities.
12. Flushing, tingling, sweating. May also produce orthostatic hypotension and tachycardia. Also may cause possible nervousness and weakness as therapy progresses.
13. Baseline assessment of symptoms of PVD and degree of pain present; take baseline vital signs and assess for tissue perfusion.

CHAPTER 26

Student Name ______________________________

Drugs Used to Treat Peripheral Vascular Disease

Learning Activities

FILL-IN-THE-BLANK

Finish each of the following statements using the correct term.

1. Major treatable causes of PVD include ____________________, cigarette smoking, and ____________________.

2. The most common form of obstructive arterial disease is ______________ ______________.

3. PVD caused by arterial vasospasm is known as ____________________ disease.

4. ____________________ and ____________________ are the only agents approved by the FDA that are specifically indicated for the treatment of intermittent claudication caused by chronic occlusive arterial disease of the limbs.

5. Patients with PVD should be taught to not elevate their extremities above the level of the ____________________ without specific orders to do so from the health care provider.

MATCHING

Match the generic drug name with its corresponding brand name. Each option will be used only once.

_____ 6. pentoxifylline

_____ 7. papaverine hydrochloride

_____ 8. isoxuprine hydrochloride

_____ 9. cilostazol

a. Trental
b. Pavagen TD
c. Vasodilan
d. Pletal

TRUE OR FALSE

Mark "T" for true and "F" for false for each statement. Correct all false statements.

_____ 10. The most cost-effective and successful forms of treatment for PVD are smoking cessation, weight reduction, exercise, and dietary modification.

_____ 11. The typical pain pattern described by a person with PVD is sharp, stabbing pain at rest.

_____ 12. PVD is often accompanied by increased blood viscosity.

_____ 13. The ACE inhibitors are used in the treatment of PVD because they cause an increase in bradykinin which is a potent vasodilator.

_____ 14. When positioning a patient who has PVD in bed, the nurse should flex the knees and place pillows in the popliteal space.

_____ 15. Part of the assessment process for PVD includes reviewing laboratory data relating to serum glucose levels and serum lipids.

_____ 16. Foot care for an individual with PVD should include regular trimming of toenails and corns.

_____ 17. Improvement in the symptoms of PVD includes reduction in frequency and degree of pain, intolerance to exercise, and an overall improvement in quality of the peripheral pulses.

_____ 18. Vasodilating agents have the potential for initiating orthostatic hypotension.

_____ 19. Flushing of the face, neck, and chest are expected side effects of vasodilators.

DRUG ACTION/SIDE EFFECTS

20. *State the action and side effects of the following drug class used to treat PVD.*

	Actions	Side Effects
CILOSTAZOL		

CHAPTER 26

Student Name____

Drugs Used to Treat Peripheral Vascular Disease

Practice Questions for the NCLEX Examination

_____ 1. Pentoxifylline works by: (Select all that apply.)
1. increasing erythrocyte flexibility.
2. decreasing the concentration of fibrinogen in the blood.
3. preventing aggregation of red blood cells and platelets.
4. increasing the viscosity of blood.

_____ 2. What is most important for the nurse to assess in the patient taking pentoxifylline for treatment of PVD?
1. Hypotension
2. Bleeding gums
3. Jaundice
4. Ulcer formation on the feet

_____ 3. When teaching a patient about isoxsuprine hydrochloride, the nurse should tell the patient to report which of the following signs/symptoms to the health care provider?
1. Flushing
2. Tachycardia
3. Sweating
4. Tingling

_____ 4. When providing patient teaching to an individual taking papaverine hydrochloride, it is most important for the nurse to tell the patient to:
1. avoid milk products when taking this medication.
2. increase consumption of foods high in vitamin C.
3. not take over-the-counter cough and cold preparations without first consulting the health care provider.
4. take this medication before bed on an empty stomach.

_____ 5. A patient asks the nurse what she can do to decrease the occurrence and severity of vasospastic attacks of Raynaud's disease. The nurse should inform the patient that: (Select all that apply.)
1. most attacks of Raynaud's disease can be stopped by the avoidance of hot temperatures.
2. tobacco use is highly associated with vasospastic attacks of Raynaud's disease.
3. it is not known what really triggers the vasospastic attacks seen with Raynaud's disease.
4. the signs and symptoms associated with Raynaud's disease are due to vasospasm of the arteries of the skin of the hands, fingers, and sometimes toes.

_____ 6. A patient receiving Trental (pentoxifylline) for the treatment of intermittent claudication should report which of the following side effects to the primary care provider? (Select all that apply.)
1. Shortness of breath
2. Intolerance to caffeine
3. Headache
4. Dyspepsia

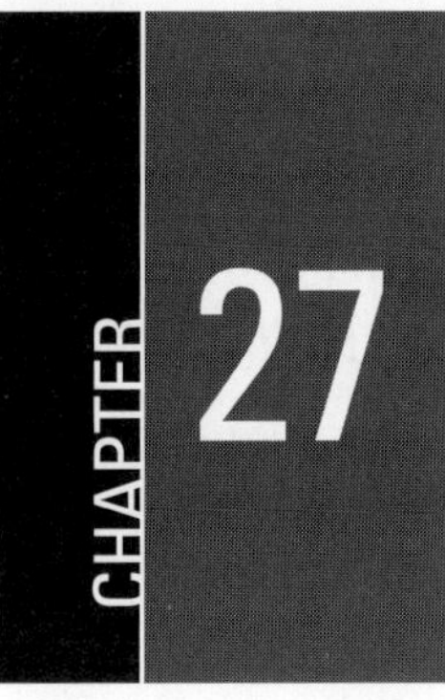

Drugs Used to Treat Thromboembolic Disorders

Review Sheet

The QUESTION column and the ANSWER column have been offset so you can cover the answer while reading the question, allowing you to assess your knowledge.

Question

1. Differentiate among thromboembolic disease, thrombosis, thrombus, and embolus.
2. Explain factors that trigger blood clot formation.
3. List factor(s) that trigger(s) the intrinsic blood clotting pathway.
4. Identify factor(s) that trigger(s) the extrinsic pathway triggers.
5. What is the difference between red and white blood clots?
6. Describe appropriate nonpharmacologic patient education for prevention and treatment of thromboembolic disease.
7. Differentiate among the drug actions of platelet inhibitors, anticoagulants, thrombolytic agents, glycoprotein IIb/IIIa inhibitors, and thromboembolic agents.
8. Summarize the nursing actions that can help in the prevention of clot formation.
9. State hydration information that should be provided to an individual for whom an anticoagulant is prescribed.
10. Identify laboratory tests used to evaluate anticoagulant therapy.

Answer

1. See textbook, p. 429.
2. See textbook, p. 429.
3. Factor XII
4. Factor VII to VIIa (factor VIIa can also activate factor X)
5. Red embolus is a venous thrombus. White thrombi develop in arteries. See also textbook, pp. 429-430.
6. See textbook, pp. 432-433.
7. Platelet inhibitors reduce arterial clot formation by inhibiting platelet aggregation. Anticoagulants prevent new clot formation. Thrombolytic agents dissolve thromboemboli already formed. Glycoprotein IIb/IIIa inhibitors prevent platelet aggregation and are specifically used for patients undergoing percutaneous coronary interventions. Thromboembolic agents either prevent platelet aggregation or inhibit a variety of steps in fibrin clot formation.
8. See textbook, pp. 431-432.
9. Adequate hydration to maintain fluidity of blood should be encouraged. Check to be certain the patient does not have coexisting disease that precludes forcing fluids.

11. Explain the desired therapeutic outcomes for platelet inhibitors.
12. List premedication assessments that should be performed before administering aspirin as a platelet inhibitor.
13. Differentiate the between the actions of low molecular weight heparins (LMWHs) and heparin.
14. Name three commonly used LMWH drugs.
15. What laboratory studies are used to monitor for adverse effects of LMWHs?
16. What drug is used as an antidote in case of heparin overdose?
17. What is the normal therapeutic range for warfarin therapy?
18. What is the antidote for hemorrhage that occurs with warfarin therapy?
19. List six fibrinolytic agents.
20. When are fibrinolytic agents administered?
21. How long a time is required before clopidogrel (Plavix) achieves full antiplatelet activity level?
22. What is the primary use of ticlopidine (Ticlid)?

10. Refer to the anticoagulant monographs in the textbook. Prothrombin time (PT) is reported as international normalized ratio (INR) and is routinely used for warfarin therapy; activated partial thromboplastin time (APTT) is most commonly used for heparin therapy.
11. Reduce the frequency of transient ischemic attacks (TIAs), strokes, and myocardial infarction.
12. Neurological assessment, gastrointestinal symptoms present, check for any concurrent anticoagulant therapy being taken; if on oral hypoglycemics, baseline serum glucose levels.
13. Heparin acts at several specific points in the coagulation pathway. LMWHs act at fewer specific steps in the coagulation pathway (factors Xa and thrombin), reducing the potential for hemorrhage. LMWHs also have a longer duration of action. Dalteparin, enoxaparin, and tinzaparin have no antiplatelet activity and only minimal effect on PT and APTT.
14. Dalteparin (Fragmin), enoxaparin (Lovenox), and tinzaparin (Innohep).
15. Periodic CBC, daily platelet counts, and periodic checking of stools for occult blood are tests used to monitor for adverse effects of LMWHs.
16. Protamine sulfate; see textbook, p. 441, for details.
17. PT is used to monitor warfarin therapy. PT is expressed as the INR. The optimal dosage of warfarin is that which prolongs the PT and maintains the INR at 2–3. In some medical conditions the INR may be maintained at 2.5–3.5.
18. In most cases of hemorrhage, the dosage of warfarin is withheld until the INR returns to therapeutic levels. In rare cases, vitamin K is administered. In cases of severe hemorrhage, a transfusion with plasma or whole blood may be required.
19. Streptokinase, urokinase, anistreplase, alteplase, reteplase, and tenecteplase.
20. Fibrinolytic agents are used to dissolve clots secondary to an MI, pulmonary or cerebral embolism, or deep vein thrombosis (DVT).
21. Three to seven days of continuous therapy are required.
22. To reduce risk of additional strokes in people who have had a stroke or TIA.

CHAPTER 27

Student Name ______________________________

Drugs Used to Treat Thromboembolic Disorders

Learning Activities

FILL-IN-THE-BLANK

Finish each of the following statements using the correct term.

1. ____________________ is the process of formation of a fibrin blood clot, and ____________________ is a small fragment of a thrombus that breaks off and circulates until it becomes trapped in a capillary, causing either ischemia or infarction to the area distal to the obstruction.

2. The ____________________ agents are used to dissolve thromboemboli, once formed.

3. While receiving anticoagulant therapy, patients must limit intake of green leafy vegetables that contain vitamin ____________________.

4. A unique property of aspirin, when compared with other salicylates, is inhibition of ____________________ aggregation with prolongation of bleeding time.

5. Enoxaprin is manufactured from heparin derived from ____________________ and should not be used in patients allergic to ____________________ by-products.

6. Subcutaneous injection of heparin is usually made into the tissue over the ____________________.

7. _____________ _____________ is the antidote for heparin.

8. The class of drugs used to dissolve recently formed thrombi is known as ____________________ agents.

9. The therapeutic effect of heparin is monitored by the use of the laboratory test known as ____________________ time.

10. The antidote for excessive bleeding during warfarin therapy is ____________________.

MATCHING

Match the generic drug name with its corresponding brand name. Each option will be used only once.

_____ 11. warfarin

_____ 12. enoxaparin

_____ 13. ticlopidine

_____ 14. clopidogrel

_____ 15. dipyridamole

a. Plavix
b. Persantine
c. Lovenox
d. Coumadin
e. Ticlid

Select the laboratory test(s) used to monitor the drug therapy listed. Some options will not be used.

_____ 16. warfarin

_____ 17. heparin

a. whole blood clotting time
b. PT or INR
c. APTT
d. bleeding time

TRUE OR FALSE

Mark "T" for true and "F" for false for each statement. Correct all false statements.

_____ 18. The pharmacologic agents used to treat thromboembolic disease act either to prevent platelet aggregation or to inhibit a variety of steps in the fibrin clot formation cascade.

_____ 19. The primary purpose of anticoagulants is to dissolve an existing clot.

_____ 20. Patients with thromboembolic disorders of the lower extremities should be positioned in bed with the knees flexed and a pillow under the popliteal space.

_____ 21. The primary therapeutic outcome from dipyridamole therapy is prevention of blood clots secondary to artificial valve placement.

_____ 22. The use of clopidogrel and aspirin concurrently is contraindicated.

_____ 23. Early studies indicate that ticlopidine is more effective in reducing the risk of strokes than aspirin, but the potential for side effects limits its use to patients who cannot tolerate aspirin therapy or who should not take aspirin.

_____ 24. Dalteparin should not be administered intramuscularly.

_____ 25. To minimize bruising after subcutaneous administration of dalteparin, rub the injection site after completing the injection.

DRUG ACTION/SIDE EFFECTS

26. *State the action and side effects of the following drug used in the treatment of thromboembolic disorders.*

	Actions	Side Effects
WARFARIN		

CHAPTER 27

Student Name______________________________

Drugs Used to Treat Thromboembolic Disorders

Practice Questions for the NCLEX Examination

_____ 1. The anti-aggregatory effect of clopidogrel persists for approximately how many days after discontinuation of therapy?
   1. 1
   2. 2
   3. 3
   4. 5

_____ 2. Which of the following herbal medicines will increase the risk for bleeding when administered with ticlopidine?
   1. St. John's wort
   2. Ginkgo
   3. Green tea
   4. Echinacea

_____ 3. Before administering dalteparin, the nurse should assess the patient for an allergy to:
   1. pork.
   2. dairy.
   3. penicillin.
   4. shellfish.

_____ 4. Which of the following procedures should the nurse follow when administering heparin subcutaneously?
   1. Check the current order and PT value before administering heparin.
   2. Inject within 1 inch of the umbilicus.
   3. Use an 18-gauge 1-inch needle for the injection.
   4. After the needle is injected into the subcutaneous skin, do not aspirate.

_____ 5. Which of the following statements is true about type II heparin induced thrombocytopenia (HIT)?
   1. Type II HIT should be suspected when the platelet count falls below $10,000/mm^3$.
   2. Type II HIT is an allergic reaction to heparin that causes aggregation of platelets.
   3. Warfarin therapy is contraindicated in patients with type II HIT.
   4. Aspirin therapy is contraindicated in patients with type II HIT.

_____ 6. Which of the following statements should the nurse include when teaching a patient about warfarin therapy?
   1. Warfarin is a potent anticoagulant that acts by inhibiting the activity of vitamin K, which is required for the activation of clotting factors in the blood.
   2. Warfarin is used to dissolve clots.
   3. Patients taking warfarin therapy will need to have their PTT blood values monitored.
   4. Protamine sulfate is the antidote for warfarin overdose.

_____ 7. Which of the following laboratory values would the nurse identify as ideal in a patient receiving warfarin therapy?
   1. Platelets at $10,000/mm^3$
   2. APTT at 4.5 to 5.5 control
   3. INR at 2 to 3
   4. Serum cholesterol of 220 mg/dL

_____ 8. Which of the following fibrinolytic agents requires concurrent use of heparin therapy?
1. Streptokinase
2. Urokinase
3. Atistreplase
4. Alteplase

_____ 9. Which of the following is a contraindication or drug interaction associated with warfarin therapy? (Select all that apply.)
1. Current phenytoin therapy
2. History of a nonoperable cerebral aneurysm
3. Recent surgery
4. Lactation

_____ 10. When administering heparin subcutaneously, the nurse should: (Select all that apply.)
1. administer the heparin deep into the fat in the abdominal area around the umbilicus.
2. rotate the injection sites.
3. not aspirate after injection.
4. avoid rubbing the injection site.

_____ 11. When teaching a patient about nutrition related to warfarin therapy, the nurse should include which of the following statements? (Select all that apply.)
1. "Limit your intake of green leafy vegetables."
2. "Drink six to eight 8-ounce glasses of water daily."
3. "Carrots are to be excluded from your diet."
4. "You must not eat more than one serving of protein a day."

_____ 12. Which of the following possible side effects of ticlopidine should be immediately reported to the primary care provider? (Select all that apply.)
1. Nosebleed
2. Easy bruising
3. Dark, tarry stools
4. Blood in the urine

_____ 13. Which of the following statements about Lovenox (enoxaprin) is true? (Select all that apply.)
1. Patients who are allergic to pork byproducts should not receive Lovenox.
2. Patients taking Lovenox are at a higher risk of hemorrhage than patients taking heparin.
3. Lovenox is administered intramuscularly.
4. No special monitoring of clotting times such as APTT are necessary for patients taking Lovenox.

Drugs Used to Treat Heart Failure

Review Sheet

The QUESTION column and the ANSWER column have been offset so that you can cover the answers while reading the questions, allowing you to assess your knowledge.

Question

1. What are the results of systolic dysfunction of the heart?
2. What is the ultimate problem associated with diastolic dysfunction of the heart?
3. What effect does the sympathetic nervous system's release of epinephrine and norepinephrine have on heart function?
4. What occurs when kidney perfusion is diminished?
5. Define the action of inotropic agents.
6. What is the action of intravenous nitroglycerin, nitroprusside, and nesiritide?
7. Why are diuretics used in the treatment of heart failure?
8. Name two common loop diuretics used in the treatment of heart failure.
9. List the six cardinal signs of heart disease and give a rationale for their occurrence.

Answer

1. The result of systolic dysfunction of the heart is inability of the heart to contract with sufficient force to pump all the blood from the heart to maintain sufficient cardiac output to meet the body's oxygenation needs.
2. Due to diastolic dysfunction of the heart, residual volume remains from the previous contraction and the left ventricle does not fill adequately prior to next contraction. Back-pressure builds up in the lungs and peripheral vasculature that results in symptoms of pulmonary congestion and peripheral edema.
3. Epinephrine and norepinephrine produce tachycardia and an increase in cardiac contractility, thereby increasing cardiac output.
4. With reduced perfusion, the kidneys conserve sodium, which increases circulating blood volume. As this progresses, there is an increase in capillary pressure, and edema results.
5. Inotropic agents increase the force of contraction of the heart as it beats, resulting in increased cardiac output to meet the body's oxygenation needs.
6. These drugs are vasodilators that reduce cardiac preload and afterload.
7. Diuretics are used in the treatment of heart failure to reduce sodium and fluid overload associated with heart failure.
8. Loop diuretics used for heart failure include furosemide (Lasix), bumetanide (Bumex), and torsemide (Demadex).

10. What classes of drugs are used to treat heart failure and what are the desired actions of each?
11. What nursing assessments should be performed at regular intervals to assess cardiac function?
12. Describe essential patient education and health promotion for patients being treated for heart failure.
13. List the nursing assessments that should be performed on a regular basis for a cardiac patient.
14. What is the desired therapeutic outcome of administering digoxin?
15. Explain why a "loading dose" or digitalization is done.

9. The six cardinal signs of heart disease are dyspnea, associated with inadequate tissue perfusion and diastolic dysfunction; chest pain, resulting from inadequate oxygen to support myocardium function; fatigue, due to depleted oxygen to body tissue; edema, because the left ventricle is not pumping adequate volumes of blood and a back-pressure builds up in the lungs (causing dyspnea) and the peripheral blood vessels, causing interstitial edema; syncope, due to insufficient oxygen to meet the brain's needs; and palpitations, caused by sympathetic nervous system's release of epinephrine and norepinephrine that produces tachycardia and dysrhythmias.
10. The drug classes used to treat heart failure and their desired actions include vasodilator drugs, which decrease peripheral resistance the heart has to pump against; inotropic drugs, which increase force of each heart contraction resulting in increased cardiac output; and diuretics, which reduce fluid volume, sodium, and peripheral resistance. ACE inhibitors reduce circulating blood volume by inhibiting secretion of aldosterone. They also promote vasodilation and minimize cellular aggregation, preventing thrombus formation.
11. Mental status, vital signs (T, P, R), blood pressure, heart and lung sounds, skin color, neck vein status, presence of clubbing, central venous pressure, abdomen size, fluid volume status, nutrition, activity and exercise tolerance, anxiety level, and laboratory tests should be checked regularly to assess cardiac function.
12. See textbook, pp. 453-454.
13. For cardiac patients, perform regular assessment of the respiratory rate, level of dyspnea seen in relation to exertional effort, and the degree of fatigue being experienced. Monitor for the occurrence of syncope and frequency of palpitations. Check for skin color, neck vein distention, pulse rate and rhythm, and blood pressure on a regularly scheduled basis. Perform auscultation and percussion of the lungs and heart. Check for the presence or absence of edema and for clubbing.
14. Digoxin slows and strengthens the heartbeat, allowing the heart to empty and fill more completely, thereby improving circulation.

16. List the common symptoms of digoxin toxicity.
17. What data should be gathered *before* administering a dose of digoxin?
18. Under what conditions should two qualified nurses check a dose of digoxin?
19. When should a blood sample be drawn to measure the level of digoxin in the blood?
20. Why should a patient taking digoxin be cautioned not to take an antacid within 2 hours of taking the digitalis without first consulting the physician?
21. What effect can the concurrent use of a digoxin and a diuretic have?
22. What is treatment for digoxin toxicity?
23. What is the action of phosphodiesterase inhibitors in the treatment of heart failure?
24. Name two phosphodiesterase inhibitors used to treat heart failure.
25. What is the action of ACE inhibitors in the treatment of heart failure?
26. Describe the premedication assessments needed for digoxin, phosphodiesterase inhibitors, and ACE inhibitors.

15. The process of digitalization allows the blood level of digoxin to be raised rapidly so the therapeutic effects can occur more rapidly. Once a therapeutic level [for digoxin (Lanoxin), 0.9–2.0 ng/mL] is achieved, the patient can be switched to a daily maintenance dose.
16. Common symptoms of digoxin toxicity include anorexia, nausea, extreme fatigue, bradycardia, weakness of arms and legs, visual disturbances, and psychiatric disturbances.
17. Before administering digoxin, apical pulse should be taken for one full minute. Consult the physician before administering the prescribed dose if the apical rate is below 60 beats per minute in an adult, or below 90 beats per minute in a child. When functioning in a nursing home environment, it may be permissible to take a radial pulse for one minute. Always check the clinical site's policies; if in doubt, take by the apical method.
18. Any time the dose requires calculation, two qualified nurses should check the dose.
19. Draw blood to measure the level of digoxin before the daily dose or at least 6–8 hours after administration of the last dose of digoxin.
20. An antacid taken with digoxin reduces the absorption of digoxin.
21. Diuretics may induce hypokalemia, which may result in signs of digoxin toxicity.
22. To treat for digoxin toxicity, stop digoxin, stop potassium-depleting diuretics and check potassium level and administer prescribed potassium if deficient. If signs of toxicity are severe and life-threatening, the antidote for digoxin, digoxin immune Fab (Digibind), may be administered.
23. Phosphodiesterase inhibitors increase the force of contraction of the myocardium, thereby increasing cardiac output (CO). They also cause relaxation of vascular smooth muscle, resulting in vasodilation that reduces preload and afterload.
24. Two phosphodiesterase inhibitors used to treat heart failure are inamrinone and milrinone (Primacor).
25. ACE inhibitors reduce afterload by blocking angiotensin II-mediated peripheral vasoconstriction promoting vasodilation; they also reduce circulating blood volume by inhibiting aldosterone, allowing excretion of excess water. They also minimize cellular aggregation, preventing thrombus formation.
26. See individual drug monographs, textbook pp. 456-460.

Student Name____________________

Drugs Used to Treat Heart Failure

Learning Activities

FILL-IN-THE-BLANK

Finish each of the following statements using the correct term.

1. ____________________ agents are used in the treatment of heart failure to increase the force of contractions, thus boosting cardiac output.
2. The two primary actions of digoxin glycosides on the heart are positive ____________________ and negative ____________________.
3. ____________________ is the term used to describe giving a loading dose of digitalis to a patient over the period of hours or days necessary to produce the desired cardiac effect.
4. The antidote for severe digoxin intoxication is ____________________.
5. ____________________ is the first of a new class of drugs, the human B-type natriuretic peptides.
6. The most commonly reported adverse effects of inamrinone therapy include ____________________ and ____________________.
7. The ____________________ pulse should be taken for ____________________ minute before administering digoxin in a hospital setting.
8. Digoxin should be scheduled (before, after) meals to prevent ______________ ______________.

MATCHING

Match the drug class with the corresponding drug. Each definition will be used only once.

_____ 9. inamrinone

_____ 10. captopril

_____ 11. nesiritide

_____ 12. digoxin

a. digitalis glycoside
b. phosphodiesterase inhibitor
c. ACE inhibitor
d. natriuretic peptide

TRUE OR FALSE

Mark "T" for true and "F" for false for each statement. Correct all false statements.

_____ 13. Nesiritide is used as a vasodilator in patients with severe heart failure who have dyspnea at rest or with minimal activity.

_____ 14. Large studies have shown that ACE inhibitors reduce morbidity and mortality associated with heart failure.

_____ 15. Inamrinone has been found to be the most effective treatment for diastolic heart failure.

_____ 16. If heart failure is acute, most therapy will be administered intravenously in a intensive care unit.

_____ 17. Inamrinone should be diluted with dextrose solutions.

DRUG ACTION/SIDE EFFECTS

18. *State the action and side effects of the following drug classes or drugs used in the treatment of heart failure.*

	Actions	Side Effects
DIGITALIS GLYCOSIDES		

CHAPTER 28

Student Name ______________________

Drugs Used to Treat Heart Failure

Practice Questions for the NCLEX Examination

_____ 1. A patient receives her daily dose of digitalis at 0800 hours. When would be the best time for the nurse to obtain the blood draw to assess serum digitalis levels?
1. 0800 hours
2. 1000 hours
3. 1200 hours
4. 1400 hours

_____ 2. Common early symptoms of digitalis toxicity in older adults include:
1. gastric irritation.
2. low blood pressure.
3. anorexia and mild nausea.
4. tachycardia.

_____ 3. Which of the following daily oral doses of digoxin should the nurse question before administering the medication?
1. 0.125 mg
2. 0.25 mg
3. 0.50 mg
4. 1.25 mg

_____ 4. Patients with heart failure should be taught to make which of the following dietary modifications?
1. Restrict sodium intake
2. Limit protein intake
3. Avoid carbohydrates
4. Drink 10 to 12 glasses of fluid daily

_____ 5. A patient with heart failure would most likely benefit from being placed in the _________ position.
1. Sims'
2. Trendelenberg
3. Semi-Fowler's
4. Lithotomy

_____ 6. Which of the following is the best indicator of fluid gain or loss in a patient with heart failure?
1. Daily weight
2. Intake and output record
3. Hematocrit and hemoglobin
4. Blood pressure

_____ 7. Which of the following statements about proper therapeutic regimen management should be included when teaching a patient with heart failure?
1. "Take your medications only on the days when you feel you need them."
2. "Report signs of digitalis toxicity such as anorexia, nausea, slow heart rate below 60 or high heart rate above 100, or changes in your mental status."
3. "Weigh yourself every 3 days."
4. "Take diuretics at bedtime for the most beneficial effect."

_____ 8. Prior to administration of digitalis, it is most important for the nurse to assess for:
1. hypokalemia.
2. hypocalcemia.
3. hypomagnesemia.
4. hyponatremia.

_____ 9. Which of the following drugs used to treat heart failure is most likely to cause thrombocytopenia?
1. Inamrinone
2. Nesiritide
3. Lanoxin
4. Enalapril

_____ 10. A patient receiving digoxin for heart failure informs the nurse that he also takes St. John's wort. It is most important for the nurse to assess the patient for:
1. altered electrolyte balance.
2. enhanced therapeutic and toxic effect of digoxin.
3. reduced therapeutic effect of digoxin.
4. increased urinary output.

_____ 11. The nurse identifies which of the following as signs and symptoms of digitalis toxicity? (Select all that apply.)
1. Anorexia
2. Vomiting
3. Bradycardia
4. Visual disturbances
5. Psychiatric disturbances

_____ 12. When administering digitalis to a child, the nurse should report findings of below ________ beats per minute to the primary health care provider.
1. 85
2. 90
3. 95
4. 100

_____ 13. Which of the following statements about milrinone (Primacor) is true? (Select all that apply.)
1. It is a negative inotropic agent.
2. Primacor causes vasoconstriction.
3. Primacor should not be infused in the same IV line as furosemide.
4. The most common side effects of this drug are dysrhythmias and hypotension.

_____ 14. Which of the following statements should the nurse include when teaching a patient about digoxin therapy for congestive heart failure? (Select all that apply.)
1. "Take your pulse for one full minute before taking the digoxin. If your pulse is fewer than 80 beats per minute, do not take the medicine."
2. "Weigh yourself daily and report a weight gain of 5 pounds or more in a 2-day period."
3. "Call your primary health care provider if you develop a cough."
4. "You will need to take these medications as lifelong treatment and adhere to them as prescribed to gain control of the disease."

Drugs Used for Diuresis

Review Sheet

The QUESTION column and the ANSWER column have been offset so you can cover the answer while reading the question, allowing you to assess your knowledge.

Question

1. Explain the therapeutic outcomes associated with diuretic therapy.
2. What laboratory tests should be performed to determine if kidney function is impaired?
3. What laboratory studies should be performed whenever a diuretic is prescribed?
4. What patient assessments should be performed on a regular basis when diuretics are being taken?
5. What is the action of a diuretic?
6. What are the six classes of diuretics?
7. Which class of diuretic has the most rapid onset of action? (List the four drugs.) What three routes of administration can be used for loop diuretics?
8. After administration of a loop diuretic using each of these routes, how soon will diuresis occur and how long will it last?
9. When would loop diuretics be prescribed?

Answer

1. The therapeutic outcomes of diuretic therapy are diuresis with reduction of edema and improvement in the symptoms of fluid overload and reduced blood pressure.
2. Check for elevated BUN and serum creatinine; also check for decreased creatinine clearance, decreased urine output, and increasing edema.
3. Check Hct, serum electrolytes, blood glucose, uric acid, BUN, and serum creatinine.
4. Assess intake and output of fluids, state of hydration, presence of edema, heart rate and rhythm, blood pressure bid or qid, and daily weights. Check for signs and symptoms of electrolyte imbalance, gastric irritation, rash, hyperuricemia, and hyperglycemia. Monitor for drug interactions (e.g., digitalis glycosides, corticosteroids, lithium).
5. Diuretics inhibit the reabsorption of sodium, increasing the loss of water.
6. The six classes of diuretic are thiazide, loop, potassium-sparing, methylxanthine, carbonic anhydrase inhibitors, and combination diuretics. Thiazides and potassium-sparing diuretics are available as combination products.
7. Loop diuretics are furosemide (Lasix), ethacrynic acid (Edecrin), bumetanide (Bumex), and torsemide (Demadex). Oral (PO), intramuscular (IM), or intravenous (IV) routes.
8. Oral: onset, 30–60 minutes; peak, 1–2 hours; duration, 6–8 hours. IM: onset, 30–40 minutes; peak, 1–2 hours; duration, 5–6 hours. IV: onset, 5 minutes; peak 15–45 minutes; duration, 2 hours.

10. Of the four loop diuretics, which is most frequently prescribed?
11. Would thiazide or loop diuretics be used when renal function is impaired?
12. What classes of diuretics can cause a loss of serum potassium (hypokalemia)?
13. What class(es) of diuretic(s) can cause an increase in serum potassium (hyperkalemia)?
14. Why would a potassium-sparing and another type of diuretic be prescribed simultaneously?
15. What actions can be taken to prevent and/or treat hypokalemia?
16. What actions can be taken to prevent hyperkalemia when potassium-sparing diuretics are prescribed?
17. Are diuretics useful for edema that occurs during pregnancy?
18. What medicine may need to be ordered for patients who have gouty arthritis who require diuretics?
19. Which type of diuretic has been associated with hearing loss when used concurrently with aminoglycoside antibiotics or cisplatin?
20. What class of antibiotics can cause hearing loss and, if combined with loop diuretics, may increase the possibility of ototoxicity?
21. After reading that diuretics can interact with digoxin to produce digoxin toxicity, what signs and symptoms would you monitor when therapy is combined?
22. What are the normal values for sodium, potassium, and chloride?
23. List six foods that are good sources of potassium.
24. Why should salicylates not be taken with furosemide for prolonged periods?
25. Describe the signs and symptoms of salicylate toxicity.

9. When rapid diuresis is needed (e.g., in pulmonary edema) or when renal function is diminished.
10. Furosemide.
11. Loop diuretics are more effective than other classes of diuretics when renal function is impaired (decreased creatinine clearance).
12. Thiazide and loop diuretics
13. Potassium-sparing diuretics
14. To prevent hypokalemia, improve diuresis, and lower blood pressure.
15. Give potassium supplements and/or increase dietary intake of foods rich in potassium.
16. Do not use salt substitutes that contain potassium. Maintain an adequate fluid intake. Do not administer potassium supplements. Use ACE inhibitors, angiotensin II receptor blockers, eplerenone, and NSAIDs with extreme caution to prevent hyperkalemia.
17. Diuretics are rarely used for edema associated with pregnancy. Diuretics cross the placental barrier and may be harmful to the fetus. Consult a physician before taking any medication during pregnancy or while breastfeeding.
18. Allopurinol
19. Loop diuretics
20. Aminoglycosides: gentamicin, tobramycin, kanamycin, amikacin, neomycin, streptomycin, netilmicin.
21. Anorexia, nausea, fatigue, blurred or colored vision, bradycardia, dysrhythmias.
22. Sodium: 135–145 mEq/L; potassium: 3.5–4.7 mEq/L; chloride: 95–105 mEq/L.
23. Dried almonds; apricots, raw; avocados, raw; bananas, raw; beans, lima (cooked, boiled); carrots, raw; cocoa, plain; potatoes (cooked, boiled).
24. The potential for salicylate toxicity may be increased if taken concurrently for several days.

26. Which class of diuretics can affect the male libido?
27. Why are potassium-sparing diuretics not used in patients with renal failure?
28. What are the signs and symptoms of circulatory overload?
29. What premedication assessments should be made before administering any type of diuretic?

25. Nausea, tinnitus, fever, sweating, dizziness, mental confusion, lethargy, and impaired hearing.
26. Potassium-sparing diuretics [e.g., amiloride (Midamor), spironolactone (Aldactone)]
27. They are usually not effective as diuretics in moderate to severe renal failure and may cause hyperkalemia.
28. Bounding, full pulse; jugular vein distention; dyspnea; frothy sputum; cough.
29. Baseline vital signs, lung sounds, weight, assessment of degree of edema, level of consciousness (LOC), muscle strength, tremors, general appearance; blood glucose levels for patients with diabetes. Baseline laboratory studies as prescribed by physician.

CHAPTER 29

Student Name ____________________

Drugs Used for Diuresis

Learning Activities

FILL-IN-THE-BLANK

Finish each of the following statements using the correct term.

1. The thiazide and loop diuretics act directly on the ____________ ____________ to inhibit the reabsorption of sodium and chloride from the lumen of the tubule.

2. ____________________ is the term used to describe excess fluid accumulation in the extracellular spaces.

3. Furosemide may inhibit the excretion of uric acid, resulting in ____________________.

4. ____________________ is a potassium-sparing diuretic that also has weak antihypertensive activity.

5. Because the chemical structure of ____________________ is similar to that of estrogenic hormones, an occasional male patient will report gynecomastia, reduced libido, and diminished erection.

6. The most common problem associated with thiazide diuretic therapy is ____________________.

7. The most frequently used loop diuretic is ____________________.

8. ____________________ is known to occur when a loop diuretic is combined with an aminoglycoside or cisplatin.

9. Diabetic patients receiving a diuretic must be checked regularly for ____________________.

10. ____________ ____________ is a loop diuretic which can be used in conjunction with 0.9% sodium chloride infusions to enhance excretion of calcium in patients with hypercalcemia.

MATCHING

Match the generic drug name with its corresponding brand name. Each option will be used only once.

_____ 11. acetazolamide

_____ 12. bumetanide

_____ 13. ethacrynic acid

_____ 14. furosemide

_____ 15. amiloride

_____ 16. triamterene

a. Dyrenium
b. Midamor
c. Lasix
d. Edecrin
e. Bumex
f. Diamox

TRUE OR FALSE

Mark "T" for true and "F" for false for each statement. Correct all false statements.

_____ 17. Diuretics are mainstays of treatment in two major diseases affecting the cardiovascular system: heart failure and hypertension.

_____ 18. Acetazolamide is used to reduce cerebral edema.

_____ 19. When a patient is overhydrated, hematocrit and hemoglobin values drop as a result of hemodilution.

_____ 20. The most appropriate time to administer diuretics to a patient is at bedtime.

_____ 21. Acetazolamide is a weak diuretic that acts by inhibiting the enzyme carbonic anhydrase within the kidney, brain, and eye.

_____ 22. Diuresis is occasionally noted when aminophylline is used in the treatment of asthma.

_____ 23. Furosemide is one of the most potent and effective diuretics currently available.

_____ 24. Patients who are diabetic and taking furosemide therapy must be monitored for the development of hypoglycemia, particularly during the early weeks of therapy.

DRUG ACTION/SIDE EFFECTS

25. *State the action and side effects of the following drug used for diuresis.*

	Actions	Side Effects
FUROSEMIDE		

CHAPTER 29

Student Name______________________________

Drugs Used for Diuresis

Practice Questions for the NCLEX Examination

_____ 1. When assessing a patient with overhydration, the nurse would expect to find:
   1. poor skin turgor.
   2. deteriorating vital signs.
   3. deeply furrowed tongue.
   4. neck vein engorgement.

_____ 2. A patient who has received IV fluids in excess of fluids excreted is likely to develop which of the following electrolyte imbalances?
   1. Hypokalemia
   2. Hyperkalemia
   3. Hyponatremia
   4. Hypernatremia

_____ 3. Patients taking potassium-sparing diuretics should be instructed to avoid:
   1. salt substitutes.
   2. chicken.
   3. sugar substitutes.
   4. milk products.

_____ 4. Ms. K. is currently taking digoxin, aminoglycosides, nonsteroidal anti-inflammatory drugs, and corticosteroids for her many medical problems. She has now been prescribed bumetanide. Which of the following statements about bumetanide therapy and these other drugs is true?
   1. The amount of digoxin will need to be increased.
   2. The potential for ototoxicity from the aminoglycosides is increased.
   3. The dose of bumetanide will need to be decreased when also taking nonsteroidal anti-inflammatory drugs.
   4. The use of corticosteroids and bumetanide may cause hyperkalemia.

_____ 5. A patient who has _________ and is taking ethacrynic acid is most at risk for the development of dizziness, deafness, and tinnitus.
   1. liver disease
   2. a hearing deficit
   3. impaired renal function
   4. a history of myocardial infarction

_____ 6. Which of the following electrolyte imbalances is most likely to develop as a result of spironolactone therapy?
   1. Hyperkalemia
   2. Hypercalcemia
   3. Hypermagnesemia
   4. Hypernatremia

_____ 7. Which of the following statements should the nurse include when teaching about diuretic therapy? (Select all that apply.)
   1. "If you are taking Aldactone, avoid the use of salt substitutes in your diet."
   2. "You should rise slowly from a lying or sitting position and lie down if you feel faint, because some diuretics cause you to develop low blood pressure in certain positions."
   3. "You should take your diuretic pill before you go to sleep."
   4. "Weigh yourself every day and call your primary health care provider if you note a one-pound weight gain in one day."

_____ 8. Which of the following cause drug interactions when used with bumetanide (Bumex)? (Select all that apply.)
1. Nonsteroidal antiinflammatory drugs
2. Corticosteroids
3. Digoxin
4. Narcotics

_____ 9. Which of the following electrolytes are most commonly altered due to Lasix therapy? (Select all that apply.)
1. Potassium
2. Sodium
3. Chloride
4. Magnesium
5. Calcium

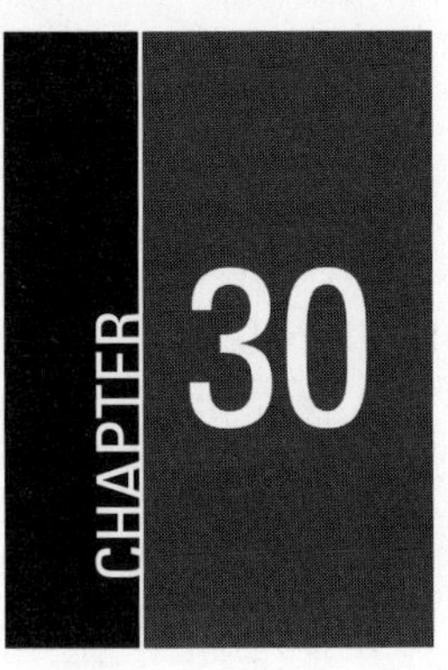

Drugs Used to Treat Upper Respiratory Disease

Review Sheet

The QUESTION column and the ANSWER column have been offset so you can cover the answer while reading the question, allowing you to assess your knowledge.

Question

1. What is allergic rhinitis?
2. What are the drugs of choice for treating allergic rhinitis?
3. What is the mechanism of action of decongestants?
4. What is a "rebound" effect associated with nasally administered decongestants?
5. Name two commonly used decongestants administered intranasally, and one administered orally.
6. Explain how to administer a nasal spray, nose drops, and medications by inhalation.
7. What response does histamine release have on the mucous membranes?
8. What is an antigen?
9. When is histamine released?
10. How do antihistamines act?
11. What side effects can be anticipated whenever an antihistamine is administered?
12. What actions should be initiated to offset the drying effects of antihistamines?
13. What patient education should accompany the use of antihistamines?

Answer

1. Inflamed nasal mucosa associated with an allergic reaction.
2. Antihistamines.
3. Decongestants are alpha-adrenergic receptor stimulants that constrict blood vessels in the nasal passages, reducing swollen tissues and obstruction.
4. Excessive or prolonged use of nasal decongestants causes a rebound swelling in the nasal passages that requires further use of nasal decongestants to unblock nasal passages. It is difficult to break this cycle, so it is particularly important not to overuse nasal decongestants.
5. Pseudoephedrine (Sudafed)—oral tablets; phenylephrine (NeoSynephrine)—nasal spray; oxymetazoline (Afrin)—nasal spray; xylometazoline (Otrivin)—nasal spray. See Table 30-1.
6. See Chapter 8, pp. 122-127.
7. Urticaria (itching), redness, and edema.
8. A substance that elicits an immunologic response such as the production of a specific antibody against that substance.
9. In cases of tissue damage (trauma), allergic reactions, and infection.
10. Histamines block the H_1 receptor sites on the target cells; they do not affect the amount or the release of histamine.
11. Sedation and dryness of mucous membranes (anticholinergic effects)
12. Consume an adequate fluid intake of 8–12 8-oz glasses daily.

14. What is the action of cromolyn sodium (Nasalcrom)?

13. Maintain adequate hydration. If the person knows he/she is going to be exposed to an allergen (e.g., pollen outdoors), take the dose 30–45 minutes prior to possible exposure to block receptors before histamine can attach. If exposure is unanticipated, take a dose immediately upon recognition of an allergic response (e.g., runny nose and burning, itchy eyes). Exercise caution when operating any power equipment or while driving because of the medicine's sedative effects.

15. What condition is treated with cromolyn sodium (Nasalcrom) that affects the upper respiratory tract?

14. Cromolyn prevents release of histamine from its storage sites, the mast cells.

16. What are the desired therapeutic outcomes from the use of respiratory antiinflammatory agents?

15. Cromolyn is used with other medications to treat severe allergic rhinitis and prevent release of histamine that causes the symptoms of allergic rhinitis.

17. When a drug monograph says that a drug produces anticholinergic effects, what does this mean?

16. Reduction in rhinorrhea, rhinitis, itching, and sneezing.

17. Blurred vision; constipation; urinary retention; dryness of mucosa of mouth, throat, and nose.

CHAPTER 30

Student Name ____________________

Drugs Used to Treat Upper Respiratory Disease

Learning Activities

FILL-IN-THE-BLANK

Finish each of the following statements using the correct term.

1. ____________________ is defined as inflammation of the nasal mucous membranes.

2. The respiratory function of the nose is to ____________________, humidify, and ____________________ the air inhaled to prepare it for the lower respiratory airways.

3. A(n) ____________________ is a physiologic reflex used by the body to clear the nasal passages of foreign matter.

4. Overuse of topical decongestants may lead to a rebound of nasal secretions known as ________________ ________________.

5. ____________________ are the drugs of choice in treating allergic rhinitis.

6. Decongestants cause the blood vessels in the nasal mucosa to ____________________.

MATCHING

Match the generic drug name with its corresponding brand name. Each option will be used only once.

_____ 7. mometasone

_____ 8. fluticasone

_____ 9. budesonide

_____ 10. fexofenadine

_____ 11. ipratropium

_____ 12. oxymetazoline

_____ 13. pseudoephedrine

_____ 14. loratidine

a. Afrin
b. Allegra
c. Sudafed
d. Atrovent
e. Claritin
f. Flonase
g. Nasonex
h. Rhinocort

TRUE OR FALSE

Mark "T" for true and "F" for false for each statement. Correct all false statements.

_____ 15. Cholinergic stimulation causes vasodilatation of the blood vessels lining the nasal mucosa, and sympathetic stimulation causes vasoconstriction.

_____ 16. The common cold is actually a bacterial infection of the upper respiratory tissues.

_____ 17. The medical term used for a runny nose is *rhinorrhea.*

_____ 18. When an antigen-antibody reaction takes place and histamine is released, it reacts with the H_1 receptors in the bronchioles resulting in bronchodilation.

_____ 19. A paradoxical effect from antihistamines often seen in children and older adults is central nervous system stimulation rather than sedation, which may cause insomnia, nervousness, and irritability.

DRUG ACTION/SIDE EFFECTS

20. *State the action and side effects of antihistamines in the treatment of upper respiratory disorders.*

	Actions	Side Effects
ANTIHISTAMINES		

CHAPTER 30

Student Name ______

Drugs Used to Treat Upper Respiratory Disease

Practice Questions for the NCLEX Examination

_____ 1. When large amounts of histamine are released, such as in a severe allergic reaction, which one of the following would the nurse expect the patient to exhibit?
1. Hypertension
2. Dry skin
3. Urticaria
4. Dilation of the bronchial tubes

_____ 2. Antihistamines reduce which of the following symptoms of allergic rhinitis? (Select all that apply.)
1. Nasal itching
2. Sneezing
3. Rhinorrhea
4. Nasal congestion

_____ 3. Sympathomimetic decongestants should be used with caution in patients with:
1. diabetes mellitus.
2. allergy to penicillin.
3. allergy to shellfish.
4. hypothyroidism.

_____ 4. When assessing a patient who is taking antihistamines, the nurse would expect the patient to display which of the following anticholinergic side effects? (Select all that apply.)
1. Diarrhea
2. Blurred vision
3. Dry mouth
4. Urinary retention

_____ 5. Which of the following statements would the nurse include when teaching patients about cromolyn sodium?
1. "Cromolyn sodium should be administered after the body receives a stimulus to release histamine."
2. "Cromolyn sodium causes bronchodilation."
3. "A 2 to 4 week course of therapy is usually required to determine clinical response."
4. "Cromolyn sodium should be discontinued when the desired therapeutic response is achieved."

_____ 6. Which of the following conditions contraindicates the use of antihistamines? (Select all that apply.)
1. Concurrent use of a monoamine oxidase inhibitor
2. Narrow-angle glaucoma
3. Peptic ulcer
4. Prostatic hypertrophy

_____ 7. Which of the following statements should the nurse include when teaching a patient about the use of topical decongestants and intranasal corticosteroids for allergic seasonal rhinitis? (Select all that apply.)

1. "Take your intranasal corticosteroid first, followed by the topical decongestant."
2. "Be sure to blow your nose thoroughly before administering the nasal therapy."
3. "Immediately discontinue the therapy if you experience nasal burning."
4. "The therapeutic effect is usually not immediate, so be sure to follow the medical regimen fully, as most patients usually do not experience full benefit of the therapy for a few days."

_____ 8. Which of the following statements about cromolyn sodium is true? (Select all that apply.)

1. Cromolyn must be taken before exposure to the stimulus that initiates an attack of allergic rhinitis.
2. Cromolyn has no direct bronchodilatory or antihistaminic activities.
3. Cromolyn does not relieve nasal congestion.
4. Patients who experience coughing when taking cromolyn should notify their primary health care provider.

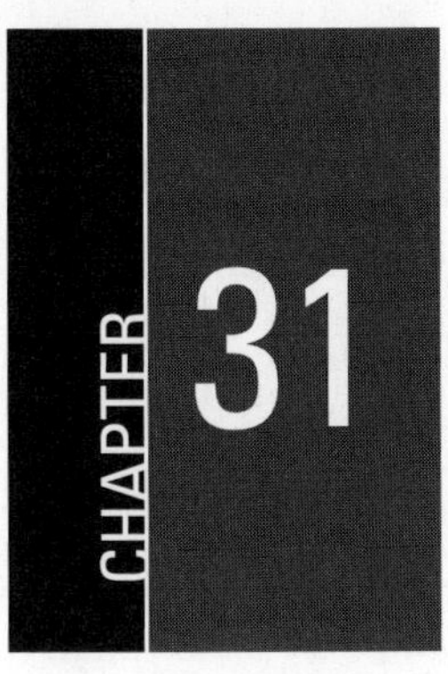

Drugs Used to Treat Lower Respiratory Disease

Review Sheet

The QUESTION column and the ANSWER column have been offset so that you can cover the answers while reading the questions, allowing you to assess your knowledge.

Question	Answer
1. Define *ventilation, perfusion,* and *diffusion.*	
2. What are the differences between obstructive and restrictive respiratory diseases?	1. Ventilation is the movement of air in and out of the lungs; perfusion is blood flow through the pulmonary arteries to the capillaries surrounding the alveoli to the pulmonary veins; and diffusion is the process by which oxygen passes across the alveolar membrane to the blood in the capillaries and carbon dioxide passes from the blood to the alveolar sacs.
3. Why are pulmonary function tests performed?	2. Obstructive disease is associated with narrowed air passages and increasing resistance to air flow (e.g., asthma, acute bronchitis). Restrictive airway disease is characterized by restricted alveolar expansion due to loss of elasticity of tissue or physical deformity of the chest itself.
4. Why is the SaO_2 ratio valuable in an assessment of respiratory function?	3. To assess ventilation and diffusion capacity of the lungs and to determine whether medicines are having a therapeutic effect.
5. What is asthma?	4. It reflects the percent of oxygen bound to the hemoglobin compared with the maximum amount of oxygen that could be attached.
6. What is bronchitis?	5. Asthma is a chronic inflammatory disease of bronchi and bronchioles.
7. What is emphysema?	6. Bronchitis is inflammation and edema with excessive mucus secretions leading to airflow obstruction.
8. What are the goals of therapy for asthma?	7. Emphysema is a disease of alveolar destruction without fibrosis.
9. What is the action of expectorants?	8. Goals are: maintain normal activity levels, maintain near-normal pulmonary function rates, prevent chronic and troublesome symptoms, prevent recurrent exacerbations, and avoid adverse effects from asthma medications.

10. What is the action of an antitussive agent?
11. What is the action of a mucolytic agent?
12. What is the purpose of administering a bronchodilator?
13. What types of drugs are known as anti-inflammatory agents?
14. What data should be collected as part of a respiratory assessment?
15. Explain desirable peak expiratory flow (PEF) used to assess the severity of asthma symptoms.
16. What dietary considerations should be made for a person with a respiratory disease?
17. How should people with known respiratory disease prevent infection?
18. What medication administration considerations should be made for the delivery of aerosol therapy to a child or older adult?
19. Cite important aspects of patient education and health promotion for individuals with a lower respiratory disease.
20. What posture does a dyspneic patient assume?
21. Describe appropriate health teaching for patients requiring respiratory therapy.
22. What is the primary action of an expectorant?
23. What precautions must be used when administering an iodine product?
24. When should SSKI not be administered?
25. What types of respiratory diseases may be treated with mucolytic agents [e.g., acetylcysteine (Mucomyst)]?
26. The patient receiving medication by inhalation should be placed in what position?
27. The patient should be instructed to exhale through _______ lips.
28. What patient teaching should be performed for a patient taking an expectorant?

9. Expectorants liquefy mucus by stimulating natural lubricant fluids.
10. Antitussives suppress the cough center in the brain.
11. Mucolytic agents reduce stickiness and viscosity of pulmonary secretions by acting directly on the mucus plug to cause dissolution.
12. It causes a widening of the opening of the bronchioles and alveolar ducts and a decrease in resistance to airflow into the alveolar sacs.
13. Corticosteroids are the most effective anti-inflammatory agents. Other agents are leukotriene modifiers, cromolyn, and nedocromil.
14. See textbook, pp. 499-500.
15. See textbook, pp. 496-497; p. 501.
16. Well-balanced diet to maintain near-normal weight. With dyspnea, eat small servings throughout day, take small bites, and eat slowly. Administer oxygen during meals as needed.
17. Good hygiene; influenza and pneumococcal vaccinations. Seek medical attention at earliest signs of suspected infection.
18. See textbook, p. 502.
19. See textbook, pp. 502-503.
20. Sits upright and leans forward from the waist, resting the elbows on the knees. When hospitalized, will be placed in a high-Fowler's position.
21. See pp. 501-503, Patient Education and Health Promotion.
22. Expectorants enhance the output of respiratory tract fluids.
23. Dilute in water or fruit juice. Use a straw placed well back on the tongue to administer iodine products; this prevents permanent staining of the teeth.
24. Do *not* give to a patient allergic to iodine or one who has hyperthyroidism, hyperkalemia, or experiences a skin eruption after taking the medication.
25. Emphysema, bronchitis, pneumonia, cystic fibrosis.
26. Sitting
27. Pursed

29. What is the desired action for giving saline solution by nebulizer?
30. What classes of antitussive agents are available?
31. What are the major drawbacks to using an opiate antitussive?
32. In what type of patient must great caution be exercised if an opiate antitussive is to be administered?
33. Give one example of an antitussive agent.
34. What premedication assessments should be made prior to administering an antitussive agent, potassium iodide, saline solutions, mucolytic agent, expectorant, anticholinergic bronchodilating agent, xanthine derivative bronchodilating agent, respiratory antiinflammatory agent, antileukotriene agents, and immunomodulators?
35. What are the four components of asthma therapy?
36. Review the premedication assessments associated with acetylcysteine therapy.
37. What types of patients benefit from beta-adrenergic bronchodilator therapy?
38. What two classes of drugs are prescribed as bronchodilators?
39. What is the drug ipratropium bromide (Atrovent) primarily used to treat?
40. How do sympathomimetic (adrenergic) agents act?
41. Which drugs are classified as xanthine derivatives?

28. Teach the patient the difference between a productive and nonproductive cough, as well as measures to combat nonproductive coughs.
29. Hydration of viscous mucus.
30. Opiate and nonopiate cough suppressants.
31. Codeine may cause dependence (rarely), respiratory depression, bronchial constriction, central nervous system (CNS) depression, and constipation.
32. Patients with preexisting pulmonary distress; people already taking sedative/hypnotics, CNS depressants, or psychotropic agents; people using alcohol.
33. Codeine
34. Antitussive agent, p. 505; potassium iodide, p. 505; saline solutions, p. 505; mucolytic agents, p. 506; expectorants, p. 503; anticholinergic bronchodilating agents, p. 508; xanthine derivative bronchodilating agents, p. 511; respiratory antiinflammatory agents, p. 512; antileukotriene agents, p. 513; immunomodulators, p. 515.
35. Patient education, environmental control, comprehensive pharmacologic therapy, and objective monitoring via regular use of a peak flow meter.
36. See textbook, p. 507.
37. Patients with diseases that cause constriction of the tracheobronchial tree, obstructing the airways.
38. Sympathomimetics and xanthine derivatives.
39. Ipratropium bromide (Atrovent) is used as a bronchodilator for long-term treatment of reversible bronchospasm associated with chronic obstructive pulmonary disease (COPD).
40. Adrenergic agents stimulate $beta_2$ receptors, causing bronchodilation. Many of the drugs also stimulate $beta_1$ receptors in the heart. Always monitor patients taking adrenergic agents for changes in cardiac function (e.g., hypertension, tachycardia), CNS stimulation (exhibited as insomnia, nervousness, anxiety, tremors), and gastrointestinal (GI) disturbances.

42. How do xanthines work?

43. What pharmacologic effects do xanthines cause?

44. How can dosages of theophylline be measured?

45. Describe the clinical uses of montelukast (Singulair), and zafirlukast (Accolate).

46. Describe premedication assessments for omalizumab (Xolair).

41. Aminophylline, theophylline, dyphylline, oxtriphylline (*Note:* all xanthine derivatives except caffeine end in "-phylline.")
42. They cause an increase in cyclic adenosine monophosphate (cAMP), a substance that is associated with bronchodilation and smooth muscle relaxation.
43. They stimulate the CNS, cause diuresis, increase gastric secretions, and stimulate the heart to beat rapidly. Always monitor patients for nausea, changes in cardiac function, and CNS stimulation.
44. Theophylline levels can be monitored by a blood test. Adult: 10–20 mcg/mL; Newborn: 6–11 mcg/mL.
45. See textbook, pp. 513-514.
46. See textbook, p. 515.

CHAPTER 31

Student Name ____________________

Drugs Used to Treat Lower Respiratory Disease

Learning Activities

FILL-IN-THE-BLANK

Finish each of the following statements using the correct term.

1. ____________________ is the movement of air in and out of the lungs; ____________________ is the process by which oxygen passes across the alveolar membrane to the blood in the capillaries, and carbon dioxide passes from the blood to the alveolar sacs.

2. Respiratory diseases are divided into two types: ____________________ and ____________________.

3. ____________ ____________ is a condition in which chronic irritation causes inflammation and edema with excessive mucus secretion leading to airflow obstruction.

4. The ____________________ liquefy mucus by stimulating the secretion of natural lubricant fluids from the serous glands.

5. ____________________ agents reduce the stickiness and viscosity of pulmonary secretions by acting directly on the mucus plugs to cause dissolution.

6. ______________-______________ respirations is a cyclic breathing pattern in which periods of deep breathing alternate with periods of apnea.

7. ____________________ agents play an important role in the treatment of asthma to reduce inflammation.

8. The ____________________ measures the ratio of actual oxygen content of hemoglobin compared with the hemoglobin's oxygen-carrying capacity.

9. ____________________ is an inflammatory disease of the bronchi and bronchioles. There are intermittent periods of acute, reversible airflow obstruction (bronchoconstriction) caused by bronchiolar inflammation and overresponsiveness to a variety of stimuli.

10. A(n) ____________________ is an instrument used to measure volumes of air during inhalation and exhalation.

11. Guaifenesin (Robitussin) is a drug known as a(n) ____________________.

12. This drug may produce a goiter when used over an extended length of time in children such as those with cystic fibrosis: ____________ ____________.

13. ____________________ is a medicine that acts by dissolving mucus by disrupting the chemical bonds.

14. ____________________ (drug class) therapy requires a period of up to 4 weeks of therapy for maximum benefits on obstructive lung disease.

15. ____________________ agents must NOT be considered as the primary treatment for an acute episode of asthma.

16. The ____________________ (drug class) relax the smooth muscle of the tracheobronchial tree.

MATCHING

Match the generic drug name with its corresponding brand name. Each option will be used only once.

_____ 17. guaifenesin

_____ 18. acetylcysteine

_____ 19. albuterol

_____ 20. metaproterenol

_____ 21. ipratropium bromide

_____ 22. montelukast

_____ 23. zafirlukast

_____ 24. omalizumab

_____ 25. cromolyn sodium

_____ 26. nedrocromil sodium

a. Xolair
b. Singulair
c. Tilade
d. Accolate
e. Proventil
f. Robitussin
g. Mucomyst
h. Alupent
i. Atrovent
j. Intal

TRUE OR FALSE

Mark "T" for true and "F" for false for each statement. Correct all false statements.

_____ 27. Stimulation of the smooth muscles of the tracheobronchial tree by the cholinergic nerves causes bronchial constriction and increased mucus secretion.

_____ 28. Asthma is a constrictive disease of the bronchi and bronchioles.

_____ 29. Emphysema is a disease of alveolar destruction with fibrosis.

_____ 30. Antitussives act by suppressing the cough center located in the trachea.

_____ 31. Fingernail clubbing is a flattening or an increase in the angle between the fingernail and the nail base of the fingers.

_____ 32. Central cyanosis indicates a general lack of oxygen in the hemoglobin.

_____ 33. Molds are often asthma triggers.

_____ 34. Spiriva is a new class of rescue medications used for the treatment of patients with chronic obstructive pulmonary disease.

_____ 35. There is no acceptable role for the use of steroids in the treatment of patients with chronic obstructive pulmonary disease.

DRUG ACTION/SIDE EFFECTS

36. *State the action and side effects of the following drug class used to treat lower respiratory disease.*

	Actions	Side Effects
MONTELUKAST		

CHAPTER 31

Student Name ______________________________

Drugs Used to Treat Lower Respiratory Disease

Practice Questions for the NCLEX Examination

_____ 1. Which of the following statements should the nurse include when teaching a patient about potassium iodide for the treatment of cough?
   1. "Do not use salt substitutes high in potassium because of potential dangerous effects from hyperkalemia."
   2. "Limit your intake of protein to prevent complications."
   3. "Maintain a maximum fluid intake of four eight-ounce glasses of fluid daily."
   4. "Double your intake of calcium products to prevent hypocalcemia."

_____ 2. Which of the following drugs is an effective cough suppressant and the standard against which other antitussive agents are compared?
   1. Dextromethorphan
   2. Acetylcysteine
   3. Guaifenesin
   4. Codeine

_____ 3. Ms. L. has been prescribed acetylcysteine for the treatment of pneumonia. The nurse tells her acetylcysteine works by:
   1. hydrating the mucus and reducing its viscosity.
   2. dissolving chemical bonds within the mucus itself, causing it to separate and liquefy, thereby reducing viscosity.
   3. producing bronchodilation by relaxing bronchial smooth muscle.
   4. reducing bronchial inflammation.

_____ 4. Which one of the following beta-adrenergic bronchodilating agents is most effective for the treatment of acute bronchospasm?
   1. Serevent
   2. Salmeterol
   3. Albuterol
   4. Formoterol

_____ 5. The patient who has ________ would most likely be particularly sensitive to beta-adrenergic bronchodilator therapy, and therefore must be observed closely when taking Proventil.
   1. Diabetes mellitus
   2. Asthma
   3. Pneumonia
   4. An allergy to eggs

_____ 6. The nurse is teaching Mr. I. how to administer 2 puffs of ipratropium bromide via inhalation. Mr. I. is asked to provide the nurse with a return demonstration. Which of the following actions by Mr. I. indicate he is in need of more teaching on proper inhalation techniques?
   1. He encloses the mouthpiece with his lips.
   2. He washes the mouthpiece with hot water.
   3. He inhales slowly through the mouthpiece and simultaneously presses the canister once.
   4. He waits 5 seconds and repeats the second inhalation.

_____ 7. Which of the following statements about the use of zafirlukast with other medications is true? (Select all that apply.)
1. Aspirin significantly decreases the activity of zafirlukast.
2. Zafirlukast increases the activity of warfarin.
3. Theophylline decreases the activity of zafirlukast.
4. Erythromycin decreases the activity of zafirlukast.

_____ 8. How should the nurse prepare to administer 150 mg of omalizumab?
1. Assess patency of the intravenous line and flush with saline before administering the omalizumab.
2. Clean the nebulizer of any unused medication.
3. Review proper inhalation techniques with use of a spacer.
4. Obtain needed equipment to dilute the medication and administer it subcutaneously.

_____ 9. Which of the following statements by the patient indicate that further teaching is needed about the proper use of cromolyn sodium for treatment of asthma?
1. "I will take the cromolyn sodium 10 to 60 minutes before exercising."
2. "I will drink plenty of water after taking the cromolyn capsule by mouth so it is absorbed."
3. "I will not use cromolyn sodium for immediate relief of asthma symptoms."
4. "I will not receive full therapeutic benefit from cromolyn sodium therapy for 2 to 4 weeks of continuous use."

_____ 10. Which of the following statements would the nurse include when teaching a patient about proper administration of a bronchodilator and steroid via metered-dose inhaler for treatment of chronic obstructive pulmonary disease?
1. "Inhale halfway, then take your medicine through the inhaler."
2. "Take your steroid first, then take the bronchodilator."
3. "Hold your breath for about 2 seconds during inhalation of the medication."
4. "Rinse your mouth with water and spit it out after you take your steroid by inhalation."

_____ 11. Children with cystic fibrosis who are on long term therapy with SSKI potassium iodide should be assessed for the development of ______ as a result of the therapy.
1. goiter
2. edema
3. tremor
4. tachycardia

_____ 12. The patient who is taking a beta-adrenergic bronchodilator should report which of the following side effects? (Select all that apply.)
1. Escalation of tension
2. Tremors
3. Palpitations
4. Dizziness

_____ 13. A patient who has been on long-term inhaled corticosteroid therapy for obstructive airway disease should be assessed for _______, because this is the most common side effect to expect with this type of therapy.
1. liver dysfunction
2. abdominal pain
3. thrush
4. constipation

Drugs Used to Treat Oral Disorders

Review Sheet

The QUESTION column and the ANSWER column have been offset so that you can cover the answers while reading the questions, allowing you to assess your knowledge.

Question

1. Summarize the major goals of treatment and drug therapy used for cold sores.
2. Summarize the major goals of treatment and drug therapy used for canker sores.
3. Summarize the major goals of treatment and drug therapy used for mucositis. Describe how a pretreatment oral mucosal assessment is completed for patients scheduled to undergo chemotherapy.
4. Summarize the major goals of treatment and drug therapy for xerostomia.
5. Explain how to perform an oral assessment.
6. Summarize the use of various types of mouthwashes.

Answer

1. The goals of treatment are to control discomfort, allow healing, prevent spread to others, and prevent complications. The cold sore should be kept moist to prevent drying. Dosasanol (Abreva) is the only FDA-approved product clinically proven to shorten healing time as well as the duration of symptoms. Local anesthetics can temporarily relieve the pain and itching and prevent drying of the lesion. Topical oral analgesics may also provide significant pain relief. Protection from the sun can help those who have cold sores that are stimulated from exposure to the sun. Secondary infections can be treated with topical antibiotic ointment.
2. The goals of treatment are similar to those for cold sores. See text for details.
3. Prevention is key in treatment of mucositis. Basic oral hygiene should be performed. See text for details on the pretreatment assessment and treatment of patients with mucositis.
4. Xerostomia is treated by changing the medicines that cause dry mouth or with artificial saliva. Patients with xerostomia should be seen on a regular basis by a dentist. Commercially available saliva substitutes are often used.
5. See text for details.

7. When lidocaine, a local anesthetic, is used as an oral spray or as a viscous solution, what precautions should be taught to the patient?

8. Describe the World Health Organization Oral Mucositis Scale.

6. The most common mouthwashes are the fluoride-containing mouthwashes used to prevent dental caries. Medicinal mouthwashes are used to reduce plaque accumulation and gingivitis. Some mouthwashes such as Peridex are antibacterial agents used to treat oral mucositis. See text for more details on these agents.
7. Do not smoke, eat, or drink for at least 30 minutes after use. Test ability to swallow before taking oral foods or drink. These products decrease normal sensations in the mouth; test temperature of foods or drinks before ingesting to prevent accidental burning of the oral mucosa.
8. See textbook, Box 32-1.

CHAPTER 32

Student Name ______________________________

Drugs Used to Treat Oral Disorders

Learning Activities

FILL-IN-THE-BLANK

Finish each of the following statements using the correct term.

1. The medical term used to describe lack of saliva is ____________________.
2. Canker sores are also known as ______________ ______________.
3. The most common form of candidiasis is often referred to as ____________________.
4. Candidiasis is a fungal infection caused by ________________ ________________.
5. If plaque is not removed within 24 hours, it begins to calcify, forming calculus or ____________________.
6. ____________________ is the general term used to describe a painful inflammation of the mucous membranes of the mouth.
7. ____________________ is the whitish-yellow substance that builds up on teeth and gum lines around the teeth.

TRUE OR FALSE

Mark "T" for true and "F" for false for each statement. Correct all false statements.

_____ 8. Antibiotics are the standard treatment used for candidiasis.

_____ 9. Tartar is the primary cause of most tooth, gum, and periodontal disease.

_____ 10. *Halitosis* is the term used to describe very foul mouth odor.

_____ 11. Docasanol is the treatment of choice for canker sores.

_____ 12. Kaopectate stirred in water may be used as a mouthwash to coat painful oral lesions for patients with stomatitis.

DRUG ACTION/SIDE EFFECTS

13. *State the actions and side effects of the following drug used to treat oral disorders.*

	Actions	Side Effects
ACYCLOVIR		

CHAPTER 32

Student Name______________________________

Drugs Used to Treat Oral Disorders

Practice Questions for the NCLEX Examination

_____ 1. How many days after receiving chemotherapy would a patient be most at risk for the development of mucositis?
1. 6
2. 10
3. 12
4. 16

_____ 2. The nurse determines that a patient who is receiving radiation therapy to her neck is in need of more teaching regarding dietary habits when the patient says:
1. "I will eat hot soup with every meal."
2. "I will avoid alcohol."
3. "I will use bland gravy and sauces on my foods."
4. "I will avoid the use of spicy foods."

_____ 3. Which of the following actions would be most effective in providing a patient with relief of symptoms caused by mucositis?
1. Avoid use of oral or parenteral analgesics for severe pain to prevent addiction.
2. Use commercially prepared mouthwashes with alcohol to stimulate salivation.
3. Perform mouth care at 6-hour intervals.
4. Use 1 tablespoon of salt or hydrogen peroxide, or 1/2 teaspoon of baking soda in 8 oz of water as a mouthwash.

_____ 4. Which of the following statements should the nurse include when teaching a patient how to care for his cold sore?
1. "Avoid exposure of the cold sore to any type of soap solution."
2. "Keep the cold sore dry to aid in healing."
3. "Cold sores are caused by bacteria, so take your antibiotics."
4. "Avoid the use of highly astringent products such as zinc sulfate in the area of the cold sore."

_____ 5. A patient has severe grade 3 mucositis as determined by the World Health Organization Oral Mucositis Scale. Which of the following medications may be ordered for the patient to treat oral mucositis? (Select all that apply.)
1. Recombinant human keratinocyte growth factor (Kepivance)
2. Milk of magnesia
3. Sucralfate suspensions
4. Viscous lidocaine

CHAPTER 33

Drugs Used to Treat Gastroesophageal Reflux and Peptic Ulcer Diseases

Review Sheet

The QUESTION column and the ANSWER column have been offset so that you can cover the answers while reading the questions, allowing you to assess your knowledge.

Question

1. What types of conditions are treated with antacids?
2. What is the difference between GERD and PUD?
3. What are the major treatment goals for GERD and PUD?
4. What premedication assessments should be made prior to beginning antacid therapy?
5. What effect does the administration of an antacid have on the pH of the gastric secretions?
6. Are antacids alkaline or acidic?
7. Describe effect(s) of the following active ingredients of antacids: simethicone, aluminum hydroxide, magnesium oxide or hydroxide, magnesium trisilicate, and calcium carbonate.
8. What ingredients in an antacid may produce constipation?
9. What ingredients in antacids may cause diarrhea?

Answer

1. Antacids decrease hyperacidity associated with peptic ulcer disease (PUD), gastroesophageal reflux disease (GERD), gastritis, and hiatal hernia.
2. See textbook, pp. 527-528.
3. See textbook, p. 528.
4. Prior to antacid therapy, check for any abnormal renal function. If present, avoid magnesium-containing products. Check bowel pattern for diarrhea or constipation. Record any gastric pain or symptoms present. If patient is pregnant or has edema, heart failure, hypertension, or salt restrictions, ensure that a low-sodium antacid is prescribed. Check scheduling of antacids in relation to other prescribed medications to avoid interactions.
5. Antacids buffer the hydrogen ion concentration, reducing the acidity of the gastric secretions and raising the pH of the gastric contents to neutralize gastric secretions.
6. Mildly alkaline.
7. Simethicone is an antiflatulent. Aluminum hydroxide, magnesium oxide or hydroxide, magnesium trisilicate, and calcium carbonate all buffer gastric acidity.
8. Calcium and aluminum products may cause constipation.

10. What ingredient(s) in antacids should not be administered to patients with renal disease?
11. Define *acid rebound.*
12. Should antacids be given on an empty stomach or with food in the stomach?
13. What types of products can produce a systemic alkaline effect?
14. Patients with chronic renal failure who have hyperphosphatemia can benefit from taking which type of antacid and why?
15. What class of antibiotics, when given with antacids (Mg, Ca, or Al types), interact to result in a decrease in the absorption of the antibiotic?
16. Because antacids alter the absorption rate of digoxin and iron compounds, what dosing schedule should be used to administer antacids when these medicines are also ordered?
17. In order to obtain the most rapid onset of action, should an antacid be administered in a liquid or a tablet form?
18. Are antacid tablets recommended for the treatment of PUD?
19. Compare the actions of antihistamines and H_2 antagonists.
20. What premedication assessments should be performed for H_2 antagonists?
21. When should the H_2 antagonist agents cimetidine (Tagamet), famotidine (Pepcid), nizatidine (Axid), or ranitidine (Zantac) be administered in relation to food intake?

9. Magnesium.
10. Magnesium should not be administered to patients with renal failure because they are unable to excrete it.
11. Acid rebound is found with calcium compounds and sodium bicarbonate; acid is neutralized followed by hypersecretion of gastric acid.
12. Given on an empty stomach, the neutralizing effects of antacids last only approximately 30 minutes. With food in the stomach, the neutralizing action is extended to 2–4 hours.
13. Sodium bicarbonate (baking soda).
14. Aluminum hydroxide and aluminum carbonate gel, because the aluminum ion binds the phosphate in the gastrointestinal tract.
15. Tetracyclines.
16. Administer 1 hour before or 2 hours after the antacid.
17. Liquid form.
18. Tablets do not contain enough antacid to be effective for treatment of peptic ulcers.
19. Antihistamines block the receptor sites on target cells (e.g., arterioles, capillaries, glands) so that the histamine cannot attach there. This prevents the symptoms of an allergic reaction such as rhinorrhea and lacrimation. To be effective, antihistamines need to be taken 30–40 minutes before exposure to allergens such as pollen or as soon as symptoms first appear. Antihistamines do not have a direct effect on gastric acid secretion. H_2 antagonists (e.g., cimetidine, famotidine, nizatidine, ranitidine) block the action of histamine on the gastric acid-secreting cells (parietal cells) in the stomach.
20. See textbook, p. 533. Assess patient's mental status to detect CNS alterations, particularly with cimetidine therapy.

22. Compare the dosage and scheduling of the H_2 antagonists.
23. If antacid therapy is continued concurrently with the use of cimetidine (Tagamet), what scheduling for the antacid should be used?
24. What advantages does famotidine (Pepcid) have when compared to cimetidine (Tagamet)?
25. How does the coating agent sucralfate (Carafate) differ from histamine H_2 antagonists?
26. List the actions of gastrointestinal prostaglandins.
27. What premedication assessments should be performed before misoprostol therapy?
28. Cite the most common side effect of misoprostol therapy.
29. How can diarrhea associated with misoprostol therapy be minimized?
30. Should misoprostol be taken during pregnancy?
31. What drugs can have altered absorption as a result of a reduction in gastric acid secretions?
32. What is the more common name for the substituted benzimidazoles?
33. What is the action of the proton pump inhibitors?
34. What are proton pump inhibitors used to treat?
35. What is the ending on the generic name of all proton pump inhibitors?

21. Cimetidine, famotidine, and ranitidine are administered with food. Nizatidine may be administered with or without food.
22. Cimetidine (Tagamet) 300 mg, 4 times per day with meals and at bedtime; famotidine (Pepcid) 40 mg once daily at bedtime or 20 mg twice daily; ranitidine (Zantac) 150 mg, twice daily or 300 mg at bedtime. Nizatidine (Axid) 300 mg, PO, once daily at bedtime or 150 mg two times daily.
23. Antacids should be administered 1 hour before or 2 hours after the H_2 antagonist.
24. Famotidine is taken once daily, does not produce gynecomastia, and has fewer significant drug interactions reported with its use.
25. Coating agents do not affect the amount of hydrochloric acid secreted; they adhere to the crater of the ulcer.
26. Gastrointestinal prostaglandins stimulate GI motility, gastric acid and pepsin secretion, and protect the stomach and duodenal lining against ulceration.
27. Determine if the patient is pregnant. This drug is a uterine stimulant and may induce a miscarriage. Check pattern of bowel elimination. Misoprostol may induce diarrhea.
28. Diarrhea
29. Take misoprostol with meals and at bedtime; avoid antacids containing magnesium (e.g., Maalox, Mylanta).
30. Discontinue if that patient is pregnant.
31. Digoxin, ketoconazole, ampicillin, and iron.
32. Substituted benzimidazoles are more commonly known as *proton pump inhibitors.*
33. Proton pump inhibitors inhibit gastric acid secretion.
34. Proton pump inhibitors are used to treat severe esophagitis, GERD, gastric and duodenal ulcers, and hypersecretory disorders, such as Zollinger-Ellison syndrome. They may also be used in combination with antibiotics (e.g., ampicillin, amoxicillin, clarithromycin) to eradicate *Helicobacter pylori*, a common cause of PUD.

36. What is the action of metoclopramide (Reglan)?

35. All generic names of proton pump inhibitors end in "-prazole."
36. Metoclopramide is a gastric stimulant; as an antiemetic it blocks dopamine in the chemoreceptor trigger zone. It increases stomach contractions, relaxes the pyloric valve, and increases peristalsis in GI tract resulting in increased rate of gastric emptying and intestinal transit.

CHAPTER 33

Student Name______________________________

Drugs Used to Treat Gastroesophageal Reflux and Peptic Ulcer Diseases

Learning Activities

FILL-IN-THE-BLANK

Finish each of the following statements using the correct term.

1. Normal pH of the stomach ranges from ______ to ______ depending on the presence of food and medications.

2. Infection of the mucous wall of the stomach by ______________ ______________ is one of the causes of peptic ulcer disease.

3. The proton pump inhibitors used in the treatment of peptic ulcer disease block the formation of __________________ acid, reducing irritation of the gastric mucosa.

4. The three types of secretory cells lining portions of the stomach include the __________________, __________________, and __________________ cells.

5. __________________ coats the ulcer crater to protect it from gastric acid secretions.

6. Hypersecretion of gastric acid after taking calcium compounds and sodium bicarbonate is called ______________ ______________.

MATCHING

Match the generic drug name with its corresponding brand name. Each option will be used only once.

_____ 7. dicyclomine

_____ 8. pantoprazole

_____ 9. omeprazole

_____ 10. lansoprazole

_____ 11. esomeprazole

_____ 12. nizatidine

_____ 13. famotidine

_____ 14. cimetidine

a. Axid
b. Prevacid
c. Tagamet
d. Bentyl
e. Prilosec
f. Nexium
g. Protonix
h. Pepcid

TRUE OR FALSE

Mark "T" for true and "F" for false for each statement. Correct all false statements.

_____ 15. The parietal cells secrete intrinsic factor needed for absorption of vitamin C.

_____ 16. The enzyme amylase digests fats, and the enzyme lipase digests carbohydrates.

_____ 17. The pain associated with peptic ulcer disease is most often noted when the stomach is empty, such as at night or between meals, and is relieved by food or antacids.

_____ 18. The antispasmodic agents used in the treatment of gastroesophageal reflux and peptic ulcer disease reduce the secretion of saliva, hydrochloric acid, pepsin, bile, and other enzymatic fluids necessary for digestion and decrease GI motility and secretions.

_____ 19. Prokinetic agents are used to treat gastroesophageal reflux disease.

_____ 20. Antacid tablets are effective in treating PUD.

_____ 21. Patients with renal failure may develop hypermagnesemia if magnesium-containing antacids are taken.

_____ 22. The pH of the stomach decreases when the hydrochloric acid content is reduced.

_____ 23. Smoking causes an increase in hydrochloric acid secretion.

_____ 24. Antacids containing magnesium may be dangerous to patients with renal disease.

DRUG ACTION/SIDE EFFECTS

25. *State the action and side effects of proton pump inhibitors used in the treatment of gastroesophageal reflux and peptic ulcer disease.*

	Actions	**Side Effects**
PROTON PUMP INHIBITORS		

CHAPTER 33

Student Name ______________________________

Drugs Used to Treat Gastroesophageal Reflux and Peptic Ulcer Diseases

Practice Questions for the NCLEX Examination

_____ 1. Which one of the following statements should the nurse include when teaching about antacid therapy?
1. For indigestion, antacids should not be administered for more than 6 weeks. If after this time you are still in discomfort, notify your primary health care provider.
2. Antacid tablets do not contain enough antacid to be effective in treating peptic ulcer disease.
3. Excessive use of magnesium antacids results in constipation.
4. A common complaint of patients using large quantities of calcium carbonate antacids is diarrhea.

_____ 2. The nurse has just administered digoxin 0.125 mg PO QD at 0900 for Mr. P. He has just been ordered to receive one tablet of Ripoan three times a day. When would be the best time for the nurse to start Mr. P. on the Ripoan therapy?
1. 0900
2. 0930
3. 1000
4. 1130

_____ 3. A 60-year-old patient with a history of chronic renal failure is on high dose cimetidine therapy for the treatment of a duodenal ulcer. It is most important for the nurse to assess the patient for what side effect of this therapy?
1. Dizziness
2. Disorientation
3. Constipation
4. Diarrhea

_____ 4. Which statement made by a patient taking misoprostol for a gastric ulcer indicates that she is in need of more teaching?
1. "To minimize diarrhea associated with misoprostol therapy, I will take magnesium-containing antacids."
2. "I will not discontinue misoprostol therapy without first consulting my health care provider."
3. "To minimize diarrhea associated with misoprostol therapy, I will take it with meals and at bedtime."
4. "I understand that I should tell my primary health care provider if I am pregnant or become pregnant while on misoprostol therapy."

_____ 5. When assessing a patient who is taking a proton pump inhibitor for GERD, which of the following findings by the nurse should be reported to the primary health care provider immediately, as it may be cause for discontinuing therapy?
1. Diarrhea
2. Muscle pain
3. Persistent vesicular rash
4. Fatigue

_____ 6. It is most important for the nurse to assess the patient on metoclopramide for which of the following before initiating this therapy?
1. Allergy to penicillins
2. History of asthma
3. History of epilepsy
4. Allergy to shellfish

_____ 7. A 75-year-old patient is being evaluated for drug therapy to treat peptic ulcer disease. The nurse would expect the patient to present with which of the following symptoms? (Select all that apply.)
1. Anorexia
2. Weight gain
3. Headache
4. Vague abdominal discomfort

_____ 8. Which of the following statement(s) are correct when discussing use of antacids for the treatment of gastrointestinal disorders? (Select all that apply.)
1. Maalox is an example of a low-sodium antacid.
2. Use of an antacid with large amounts of magnesium usually results in constipation.
3. Calcium carbonate and sodium bicarbonate may cause rebound hyperacidity.
4. Patients with renal failure should not use large quantities of antacids containing magnesium.

Drugs Used to Treat Nausea and Vomiting

Review Sheet

The QUESTION column and the ANSWER column have been offset so that you can cover the answers while reading the questions, allowing you to assess your knowledge.

Question

1. What is an antiemetic?
2. What seven classes of drugs are used to treat nausea and vomiting?
3. What is the mechanism of action for the seven drug classes used to treat nausea and vomiting?
4. Name the most widely used antiemetic in the dopamine antagonist class used to treat nausea and vomiting associated with surgery, radiation, and cancer chemotherapy.
5. What is the action of metoclopramide (Reglan) on the gastrointestinal tract that makes it useful as an antiemetic?
6. When is ondansetron (Zofran) administered in relation to chemotherapy?
7. What drugs are recommended for nausea and vomiting associated with pregnancy?
8. What herbal medicine is used by some cultures to treat pregnancy-induced nausea and vomiting?
9. What are the usual nursing implementations used for an adult and for an infant experiencing nausea and vomiting?
10. What are the usual premedication assessments performed for any antiemetic?
11. Define *postoperative nausea and vomiting (PONV), motion sickness, hyperemesis gravidarum, psychogenic vomiting, anticipatory vomiting, radiation-induced nausea and vomiting,* and *chemotherapy-induced vomiting.*

Answer

1. A medication used to prevent nausea and vomiting.
2. Dopamine antagonists, serotonin antagonists, anticholinergic agents, corticosteroids, benzodiazepines, cannabinoids, and neurokinin-1 receptor antagonists.
3. See sections labeled "Action" for each drug class.
4. Prochlorperazine (Compazine)
5. Metoclopramide is thought to work as an antiemetic by blocking dopamine in the chemoreceptor trigger zone. It has also been suggested that it inhibits serotonin when administered in higher doses.
6. Ondansetron (Zofran) is administered 30 minutes before chemotherapy and at 4-hour intervals after chemotherapy for two doses.
7. Administration of meclizine, cyclizine, or dimenhydrinate is recommended first for nausea and vomiting associated with pregnancy.
8. Ginger.
9. See textbook, pp. 547-548.
10. See textbook, p. 554.

12. Summarize drug therapy for the treatment of postoperative nausea and vomiting, motion sickness, nausea and vomiting in pregnancy, psychogenic vomiting, anticipatory nausea and vomiting, chemotherapy-induced nausea and vomiting, delayed emesis, and radiation-induced nausea and vomiting.

11. See textbook, pp. 543-545.

12. See textbook, pp. 545-547.

CHAPTER 34

Student Name ____________________

Drugs Used to Treat Nausea and Vomiting

Learning Activities

FILL-IN-THE-BLANK

Finish each of the following statements using the correct term.

1. ____________________ is the involuntary labored, spasmodic contractions of the abdominal and respiratory muscles without the expulsion of gastric contents.
2. Nausea and vomiting associated with motion are thought to result from stimulation of the ____________________ system of the ear, with subsequent transmission of this stimulus to the vestibular network located near the vomiting center.
3. A pregnant woman with severe persistent vomiting that interferes with nutrition, fluid, and electrolyte balance may be experiencing ______________ ______________, a condition in which starvation, dehydration, and acidosis are superimposed on the vomiting syndrome.
4. Most agents used to reduce nausea and vomiting from motion sickness are chemically related to ____________________.
5. In many cultures, the herb ____________________ is used to treat pregnancy-induced nausea and vomiting.
6. Drugs used to treat nausea and vomiting are referred to as ____________________ agents.

MATCHING

Match the generic drug name to its corresponding brand name. Each option will be used only once.

_____ 7. prochlorperazine

_____ 8. thiethylperazine

_____ 9. trimethobenzamide

_____ 10. ondansetron

_____ 11. meclizine

a. Tigan
b. Torecan
c. Antivert
d. Compazine
e. Zofran

TRUE OR FALSE

Mark "T" for true and "F" for false for each statement. Correct all false statements.

_____ 12. There are several physiologic mechanisms of nausea and vomiting, but none are well-understood.

_____ 13. Pain not treated with appropriate analgesia induces nausea and vomiting.

_____ 14. Older adults between the ages of 60-70 years have the highest incidence of postoperative nausea and vomiting based on age groups.

_____ 15. Patients under nitrous oxide anesthesia have a higher incidence of nausea and vomiting than do those under halothane, enflurane, or isoflurane.

_____ 16. Antiemetic agents are generally more effective if administered before the onset of nausea, rather than after it has started.

DRUG ACTION/SIDE EFFECTS

17. *State the action and side effects of the serotonin antagonists used to treat nausea and vomiting.*

	Actions	Side Effects
SEROTONIN ANTAGONISTS		

CHAPTER 34

Student Name______________________________

Drugs Used to Treat Nausea and Vomiting

Practice Questions for the NCLEX Examination

_____ 1. Which one of the following statements about phenothiazine therapy for the treatment of nausea and vomiting is true?
1. Phenothiazines often cause hypertension.
2. Phenothiazines are safe to use in patients with seizure disorders.
3. A rash is a common side effect of phenothiazine therapy and does not need to be reported to the primary care provider.
4. Phenothiazines may suppress the cough reflex.

_____ 2. A patient who has just undergone an open exploratory abdominal laparotomy is ordered 200 mg of trimethobenzamide IM 3 to 4 times daily, along with her patient controlled analgesic pump. Which of the following statements about administration of this drug is true?
1. Do not use in patients allergic to benzocaine or local anesthetics.
2. Use a one-half inch needle to administer this medication.
3. Inject into the deltoid region.
4. Inject into the vastus lateralis.

_____ 3. A patient with a history of motion sickness is scheduled to be transported to another health care facility located about 90 minutes away. The primary care provider has ordered dimenhydrinate 100 mg by mouth for the patient. The patient is scheduled to depart at 0900. When should the nurse administer the dimenhydrinate for it to be most effective?
1. 0700
2. 0730
3. 0830
4. 0900

_____ 4. Which of the following agents used to treat nausea and vomiting are considered Schedule II controlled substances?
1. Cannabinoids
2. Anticholinergic agents
3. Dopamine antagonists
4. Serotonin antagonists

_____ 5. A patient is experiencing involuntary, labored, spasmodic contractions of the abdominal and respiratory muscles without the expulsion of gastric contents. The patient is experiencing:
1. constipation.
2. retching.
3. vomiting.
4. diarrhea.

_____ 6. Which of the following are expected side effects of anticholinergic agents used for the treatment of motion sickness? (Select all that apply.)
1. Diarrhea
2. Urinary retention
3. Blurred vision
4. Dry mouth

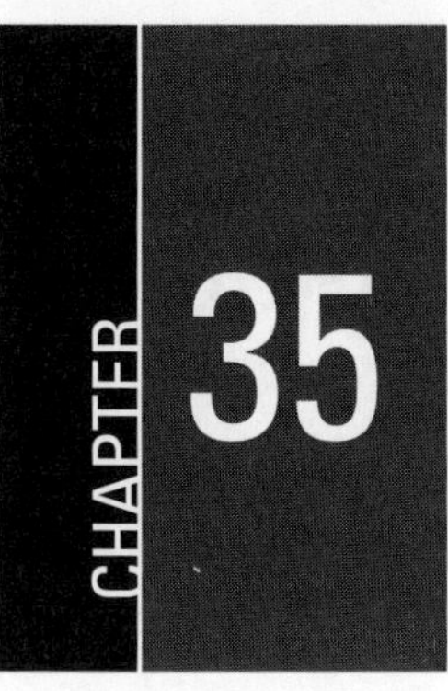

Drugs Used to Treat Constipation and Diarrhea

Review Sheet

The QUESTION column and the ANSWER column have been offset so that you can cover the answers while reading the questions, allowing you to assess your knowledge.

Question

1. What is the mechanism of action of:
   a. contact or stimulant laxatives?
   b. saline laxatives?
   c. lubricant or emollient laxatives?
   d. bulk-forming laxatives?
   e. fecal softeners?

2. What is the onset of action for:
   a. contact or stimulant laxatives?
   b. saline laxatives?
   c. lubricant or emollient laxatives?
   d. bulk-forming laxatives?
   e. fecal softeners?

3. When administering fecal softeners, what factors must be considered to promote the action of these laxative agents?

4. Differentiate between the action of systemic and local antidiarrheal agents.

5. What premedication assessments should be performed before administration of an antidiarrheal agent?

6. Examine Table 35-1 to identify the names and types of laxatives commonly prescribed and Table 35-2 for antidiarrheals prescribed.

Answer

1. a. Promote peristalsis by irritation.
   b. Attract water into intestines from surrounding tissues, promote peristalsis.
   c. Lubricate intestinal wall and soften the stool; peristalsis does not appear to be increased.
   d. Cause water to be retained in stool, thus increasing bulk that stimulates peristalsis.
   e. Draw water into stool causing it to soften. No stimulation of peristalsis.

2. a. 6–10 hours orally; 60–90 minutes rectally
   b. 1–3 hours
   c. 6–8 hours
   d. 12–24 hours, up to 72 hours
   e. up to 72 hours

3. Adequate fluid intake is essential.

4. Systemic: Decrease peristalsis and GI motility via the autonomic nervous system, allowing the mucosal lining to absorb nutrients, water, and electrolytes and leaving a formed stool from the residue remaining in the colon. Local: Adsorb excess water to cause a formed stool and to adsorb irritants or bacteria that cause diarrhea.

5. Take medication history and examine for drugs that may be contributing to the diarrhea; review for precipitating factors.

6. See textbook, pp. 565-566.

CHAPTER 35

Student Name____

Drugs Used to Treat Constipation and Diarrhea

Learning Activities

FILL-IN-THE-BLANK

Finish each of the following statements using the correct term.

1. ____________________ is the infrequent, incomplete, or painful elimination of feces.

2. ____________________ is an increase in the frequency or fluid content of bowel movements.

3. Chronic diarrhea may be one of the first symptoms of cancer of the ______________ or ________________.

4. Unless contraindicated by coexisting conditions, such as heart failure and/or renal disease, patients with constipation or diarrhea should have a scheduled fluid intake of at least _______ mL per day.

5. ____________________ are chemicals that act to promote the evacuation of the bowel.

MATCHING

Match the generic drug name with its corresponding brand name. Each option will be used only once.

_____ 6. diphenoxylate with atropine

_____ 7. opium

_____ 8. bismuth subsalicylate

_____ 9. difenoxin with atropine

a. Motofen
b. Pepto-Bismol
c. Paregoric
d. Lomotil

TRUE OR FALSE

Mark "T" for true and "F" for false for each statement. Correct all false statements.

_____ 10. Anemia can be one of the diseases that contributes to the development of constipation.

_____ 11. Habitual constipation leads to an increased incidence of hemorrhoids.

_____ 12. Using laxatives or enemas daily should be avoided because they decrease the muscular tone and mucus production of the rectum and may result in water and electrolyte imbalance.

_____ 13. Daily bowel movements are necessary for good health.

_____ 14. Diarrhea is a symptom and not a disease.

DRUG ACTION/SIDE EFFECTS

15. *State the action and side effects of the antidiarrheal agents.*

	Actions	Side Effects
ANTIDIARRHEALS		

CHAPTER 35

Student Name________________________________

Drugs Used to Treat Constipation and Diarrhea

Practice Questions for the NCLEX Examination

_____ 1. A patient who is at 30 weeks gestation complains to her primary care provider that she is extremely constipated and in need of assistance. Which of the following laxatives is most likely to be ordered for this patient?
1. Stimulant laxative
2. Saline laxative
3. Bulk-forming laxative
4. Polyethylene glycol-electrolyte solution

_____ 2. Which one of the following patients would most likely benefit from the effects of a laxative?
1. 27-year-old who has colitis
2. 49-year-old diagnosed with appendicitis
3. 34-year-old paraplegic
4. 65-year-old with gastritis

_____ 3. Which of the following medications would a 55-year-old patient recovering from a recent myocardial infarction likely receive to prevent constipation or straining at stool?
1. Stool softener
2. Saline laxative
3. Stimulant laxative
4. Bulk-forming laxative

_____ 4. A patient experiencing diarrhea with extreme pain would likely receive which of the following drugs to inhibit peristalsis and assist with the pain she is experiencing?
1. Lomotil
2. Paregoric
3. Imodium
4. Motofen

_____ 5. Which of the following antidiarrheal agents has the potential to cause a hypertensive crisis when administered with a monoamine oxidase inhibitor?
1. Bismuth subsalicylate
2. Lactobacillus acidophilus
3. Loperamide
4. Diphenoxylate with atropine

_____ 6. Which of the following statements about diarrhea is correct? (Select all that apply.)
1. It may be a defense mechanism to rid the body of infecting organisms or irritants.
2. Diarrhea is usually self-limiting.
3. It is the last symptom to develop with cancer of the colon.
4. Diarrhea is never chronic in nature.

_____ 7. The nurse may administer bisacodyl with which of the following drugs? (Select all that apply.)
1. Acetaminophen
2. Cimetidine
3. Lasix
4. An antacid

_____ 8. Which of the following statements about bulk-producing laxatives are true? (Select all that apply.)
1. Bulk-producing laxatives must be administered with a full glass of water.
2. The onset of action is usually 12 to 24 hours.
3. Bulk-forming laxatives are usually considered to be the safest laxative.
4. The laxative causes water to be retained within the stool.

CHAPTER

36 Drugs Used to Treat Diabetes Mellitus

Review Sheet

The QUESTION column and the ANSWER column have been offset so that you can cover the answers while reading the questions, allowing you to assess your knowledge.

Question

1. Diabetes mellitus is a group of diseases characterized by ____________________.
2. Summarize type 1 diabetes mellitus
3. Summarize type 2 diabetes mellitus.
4. Name some other types of diabetes that are a part of other diseases having features not generally associated with the diabetic state.

Answer

1. Diabetes mellitus is a group of diseases characterized by hyperglycemia (fasting plasma glucose >125 mg/dL) and abnormalities in fat, carbohydrate, and protein metabolism which lead to microvascular, macrovascular, and neuropathic complications.
2. Type 1 diabetes mellitus, formerly known as insulin-dependent diabetes mellitus (IDDM), affects 5% to 10% of the population. It is caused by an autoimmune destruction of the beta cells in the pancreas. It occurs more frequently in juveniles, but patients can become symptomatic for the first time at any age. The onset of this form of diabetes usually has a rapid progression of symptoms characterized by polydipsia, polyphagia, polyuria, increased frequency of infections, loss of weight and strength, irritability, and often ketosis. Since there is no insulin secretion from the pancreas, the patient requires administration of exogenous insulin.
3. Type 2 diabetes mellitus, formerly known as non-insulin–dependent diabetes mellitus (NIDDM), represents about 90% of the diabetic population. It is characterized by a decrease in beta cell activity, insulin resistance, or an increase in glucose production by the liver. Over time, the beta cells of the pancreas fail and exogenous insulin may be required. Most people with type 2 DM also have metabolic syndrome, also known as insulin resistance syndrome and syndrome X. The onset of type 2 DM is usually more insidious than that of type 1 DM. The pancreas still maintains some capability to produce and secrete insulin.

5. Summarize gestational diabetes mellitus.
6. What is impaired glucose tolerance (IGT) or impaired fasting glucose (IFG)?
7. "Polydipsia" is ____________________.
8. "Polyuria" is ____________________.
9. What are the symptoms of neuropathies?
10. What is the immediate goal for treatment of diabetes mellitus?
11. What does the treatment of type 2 diabetes mellitus require?
12. Name the four groups of oral antidiabetic agents.
13. What laboratory values of the fasting plasma glucose (FPG) are considered normal, impaired, or result in a diagnosis of type 1 diabetes mellitus?
14. What are the recommended guidelines for glucose levels while exercising?
15. What are the usual causes of hypoglycemia?
16. When should ketone testing of the urine be performed?
17. What is the difference between the glycosylated hemoglobin and fructosamine tests to measure glucose?

4. Pheochromocytoma, acromegaly, and Cushing's syndrome. Others include malnutrition, infection, drugs and chemicals that induce hyperglycemia, defects in insulin receptors, and certain genetic syndromes.
5. Gestational diabetes mellitus occurs when women have abnormal glucose tolerance during pregnancy.
6. IGT or IFG is used to describe those patients who are often euglycemic in their daily living, but develop hyperglycemia when challenged with an oral glucose tolerance test. This intermediate state between normal glucose homeostasis and diabetes is now known as *prediabetes.*
7. Increased thirst.
8. Increased frequency of urination.
9. Numbness and tingling of extremities (paresthesia), loss of sensations, postural hypotension, impotence, and difficulty controlling urination.
10. The primary treatment goal of type 1 and type 2 diabetes is normalization of blood glucose levels.
11. Oral antidiabetic agents are used in the therapy of type 2 diabetes. They are recommended only for those patients whose diabetes cannot be controlled by diet alone and who are not prone to develop ketosis, acidosis, or infections. Patients most likely to benefit from treatment are those who have developed diabetes after 40 years of age and who require less than 40 units of insulin per day.
12. Secretogogues, biguanide, thiazolidinediones, and the alpha-glucosidase inhibitors.
13. FPG less than 100 mg/dL = normal fasting glucose
    FPG at 100 mg/dL or greater but less than 126 mg/dL = impaired fasting glucose (IFG)
    See Table 36-2 for criteria for the diagnosis of diabetes mellitus.
14. Individuals should not exercise with glucose level above 250 mg/dL or less than 100 mg/dL.
15. Too much insulin, insufficient food intake to cover insulin taken, imbalances from diarrhea and vomiting, or excessive exercise without additional carbohydrate intake are common causes of hypoglycemia.
16. When serum glucose is 240 mg/dL or above, test for the presence of ketones.

18. What signs and symptoms result from peripheral vascular disease?
19. What types of visual complications are people with diabetes mellitus more susceptible to?
20. How often should people with diabetes mellitus have an eye exam?
21. How can complications of diabetes affecting the kidneys be identified?
22. What is the source of endogenous insulin? What are the primary animal sources of exogenous insulins?
23. What methods are used to produce human exogenous insulin?
24. Is insulin required for glucose transport into the brain or liver tissue?
25. Why can't insulin be administered orally?
26. Differentiate among *onset, peak*, and *duration* in relation to insulin therapy.
27. What are the most rapid-acting forms of insulin manufactured today?
28. Do short-acting, intermediate-acting, and long-acting insulins differ in terms of onset, peak, and duration of action?
29. How far in advance of a meal should a rapid-acting insulin be administered?
30. How far in advance of a meal should a short-acting insulin be administered?
31. Examine Table 36-6 in the textbook and identify compatibility of insulin combinations.

17. The glycosylated hemoglobin measures glucose control over the previous 8–10 weeks, while the fructosamine test measures the amount of glucose bonded to the protein fructosamine over the previous 1–3 weeks. Each has a benefit in measuring glucose control.
18. Cyanosis or reddish-blue discoloration in the hands, feet, and legs. Pallor and coolness in the feet and legs. Ulcerations may develop. When any circulatory impairment is found, pedal and radial pulses should be checked at least every 4 hours.
19. Blurred vision may occur with hyperglycemia. With advanced diabetes mellitus, there are changes in small blood vessels in the eyes (microangiopathies). Retinal hemorrhages, degeneration of retinal vascular tissue, cataracts, and blindness may also occur.
20. Regular eye exams to detect changes in the eye should be performed at least annually and more often as deemed appropriate by the HCP.
21. Presence of proteinuria, elevated serum creatinine, and blood urea nitrogen. People with diabetes mellitus are more likely to have urinary tract infections.
22. Endogenous insulin is produced by the beta cells of the pancreas. Synthetic insulin is the primary source of insulin for recently diagnosed diabetics. Beef and pork pancreas are the primary animal sources of exogenous insulin, but fish and sheep pancreas have been used as well.
23. Most common source of human insulin production is with recombinant DNA.
24. No
25. Insulin is destroyed by the proteolytic enzymes in the gastrointestinal tract.
26. Onset is the time required for the initial effect of insulin to occur. Peak is the time of the maximum effect of insulin. Duration is the length of time insulin remains active.
27. The most rapid-acting insulins are the insulin analogs, new synthetic forms called Lispro, Aspart, and Glulisine.
28. Yes. See Table 36-5.
29. Rapid-acting (Aspart and Lispro) are given 10–15 minutes before a meal.
30. Short-acting (Humulin R, Novolin R) are given 30 minutes before a meal.

32. What are the major advantages of insulin glargine and detemir?
33. How should insulin be stored?
34. What does "U-100" mean?
35. What kind of syringe is used to measure U-100 insulin?
36. What is the only type of insulin used intravenously?
37. Why is it important to teach the patient to rotate insulin sites within one area before proceeding to the next area on a rotation schedule?
38. What effect does the long-term use of one injection site have on insulin absorption?
39. With increased activity and exercise, what adjustment may be required in the insulin dose?

31. See Table 36-6.
32. Insulin glargine and detemir are biosynthetic long-acting insulins. They are absorbed from the subcutaneous tissue in a uniform manner without large fluctuations in insulin levels, reducing the possibility of hypoglycemic reactions. Either product is usually injected in the evening to serve as a 24-hour basal source of insulin for the body.
33. It is recommended that insulin be neither allowed to freeze nor heated above a temperature of 98°F. A general rule of thumb is that the bottle of insulin should be stored in the refrigerator (not the freezer) until opened. Because patients find it uncomfortable to inject cold insulin, the bottle may then be kept at room temperature until gone. It is recommended that once an insulin vial is opened, it should be discarded in 30 days. Even though the insulin has not "gone bad," there is concern that the contents are no longer sterile and that the vial may become a reservoir for infection, especially in patients who reuse needles. At sustained temperatures above room temperature, insulins lose potency rapidly.
34. U-100 means 100 units of insulin are contained in 1 mL of solution.
35. An insulin syringe calibrated in 100 units has been available for years; however, because U-100 = 100 units in 1 mL, a tuberculin syringe could also be used to accurately measure the dosage.
36. Regular insulin.
37. To prevent hypertrophy or atrophy of subcutaneous tissue.
38. Absorption is prolonged and control of glucose may require an increase in the insulin dose. If switching from an injection site that has been used repeatedly to one used infrequently, the dose of insulin may need to be decreased to prevent hypoglycemia. Each patient is somewhat variable, but patients may become hypoglycemic. A snack may be required to cover the action of the insulin, or the insulin dose could be reduced if the increased activity can be anticipated.

40. When are patients who are receiving rapid-acting, short-acting, intermediate-acting, or long-acting insulin most likely to develop hypoglycemia if the dose is excessive or meals are not taken as planned?
41. When are blood or urine tests for glucose performed in relation to meals and insulin administration?
42. Differentiate between the symptoms of hypoglycemia and hyperglycemia.
43. What are the treatments for hypoglycemia and hyperglycemia?
44. If uncertain whether a patient is hypoglycemic or hyperglycemic, what action should be taken?
45. Why do allergic reactions to insulins occur?
46. What complications are associated with diabetes mellitus?

39. Because of risk of hypoglycemia, the insulin dose could be reduced if increased activity can be anticipated.
40. If the patient injects insulin at 7 AM, rapid-acting insulin may induce hypoglycemia within 1–3 hrs; short-acting insulin: occurs before lunch; intermediate-acting insulin: between 3 PM and supper; and long-acting insulin: between 2 AM and breakfast.
41. 1/2 hour ac and hs
42. Hypoglycemia: rapid onset, nervousness, tremors, headache, apprehension, sweating, hunger, double or blurred vision, lack of coordination, unconsciousness. Hyperglycemia: gradual onset, increased thirst, headache, nausea and vomiting, rapid pulse, shallow respirations, acetone odor on breath, unconsciousness.
43. Hypoglycemia: If conscious and able to swallow: 2–4 oz fruit juice with 2 teaspoons sugar or honey added, or 1 cup skim milk, 4 oz nondiet soft drink, or piece of candy (not chocolate), or frosting added. If unable to swallow: 20–50 mL glucose 50% IV. Hyperglycemia: Hospitalize the patient, identify the cause, hydrate the patient and give insulin IV; stabilize electrolytes, especially potassium. See also drug monograph for glucagon.
44. Treat for hypoglycemia.
45. Allergy may be caused by a protein from the animal source of insulin (e.g., pork, beef) or from the protein modifiers used to extend the duration of insulin (e.g., isophane). An acute reaction with a rash over the entire body is a rare, but possible, symptom of an anaphylactic reaction that must be treated with antihistamines, epinephrine, and steroids. Allergic reactions can be minimized by changing to an insulin without protein modifiers or to insulins derived from biosynthetic (nonanimal) sources; by using unscented alcohol swabs. Local irritation can be minimized by using disposable syringes and needles and by checking the patient's injection technique.

47. Describe the procedure for mixing two insulins in the same syringe.
48. What effect does the administration of beta-adrenergic blocking agents concurrent with insulin have on symptoms of hypoglycemia?
49. What drug class does the drug metformin (Glucophage) belong to and what is its mechanism of action?
50. How do oral hypoglycemic agents differ from insulin?

46. Microvascular complications are those that arise from destruction of capillaries in eyes, kidneys, and peripheral tissues. Macrovascular complications are those associated with atherosclerosis of middle to large arteries such as those in the heart and brain. Comorbid diseases that often arise include hypertension; cardiovascular disease leading to myocardial infarction and stroke; retinopathy leading to blindness; renal disease leading to end-stage renal disease and the need for dialysis; peripheral arterial disease leading to nonhealing ulcers, infections, and lower extremity amputations; neuropathies with sexual dysfunction, bladder incontinence, paresthesias, and gastroparesis; and periodontal disease with loss of teeth.
47. See the text for details.
48. Beta-adrenergic blocking agents mask the signs of hypoglycemia.
49. Metformin represents a class of oral antidiabetic agents known as the *biguanides*. Metformin decreases hepatic glucose production by inhibiting glucogenolysis and gluconeogensis, reduces absorption of glucose from the small intestine, and increases insulin sensitivity improving glucose uptake in peripheral muscle and adipose cells. It may also stimulate glucose metabolism by anaerobic glycolysis. The net result is a significant decrease in fasting and postprandial blood glucose and hemoglobin A1C concentrations. Insulin must be present for metformin to be active, and therefore is not effective in type 1 diabetes.

51. Which type of diabetes mellitus requires treatment with insulin and which type may be treated with oral hypoglycemic agents?

50. For sulfonylurea oral hypoglycemic agents (e.g., chlorpropamide [Diabinese], tolazamide [Tolinase], and others), and meglitinide oral hypoglycemic agents (repaglinide and nateglinide) to be effective, the diabetic patient must still have beta cells in the pancreas that are capable of producing insulin. These agents act by stimulating the release of insulin from the beta cells. Oral hypoglycemic agents are not an oral form of insulin. The biguanide oral antidiabetic [e.g., metformin (Glucophage)], does not stimulate release of insulin from the pancreas; the mechanism of its action is as stated in the answer to question 49.

For thiazolidinedione (TZDs) oral antidiabetic agents, (pioglitazone [Actos] and rosiglitazone [Avandia]), the blood glucose is lowered by increasing the sensitivity of muscle and fat tissue to insulin, allowing more glucose to enter the cells in the presence of insulin metabolism. The antihyperglycemic agents (acarbose [Precose] and miglitol [Glyset]) inhibit the pancreatic alpha-amylase and gastrointestinal alpha-glycoside hydrolase enzymes used in the digestion of sugars resulting in delayed glucose absorption and lowering of postprandial hyperglycemia.

Exenatide is the first of a new type of agent called incretin-mimetic agents. In normal physiology, proteins known as incretin peptides are released from L-cells located in the distal ileum and colon in response to ingestion of carbohydrates and fats. The incretins help control blood glucose by enhancing insulin secretion, suppressing glucagons secretion from the liver, suppressing glucose output from the liver, delaying gastric emptying, thus slowing carbohydrate and lipid absorption, reducing postprandial hyperglycemia, reducing appetite, and maintaining beta cell function. Pramlintide is a synthetic analogue of amylin. Amylin is a protein secreted from pancreatic cells with insulin in response to food intake. Patients with a deficiency of insulin also have a deficiency of amylin. Amylin and pramlintide reduces postprandial glucose by suppressing glucagon secretion from the liver, suppressing glucose output from the liver, delaying gastric emptying, thus slowing carbohydrate and lipid absorption, reducing postprandial hyperglycemia, and suppressing the appetite with subsequent potential weight reduction.

52. For what type of allergy should you check the chart and the patient before initiating therapy with a sulfonylurea oral hypoglycemic agent?
53. What is the effect of sulfonylurea hypoglycemic agents combined with ethanol on blood glucose levels?
54. When should a diabetic patient perform urine testing for ketones?
55. What are the therapeutic outcomes expected from a biguanide oral antidiabetic agent, sulfonylurea oral hypoglycemic agents, meglitinide oral hypoglycemic agents, thiazolidinedione oral antidiabetic agents, alpha-glucosidase inhibitor agents, incretin-mimetic agents, and amylinomimetic agents?
56. What side effects can be expected with acarbose (Precose) and miglitol (Glyset)?
57. What affect can acarbose and miglitol have on digoxin absorption?
58. What is the action of glucagon?

51. Type 1 diabetes mellitus uses insulin; type 2 diabetes mellitus may be treated with diet and oral hypoglycemic agents. In certain cases, type 2 diabetes mellitus may also be treated with low doses of insulin.
52. Sulfonamides. The patient who is allergic to sulfonamides may also be allergic to sulfonylureas.
53. Hypoglycemia. Also may result in an Antabuse-like reaction manifested by facial flushing, pounding headache, breathlessness, and nausea.
54. Perform urine testing for ketones whenever the blood glucose is 240 mg/dL or above and whenever under stress or having an infection. Perform at least four times daily under these circumstances.
55. More appropriate control of FPG and glycosylated hemoglobin concentration with fewer long-term complications from poorly controlled type 2 diabetes
56. Abdominal cramps, diarrhea, flatulence. Resolves with continued use of acarbose or miglitol.
57. These drugs may inhibit digoxin absorption.
58. Glucagon breaks down stored glycogen to glucose to be used as an energy source.

CHAPTER 36

Student Name ____________________

Drugs Used to Treat Diabetes Mellitus

Learning Activities

FILL-IN-THE-BLANK

Finish each of the following statements using the correct term.

1. The category of diabetes mellitus reserved for women who show abnormal glucose tolerance during pregnancy is called ____________ diabetes mellitus.

2. ____________ is a hormone produced in the beta cells of the pancreas and is a key regulator of metabolism.

3. The most rapidly acting insulins are the insulin analogs, new synthetic forms called ____________, ____________, and ____________.

4. ____________ insulin is the only dosage form of insulin that is approved to be injected by both intravenous and subcutaneous routes of administration.

5. ____________ is a hormone secreted by the alpha cells of the pancreas that breaks down stored glycogen to glucose, resulting in elevated blood glucose levels.

6. The ____________ are nonsulfonylurea oral hypoglycemic agents that lower blood glucose by stimulating the release of insulin from the beta cells of the pancreas.

7. Insulin is required to transport glucose into skeletal and heart muscle and fat. It is not required for glucose transport into the ____________.

8. ____________ of the skin can be prevented by rotating the insulin injection sites.

MATCHING

Match the generic drug name with its corresponding brand name. Each option will be used only once.

_____ 9. tolbutamide

_____ 10. chlorpropamide

_____ 11. tolazamide

_____ 12. glyburide

_____ 13. glimepiride

_____ 14. glipizide

_____ 15. rosiglitazone

_____ 16. repaglinide

a. Prandin
b. Glynase
c. Orinase
d. Avandia
e. Amaryl
f. Tolinase
g. Diabinese
h. Glucotrol

TRUE OR FALSE

Mark "T" for true and "F" for false for each statement. Correct all false statements.

_____ 17. Diabetes mellitus is a group of diseases characterized by hyperglycemia resulting from defects in insulin secretion, insulin action, or both.

_____ 18. Type 2 diabetes mellitus was formerly known as insulin dependent diabetes mellitus (IDDM).

_____ 19. Type 1 diabetes mellitus occurs only in juveniles.

_____ 20. In Type 2 diabetes mellitus, the pancreas is not able to produce or secrete any insulin.

_____ 21. Insulin is not required for glucose transport into the brain tissue.

_____ 22. Insulin must always be stored in the refrigerator.

_____ 23. Rotation of injection sites of subcutaneous insulin is important to avoid atrophy or hypertrophy of subcutaneous fat tissue.

DRUG ACTION/SIDE EFFECTS

24. *State the action and side effects of acarbose in the treatment of diabetes mellitus.*

	Actions	Side Effects
ACARBOSE		

CHAPTER 36

Student Name______________________

Drugs Used to Treat Diabetes Mellitus

Practice Questions for the NCLEX Examination

_____ 1. A nurse administers 4 units of Lispro insulin to a patient at 0800. At what time would the patient be most at risk for the development of hypoglycemia?
1. 1000
2. 1200
3. 1400
4. 1600

_____ 2. Which of the following statements from a patient with diabetes indicates that further teaching is needed regarding insulin administration and storage?
1. "I will keep insulin I am using at room temperature."
2. "I will freeze unopened insulin bottles until I need to use them."
3. "I will roll the NPH insulin bottle between my hands before administration."
4. "I do not need to roll the Regular insulin in my hands before administration."

_____ 3. Which of the following drugs when taken with insulin is most likely to induce hypoglycemia, or may mask many of the symptoms of hypoglycemia?
1. Opioids
2. Calcium channel blockers
3. Nonsteroidal antiinflammatory agents
4. Beta-adrenergic blocking agents

_____ 4. Which of the following statements about metformin is true?
1. Metformin stimulates the release of insulin from the pancreas.
2. Metformin will not cause hypoglycemia.
3. Patients taking metformin are at high risk for rapid weight gain.
4. Patients taking metformin require blood work to assess a rapid rise in triglycerides as a result of metformin therapy.

_____ 5. A patient with ________________ is most likely to benefit from treatment with sulfonylurea oral hypoglycemic agents.
1. type 1 diabetes mellitus
2. type 2 diabetes mellitus that is not controlled by diet and exercise
3. newly diagnosed diabetes who is 18 months old
4. a current regimen of 60 units of insulin a day

_____ 6. Which of the following drugs lowers blood glucose by increasing the sensitivity of muscle and fat tissue to insulin, allowing more glucose to enter the cells in the presence of insulin for metabolism?
1. Meglitinide oral hypoglycemic agents
2. Sulfonylurea oral hypoglycemic agents
3. Biguanide oral antidiabetic agents
4. Thiazolidinedione oral antidiabetic agents

_____ 7. It is important for the nurse to inform female patients with diabetes that an alternative method of birth control should be used when taking which of the following oral hypoglycemic agents?
1. Meglitinides
2. Sulfonylureas
3. Biguanides
4. Thiazolidinediones

_____ 8. The most common side effect to expect in a patient taking acarbose for type 2 diabetes mellitus is: (Select all that apply.)
1. dizziness.
2. abdominal cramps.
3. rash.
4. headache.
5. diarrhea.
6. flatulence.

_____ 9. When teaching the patient with type 2 diabetes mellitus about health promotion, which of the following statements should the nurse include? (Select all that apply.)
1. "If you feel sick, cut your insulin dose by half."
2. "If your blood glucose is greater than 240 mg/dL, you should test your urine for ketones."
3. "Notify your primary health care provider immediately if you are unable to keep anything down."
4. "Extra insulin is often needed to meet the demands of illness, so be aware of the development of hyperglycemia which is common in patients with acute illness, injury, or surgery."

_____ 10. Which of the following statements about biosynthetic long-acting insulins glargine and detemir are correct? (Select all that apply.)
1. They have a very high risk of hypoglycemic reactions because of large fluctuations in insulin levels.
2. These drugs are always administered first thing in the morning.
3. They provide a 48-hour basal source of insulin for the body.
4. Neither insulin glargine or detemir should be mixed with other insulins.

_____ 11. Which of the following side effects of the incretin-mimetic agent exenatide are usually mild to moderate and tend to resolve with continued therapy? (Select all that apply.)
1. Nausea
2. Vomiting
3. Diarrhea
4. Hypoglycemia

_____ 12. Which of the following insulins is Regular insulin compatible with? (Select all that apply.)
1. NPH
2. Lente
3. Glargine
4. Detemir

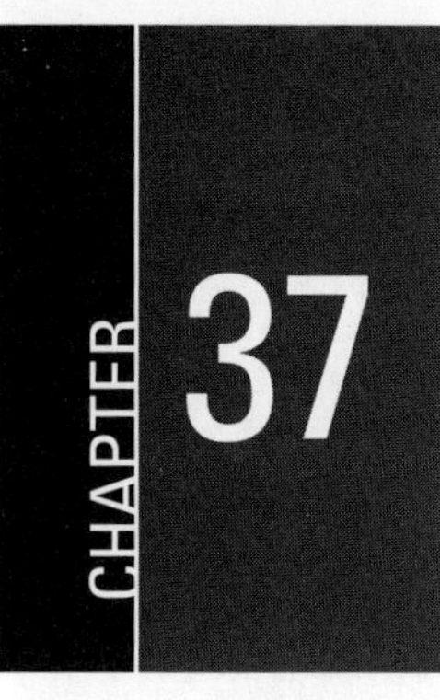

Drugs Used to Treat Thyroid Disease

Review Sheet

The QUESTION column and the ANSWER column have been offset so that you can cover the answers while reading the questions, allowing you to assess your knowledge.

Question

1. What glands regulate the function of the thyroid gland?
2. What body functions are regulated by the thyroid gland?
3. What is another name for myxedema?
4. Excessive thyroid secretion results in what conditions?
5. What is a normal thyroid state called?
6. Thyroid replacement hormones are used to replace what hormones secreted by the thyroid gland?
7. What focused assessment should be performed by the nurse when a patient has hypothyroid or hyperthyroid disorders?
8. If a patient has hypothyroidism, what change in his or her weight over the past few months could be anticipated?
9. A patient with hyperthyroidism may require what dietary changes?
10. What type of environment does a patient with hypothyroidism or hyperthyroidism need?
11. List the thyroid hormone replacement products' brand names and ingredients.
12. Of the thyroid products available, which has the most rapid onset of action?
13. Are thyroid replacement hormones given to a patient with hypothyroidism or hyperthyroidism?

Answer

1. Hypothalamus and anterior pituitary gland.
2. Growth and maturation; carbohydrate, protein, and lipid metabolism; thermal regulation; cardiovascular function; lactation; and reproduction are all processes affected by thyroid function.
3. Hypothyroidism in adult patients.
4. Hyperthyroidism, also known as *thyrotoxicosis*.
5. Euthyroid state.
6. Liothyronine (T_3) and levothyroxine (T_4).
7. See textbook, pp. 605-606.
8. Weight gain.
9. Increase in calories to meet metabolic needs—as much as 4000 to 5000 calories daily.
10. Hypothyroidism = warm environment; hyperthyroidism = cool environment
11. Levothyroxine (T_4)—(Synthroid, Levoxyl)
    Liothyronine (T_3)—(Cytomel)
    Liotrix (T_3, T_4)—(Thyrolar)
    Thyroid USP
12. Liothyronine (T_3) (Cytomel).

14. List the signs and symptoms of hypothyroidism and hyperthyroidism.
15. What are the three products available to treat hyperthyroidism?
16. State the action of propylthiouracil and methimazole.
17. Describe the desired therapeutic outcome(s) for antithyroid medications.
18. What are the side effects to assess when propylthiouracil or methimazole are administered?
19. What laboratory studies should be performed at periodic intervals for people taking propylthiouracil?
20. Would a patient with hyperthyroidism be more likely to require a smaller or larger dose of a digitalis glycoside?

13. Hypothyroidism.
14. See textbook, pp. 604-605.
15. Radioactive iodine (^{131}I), propylthiouracil (PTU, Propacil), and methimazole (Tapazole).
16. Propylthiouracil (PTU) and methimazole block the synthesis of T_3 and T_4 in the thyroid gland; the drugs do not destroy T_3 and T_4 already produced.
17. The primary therapeutic outcome expected from propylthiouracil or methimazole is a gradual return to normal thyroid metabolic function.
18. Skin eruptions, pruritus, headaches, salivary or lymph node enlargement, sore throat, purpura, jaundice, and progressive weakness.
19. RBC, WBC, and differential counts.
20. A larger dose.

CHAPTER 37

Student Name____________________

Drugs Used to Treat Thyroid Disease

Learning Activities

FILL-IN-THE-BLANK

Finish each of the following statements using the correct term.

1. ____________________ is a hypothyroidism that occurs during adult life.

2. Excessive formation of thyroid hormones and their secretion into the circulatory system causes hyperthyroidism, also known as ____________________.

3. Thyroid gland function is regulated by the ____________________ and the ________________ ________________ gland.

4. The historical name for congenital hypothyroidism is ____________________.

5. The characteristic eye changes of patients with hyperthyroidism including edema of the tissues around the eyeballs is referred to as ____________________.

MATCHING

Match the generic drug name with its corresponding brand name. Each option will be used only once.

_____ 6. levothyroxine

_____ 7. liotrix

_____ 8. liothyronine

a. Thyrolar
b. Synthroid
c. Cytomel

TRUE OR FALSE

Mark "T" for true and "F" for false for each statement. Correct all false statements.

_____ 9. A patient diagnosed with hypothyroidism will have high serum levels of circulating T_3 and T_4 hormones.

_____ 10. The thyroid gland is a large, reddish, ductless gland in front of and on either side of the trachea.

_____ 11. The thyroid hormones are triiodothyronine and thyroxine.

_____ 12. Congenital hypothyroidism is a very common disorder found today.

_____ 13. Myxedema may be caused by excessive use of antithyroid drugs used to treat hyperthyroidism.

_____ 14. Hyperthyroidism is a condition caused by excessive production of thyroid hormone.

_____ 15. Thyroid replacement hormones block the release of T_3 and T_4 in the body, thereby making the hormones available for metabolic functioning.

_____ 16. Baseline premedication assessments prior to initiation of thyroid replacement hormones are vital signs, weight, bowel elimination pattern, and laboratory studies to identify thyroid hormone levels.

_____ 17. The hypothyroid patient will be hyperactive.

_____ 18. The resting pulse rate of a hyperthyroid patient upon awakening will be low.

_____ 19. A patient with hypothyroidism would show dramatic weight loss as one of their symptoms.

DRUG ACTION/SIDE EFFECTS

20. *State the action and side effects of thyroid replacement hormones used in the treatment of hypothyroidism.*

	Actions	Side Effects
THYROID REPLACEMENT HORMONES		

CHAPTER 37

Student Name______________________________

Drugs Used to Treat Thyroid Disease

Practice Questions for the NCLEX Examination

_____ 1. Which one of the following manifestations would the nurse expect to find upon assessing a patient who has been diagnosed with hyperthyroidism?
1. Cardiac enlargement
2. Constipation
3. Subnormal body temperature
4. Puffy face

_____ 2. Ms. W. has been ordered thyroid replacement therapy to treat hypothyroidism. She has no thyroid function. She is also diabetic and is on insulin therapy. Ms. W. has multiple medical conditions requiring her to receive warfarin, digoxin, and estrogen therapy. Which of the following statements about Ms. W. and her therapeutic regimen is true? With the addition of thyroid replacement therapy, Ms. W.:
1. will most likely require a decreased dosage of the warfarin.
2. is at high risk for the development of hyperglycemia.
3. will most likely require an increased dosage of digoxin.
4. may require a decreased dosage of thyroid hormone because of the estrogen therapy.

_____ 3. Which of the following statements about iodine-131 is true? (Select all that apply.)
1. It is administered intravenously.
2. It has no color.
3. It is radioactive.
4. It is used to treat hypothyroidism.

_____ 4. A patient who has been diagnosed with hyperthyroidism has been taught about proper nutritional habits to follow. Which of the following patient statements indicate the patient is in need of additional teaching?
1. "I will limit my fluid intake to three 8-ounce glasses of water a day."
2. "I will eat a high-calorie diet, about 4000 to 5000 calories a day."
3. "I will avoid caffeinated cola."
4. "I will avoid chocolate."

_____ 5. A patient who has undergone a thyroidectomy is at greatest risk for the development of which electrolyte disturbance?
1. Hyponatremia
2. Hypokalemia
3. Hypochloremia
4. Hypocalcemia

_____ 6. Which of the following are signs and/or symptoms of hyperthyroidism? (Select all that apply.)
1. Bradycardia
2. Anxiety
3. Weight loss
4. Abdominal cramping

_____ 7. Which of the following medications has drug interactions with propylthiouracil? (Select all that apply.)
1. Acetaminophen
2. Warfarin
3. Digoxin
4. Lasix

_____ 8. Which of the following statements about myxedema is correct? (Select all that apply.)
1. The onset of symptoms is usually mild and vague.
2. It is sometimes seen in patients after radiation exposure.
3. Weight loss is a common complication of myxedema.
4. Hypertension is a common finding.

Corticosteroids

Review Sheet

The QUESTION column and the ANSWER column have been offset so that you can cover the answers while reading the questions, allowing you to assess your knowledge.

Question

1. Define *corticosteroids.*
2. For what types of illnesses are glucocorticoids frequently prescribed?
3. What endogenous hormone is known as a glucocorticoid?
4. Do exogenous corticosteroids cure disease?
5. What side effects may be observed with the administration of glucocorticoids?
6. What time of day is best to administer glucocorticoids?
7. Why do corticosteroids and diuretics produce or enhance hypokalemia when given simultaneously?
8. Why must patients taking corticosteroids be cautioned to avoid contact with people with infections?

Answer

1. Hormones secreted by the adrenal cortex of the adrenal gland.
2. To treat diseases or disorders that are inflammatory or allergic in nature. Glucocorticoids have anti-inflammatory, antiallergenic, and immunosuppressant activity. They may also be used to reduce nausea and vomiting associated with chemotherapy.
3. Cortisol.
4. Exogenous corticosteroids do not cure disease unless the adrenal glands have been surgically removed and corticosteroids are used for replacement therapy. Usually, steroids provide relief of symptoms without treating the underlying disease.
5. Hyperglycemia, glycosuria (corticosteroids stimulate formation of glucose while decreasing use of glucose by the body); electrolyte imbalances and fluid accumulation due to mineralocorticoid effects that cause sodium and water retention and potassium and hydrogen excretion; increased susceptibility to infection; peptic ulcer formation by decreasing the protective secretions of the gastric mucosa; delayed wound healing because of protein breakdown; visual changes, cataracts; osteoporosis—inhibits bone formation and growth; see textbook, pp. 620-622.
6. Between 6 AM and 9 AM to minimize suppression of normal adrenal function.
7. Diuretics (except potassium-sparing diuretics) and corticosteroids cause the loss of potassium.

9. What instructions should be given to a patient taking corticosteroids?
10. What baseline assessments should be completed for patients taking any type of corticosteroids?
11. Review the signs and symptoms of Addison's disease and Cushing's disease and contrast these with the signs and symptoms of adrenocortical excess and deficiency.
12. What effect do glucocorticoids have on blood glucose levels?
13. What type of health teaching should be done for a client receiving steroid therapy?
14. What is the major glucocorticoid secreted by the adrenal cortex?
15. Why is an alternate-day schedule for administration of corticosteroids used?
16. What effect do corticosteroids have on potassium balance?

8. Corticosteroids diminish the production of antibodies, resulting in a suppressed immune system, making the patient susceptible to infection. The anti-inflammatory properties of these drugs also mask the presence of infection. Even the slightest signs and symptoms of an infection may indicate the presence of a major infection.
9. See textbook, pp. 617-618.
10. Daily weight; blood pressure in supine and sitting position; intake and output for hospitalized patients; electrolyte studies, especially sodium and potassium; check mental status; blood glucose; signs and symptoms of infection; signs and symptoms of ulcers.
11. See a general medical/surgical nursing text.
12. Hyperglycemia.
13. Identification bracelet, *do not* suddenly discontinue drug therapy. See textbook for specific drug therapy prescribed by reviewing the drug monograph.
14. Cortisol.
15. Alternate-day schedule, between 6 AM and 9 AM, minimizes suppression of normal adrenal function. Also administer with meals to minimize gastric irritation.
16. Enhance loss of potassium. Be especially alert when diuretics such as furosemide, thiazides, bumetanide, and other non-potassium–sparing diuretics are prescribed concurrently.

Student Name______________________________

Corticosteroids

Learning Activities

FILL-IN-THE-BLANK

Fill in each of the following statements using the correct term.

1. The mineralocorticoids consist of ________________ and ________________.
2. ____________________ are hormones secreted by the adrenal cortex of the adrenal gland.
3. The two most common electrolyte disturbances associated with corticosteroid therapy are ____________________ and ____________________.
4. The major glucocorticoid of the adrenal cortex is ____________________.
5. Glucocorticoids are most frequently prescribed because of their ____________________ and ____________________ properties.

MATCHING

Match the generic drug name with its corresponding brand name. Each option will be used only once.

_____ 6. desoximetasone

_____ 7. prednisolone

_____ 8. dexamethasone

_____ 9. methylprednisolone

_____ 10. betamethasone

a. Prelone
b. Solu-Medrol
c. Celestone
d. Topicort
e. Decadron

TRUE OR FALSE

Mark "T" for true and "F" for false for each statement. Correct all false statements.

_____ 11. The glucocorticoids maintain fluid and electrolyte balance.

_____ 12. Mineralocorticoids regulate carbohydrate, fat, and protein metabolism.

_____ 13. Patients receiving corticosteroid therapy have higher incidence of peptic ulcer disease.

_____ 14. Corticosteroid therapy may induce hyperglycemia, particularly in prediabetic or diabetic patients.

_____ 15. Corticosteroids are secreted from the adrenal medulla.

_____ 16. Psychotic behavior may be seen during corticosteroid therapy.

_____ 17. Glucocorticoids taken for long-term therapy may produce cataracts.

_____ 18. Corticosteroid therapy does not mask the signs and symptoms of infection.

_____ 19. To minimize suppression of normal adrenal function, corticosteroids may be administered on alternate days.

_____ 20. Corticosteroids should not be discontinued abruptly.

_____ 21. Glucocorticoids should be administered between 6 PM and 9 PM to maintain normal adrenal function.

_____ 22. The major glucocorticoid secreted by the adrenal cortex is cortisol.

DRUG ACTION/SIDE EFFECTS

23. *State the action and side effects of glucorticoids.*

	Actions	Side Effects
GLUCOCORTICOIDS		

CHAPTER 38

Student Name________________________________

Corticosteroids

Practice Questions for the NCLEX Examination

_____ 1. It is most important for the nurse to assess for which of the following side effects in a patient taking fludrocortisone therapy for the treatment of Addison's disease?
1. Allergy
2. Sodium depletion
3. Potassium depletion
4. Hypotension

_____ 2. After a recent exacerbation of rheumatoid arthritis, the patient is taught by the nurse about the current use of glucocorticoids. Which of the following statements by the patient indicates more teaching is necessary?
1. "This drug has cured my disease."
2. "This drug is relieving the inflammation associated with rheumatoid arthritis."
3. "My fingers will not change back to normal shape due to this drug treatment."
4. "I need be aware that I am more susceptible to infections when taking these drugs."

_____ 3. A patient is ordered alternate-day therapy with methylprednisolone for treatment of lupus erythematosus, and it is anticipated that she will require long-term treatment with this medication. For the medication to be most effective, the nurse should instruct the patient to administer the once-daily methylprednisolone at what time?
1. 0800
2. 1200
3. 1400
4. 1600

_____ 4. When children are on prolonged glucocorticoid therapy, it is most important to monitor their:
1. weight.
2. skeletal growth.
3. urinary output.
4. cognitive development.

_____ 5. Patients receiving long-term therapy with glucocorticoids are at highest risk for the development of which one of the following visual disturbances?
1. Presbyopia
2. Glaucoma
3. Cataracts
4. Retinal detachment

_____ 6. Patients taking corticosteroid therapy should be instructed to call and report which of the following symptoms to the health care provider? (Select all that apply.)
1. Dyspnea
2. Productive cough
3. Worsening fatigue
4. Angina

_____ 7. Which of the following statements regarding dietary modifications for patients on corticosteroid therapy are correct? (Select all that apply.)
1. A high-sodium diet is needed when taking corticosteroids.
2. A low-potassium diet is needed when taking corticosteroids.
3. Potassium restrictions are needed for patients taking aldactone.
4. Salt substitutes are high in potassium.

_____ 8. Which of the following are expected findings when glucocorticoids are used for the treatment of rheumatoid arthritis? (Select all that apply.)
1. Relief of pain
2. Elevated sedimentation rates
3. Normalization of preexisting joint deformities
4. Increased energy

Gonadal Hormones

Review Sheet

The QUESTION column and the ANSWER column have been offset so that you can cover the answers while reading the questions, allowing you to assess your knowledge.

Question

1. What is another name for the male sex hormones?
2. What male characteristics are attributed to androgens?
3. When androgens are given to females, what effects can be anticipated?
4. Describe the effect of the administration of testosterone to boys before completion of bone growth.
5. When would androgens be prescribed for females?
6. Why is testosterone derived naturally from animal testes not administered orally?
7. What type of testosterone can be administered orally?
8. Review the uses and effects of estrogens on the body systems.
9. What are the side effects to expect and those to report for people taking estrogen products?
10. What are progestins used to treat?
11. What happens to the progesterone level if fertilization does not take place?
12. What premedication assessments should be performed prior to therapy with estrogens, progestins, and androgens?
13. What effect can androgen therapy have on calcium in patients being treated for breast cancer?
14. Identify common estrogen, progestin, and androgen medications.

Answer

1. Androgens; testosterone is the primary hormone.
2. Normal growth and development of male sex organs and secondary sex characteristics (e.g., growth and maturation of prostate, seminal vesicles, penis, and scrotum; development and distribution of male hair on the body; deepening of the voice).
3. Masculinization, if given in sufficient doses (e.g., deepening voice, hirsutism, acne, menstrual irregularity); electrolyte imbalance of Na^+, K^+, Cl^-, and Ca^{++}; gastric irritation.
4. May cause premature closure of the epiphyseal line, inhibiting normal bone growth.
5. In some types of breast cancer.
6. It is rapidly inactivated by the liver.
7. Synthetic forms (e.g., methyltestosterone, fluoxymesterone).
8. See textbook, pp. 625-627.
9. Expect: weight gain, edema, breast tenderness, nausea; report: hypertension, hyperglycemia, thrombophlebitis, breakthrough vaginal bleeding.
10. Secondary amenorrhea, breakthrough bleeding, endometriosis, and when combined with estrogen, used as an oral contraceptive.
11. Progesterone production drops and menstruation occurs.
12. See textbook: estrogens, p. 626; progestins, p. 628; androgens, p. 629.
13. Hypercalcemia.
14. Examine Tables 39-1, 39-2, and 39-3.

CHAPTER 39

Student Name ______________________

Gonadal Hormones

Learning Activities

FILL-IN-THE-BLANK

Finish each of the following statements using the correct term.

1. In addition to producing sperm, the testes produce ____________________, the male sex hormone.

2. ____________________ are other steroid hormones that produce masculinizing effects.

3. ____________________ is the female hormone that is thought to be associated mainly with body changes that favor the implantation of the fertilized ovum, continuation of pregnancy, and preparation of the breasts for lactation.

4. The gonads are called the ____________________ in males, and the ____________________ in females.

5. Androgen therapy in females produces ____________________.

MATCHING

Match the generic drug name with its corresponding brand name. Each option will be used only once.

_____ 6. estradiol

_____ 7. norethindrone

_____ 8. testosterone pellets

_____ 9. conjugated estrogens

_____ 10. norgestrel

a. Aygestin
b. Estrace
c. Premarin
d. Testopel
e. Ovrette

TRUE OR FALSE

Mark "T" for true and "F" for false for each statement. Correct all false statements.

_____ 11. Patients with diabetes mellitus who receive gonadal hormones may experience alterations in the blood glucose levels.

_____ 12. The use of estrogens during early pregnancy is contraindicated.

_____ 13. Male children receiving androgens must have the effects of the drug monitored by periodic x-ray of long bones.

DRUG ACTION/SIDE EFFECTS

14. *State the action and side effects of progestins.*

	Actions	Side Effects
PROGESTINS		

CHAPTER 39

Student Name____

Gonadal Hormones

Practice Questions for the NCLEX Examination

_____ 1. Patients taking androgen therapy are most likely to develop which of the following electrolyte disturbances?
1. Hyperkalemia
2. Hypernatremia
3. Hypocalcemia
4. Hypochloremia

_____ 2. Which of the following are indications of androgen overdose in male patients? (Select all that apply.)
1. Gynecomastia
2. Hypertension
3. Excessive sexual stimulation
4. Priapism

_____ 3. Patients taking androgens for the treatment of breast cancer are most at risk for the development of which electrolyte disturbance?
1. Hyperkalemia
2. Hypercalcemia
3. Hypernatremia
4. Hyperchloremia

_____ 4. A patient taking concurrent phenytoin and estrogens should be taught to recognize which of the following signs that indicate phenytoin toxicity? (Select all that apply.)
1. Headache
2. Nystagmus
3. Sedation
4. Lethargy

_____ 5. Which of the following patient statements indicates that additional teaching about the side effects of estrogen therapy is needed?
1. "Weight gain is an expected side effect of estrogen therapy."
2. "Breast tenderness is to be expected when I start this drug."
3. "Low blood pressure is a common side effect of estrogen therapy."
4. "If I experience any breakthrough bleeding between my menstrual periods, I will notify my primary care provider immediately."

_____ 6. Estrogen products are used for: (Select all that apply.)
1. relieving hot flash symptoms of menopause.
2. acne treatment in males.
3. advanced prostate cancer.
4. osteoporosis.

_____ 7. A female patient who has been prescribed estrogen therapy should be taught to inform their primary care provider if which of the following side effects are experienced when the medication is first started?
1. Breakthrough bleeding
2. Weight gain
3. Breast tenderness
4. Nausea

Drugs Used in Obstetrics

Review Sheet

The QUESTION column and the ANSWER column have been offset so that you can cover the answers while reading the questions, allowing you to assess your knowledge.

Question

1. Identify the factors that need to be assessed during prenatal management of a pregnant woman and during and following normal labor and delivery.
2. Describe nursing assessments and interventions needed for the pregnant patient experiencing potential obstetrical complications [e.g., infection; hyperemesis gravidarum; miscarriage; abortion; pregnancy-induced hypertension (PIH); hemolysis, elevated liver enzymes, low platelet syndrome (HELLP); and bleeding disorders].
3. How is preterm labor defined?
4. What is the fetal fibronectin test?
5. State the methods and time parameters of each approach to the termination of a pregnancy.
6. Cite the recommended times of administration for RhoGAM (human) and rubella vaccine in relation to pregnancy.

Answer

1. See textbook, pp. 633-637.
2. See text (pp. 634-635) for details of the following categories: miscarriage, placental separation and abortion, PIH, HELLP, etc.
3. See textbook, p. 635.
4. A fetal fibronectin test may be ordered to assess the presence of preterm labor in patients whose presenting symptoms are questionable, so that early interventions can be initiated when indicated to prevent preterm delivery. This test is for women with intact membranes and cervical dilatation of less than 3 cm.
5. Before 12 weeks gestation: dilatation and evacuation (D&E); 12–20 weeks gestation: saline or prostaglandin administered intra-amniotically, intramuscularly, or by vaginal suppository; intrauterine fetal death after 20 weeks gestation: prostaglandin suppositories with or without oxytocin augmentation.

7. Describe the nursing assessments and interventions used for PIH.

6. *Previous immunization.* Although there is no need to administer RhoGAM to a woman who is already sensitized to the Rh factor, the risk is no more than that when given to a woman who is not sensitized. When in doubt, administer RhoGAM.
   Before administration:
   1. Never administer the IGIM full dose or microdose products intravenously. (The IGIV full dose product may be administered intramuscularly or intravenously).
   2. *Never* administer to a neonate.
   3. *Never* administer to an Rh-negative patient who has been previously sensitized to the Rh antigen.
   4. *Confirm* that the mother is Rh negative.

   Pregnancy. Postpartum prophylaxis—one standard dose vial of IGIM intramuscularly or one standard dose vial of IGIV intramuscularly or intravenously. Additional vials may be necessary if there was unusually large fetal-maternal hemorrhage.
   Antepartum prophylaxis—one standard dose vial IM at about 28 weeks gestational age. This must be followed by another vial administered within 72 hours of delivery. After amniocentesis, miscarriage, abortion, or ectopic pregnancy—less than 13 weeks of gestation: one microdose vial IM within 72 hours; 13 or more weeks of gestation: one standard dose vial IM within 72 hours.
   Transfusion accident. Rh-negative, premenopausal women who receive Rh-positive red cells by transfusion: one standard dose vial IM for each 15 mL of transfused packed red cells.
   Idiopathic thrombocytopenic purpura:
   Before administration:
   1. *Confirm* that the mother is Rh positive.
   2. *Follow* manufacturer's instructions on dilution and administration of Rho[D] IGIV.

   IV—Initial dose: 250 units/kg as a single injection. Additional doses are dependent upon response.
   Rubella vaccine should be given to a patient whose rubella titer is low, immediately after pregnancy. She should be counseled to use birth control for at least the next 3 months.

8. State the purpose of administering glucocorticoids to certain women in preterm labor.
9. Summarize the care needs of the pregnant woman during normal labor and delivery.
10. Identify the name, dosage, route of administration, and correct time for administering oxytocic agents.
11. Describe the normal sequence of changes in the appearance of lochia during the postpartum period.
12. Summarize the immediate nursing care needs of the newborn infant following delivery.
13. Discuss the rationale for inspection of the placenta and cord following delivery of the newborn.
14. Summarize the Centers for Disease Control recommendations for prophylaxis of ophthalmia neonatorum.
15. Identify assessment data essential in detecting postpartum hemorrhage.

7. Take vital signs at regularly scheduled intervals and compare with baseline readings. Report elevations of systolic pressure of 30 mm Hg or more above the previous readings, or systolic blood pressure of 140 mm Hg or more, or diastolic pressure of 90 mm Hg or more. Edema may be present: monitor I & O and check state of hydration. Intake of 1000 mL more than the output over the preceding 24 hours is generally allowed. Perform assessment of edema: daily weights, report a weight gain of 2 or more pounds in any 1-week period. Discourage the heavy use of salt. Monitor urine for the presence of protein. Electrolyte studies should be done at regular intervals. Hematocrit will become elevated as the patient becomes dehydrated. Information from the serum estriols and L/S ratio give indications of fetal maturity. Seizure precautions: monitor for drowsiness, hyperreflexia, visual disturbances, or severe pain. Report any of these symptoms immediately. Give prescribed medications (e.g., sedatives, antihypertensives, anticonvulsants). Observe for complications (e.g., started labor, pulmonary edema, heart failure).
8. Glucocorticoids are administered IM to the woman in preterm labor to accelerate fetal lung maturation and to minimize hyaline membrane disease.
9. See textbook, p. 639, for summary of normal labor and delivery needs.
10. See textbook, pp. 647-648, for a discussion of oxytocic agents.
11. Blood-red immediately after delivery, progressing to a more watery or pinkish color.
12. See text discussion: Immediate Neonatal Care, pp. 639-640.
13. Verify presence of one vein and two arteries in the cord and inspect the placenta to be certain it is intact and no fragments or pieces have been retained.
14. See textbook, p. 640, for acceptable agents that prevent gonococcal ophthalmia neonatorum and chlamydial ophthalmia neonatorum.

16. State the drug actions and nursing assessments needed to monitor therapeutic response and development of side effects to expect or report from uterine stimulants, uterine relaxants, clomiphene citrate, magnesium sulfate, RhoGAM, and erythromycin or tetracycline ophthalmic ointment.
17. List premedication assessments needed prior to an oxytocin infusion.
18. What are signs and symptoms of fetal distress?
19. If fetal distress occurs during oxytocin therapy, what actions should be taken immediately?
20. State the primary clinical indications for use of uterine stimulants.
21. Describe specific nursing concerns and appropriate nursing actions when uterine stimulants are administered for induction of labor, augmentation of labor, and postpartum atony and hemorrhage.
22. Explain the limitations of the use of oxytocin for the purpose of initiating a therapeutic abortion.
23. Review the procedure for insertion of vaginal suppositories.

15. Fundus height and firmness, lochia color and amount, vital signs.
16. See individual drug monographs for details.
17. Maternal vital signs, especially blood pressure and pulse rate; mother's hydration status including urine output and I & O. (This will form baseline data for subsequent monitoring during drug therapy.) Monitor characteristics of uterine contractions (e.g., frequency, rate, duration, and intensity); report duration over 90 seconds. Monitor fetal heart rate and rhythm. Perform reflex testing as specified in drug monograph. Check amount and characteristics of vaginal discharge.
18. Normal fetal heart rate (120–160 beats/min); report bradycardia (below 120) or tachycardia (over 160)
19. Slow oxytocin infusion to lowest rate in accordance with hospital policy. Turn mother to left lateral position, administer O_2 by mask or cannula, call the health care provider immediately.
20. Four primary clinical uses: (1) induction or augmentation of labor; (2) control of postpartum atony and hemorrhage; (3) control of postsurgical hemorrhage (e.g., C-section); and (4) induction of therapeutic abortion.
21. Induction of labor: check vital signs every 15 minutes, use an infusion pump, monitor contractions (e.g., frequency, duration, and intensity), and fetal heart tones. Monitor for fetal distress (fetal heart rate of 160 bpm followed by bradycardia below 120 bpm). If fetal distress occurs, reduce oxytocin infusion to the slowest rate, turn mother to left lateral position, and administer oxygen. Monitor I & O of all patients receiving oxytocin and report accumulation of water by the body, known as "water intoxication."
22. Uterine smooth muscle is not very responsive to oxytocin stimulation until late in the third trimester.

24. Differentiate among the uses and actions on the uterus of dinoprostone, ergonovine maleate, methylergonovine maleate, and oxytocin.
25. Identify specific nursing assessments, interventions, and evaluation criteria used during the administration of uterine stimulants.
26. Compare the effects of methylergonovine maleate and ergonovine maleate on lactation.
27. Identify specific actions, dosage and administration, and nursing assessments needed during the use of oxytocin therapy.
28. What is the effect of oxytocin on fluid balance?
29. Compare the effects of uterine stimulants and uterine relaxants on the pregnant uterus.
30. Review the effects of adrenergic agents on beta$_1$ and beta$_2$ receptors and identify the relationship of these actions to the side effects to report when adrenergic agents are used to inhibit preterm labor.
31. What are the effects of adrenergic agents on serum glucose and electrolyte balance?

23. See Administration of Vaginal Medications in Chapter 8.
24. Dinoprostone: uterine smooth muscle stimulant. Used during pregnancy to increase the frequency and strength of uterine contractions and produce cervical softening and dilatation. Used to expel uterine contents in cases of intrauterine fetal death, benign hydatidiform mole, missed spontaneous miscarriage, and second trimester abortion.
    Ergonovine maleate, methylergonovine maleate: both stimulate contractions of the uterus. Cannot be used for induction of labor because they cause sudden, intense uterine activity. Used in postpartum patients to control bleeding and maintain uterine firmness.
    Oxytocin: stimulates smooth muscle of the uterus, blood vessels, and mammary glands. Can be used during the third trimester to initiate labor. Drug of choice to induce labor at term or to augment uterine contractions during first and second stages of labor.
25. See number 21.
26. Do not use ergonovine in patients who wish to breastfeed. Methylergonovine may be used.
27. Observe the rate of infusion of oxytocin and the fetal monitor for measurement of contractions. Assess for nausea, vomiting, fetal distress, hypertension or hypotension, seizure activity, and water intoxication.
28. Oxytocin can alter fluid balance by stimulating antidiuretic hormone, causing the body to accumulate water. Signs and symptoms include drowsiness, listlessness, headache, confusion, oliguria, edema, and in extreme cases, seizures.
29. Uterine stimulants increase uterine activity. Uterine relaxants are used to delay or prevent labor and delivery in selected patients.
30. Adrenergic or sympathetic control
    Beta$_1$: increase rate and force of heart contractions.
    Beta$_2$: relaxation of smooth muscles in bronchi, uterus, gastrointestinal tract, and peripheral vascular area. Monitor for tachycardia and hypotension.

32. Describe specific assessments needed before and during the use of terbutaline.
33. What are the baseline laboratory studies needed before the initiation of terbutaline therapy?
34. Describe the potential effects of terbutaline on the neonate.
35. For what clinical condition is clomiphene citrate used?
36. Identify the preliminary screening needed before initiation of clomiphene citrate therapy.
37. What safety precautions are needed in the event that visual disturbances occur with the use of clomiphene citrate?
38. At what specific time during the menstrual cycle can ovulation be anticipated with the use of clomiphene citrate?
39. What is the action of magnesium sulfate on the central nervous system?
40. What is the normal range of blood levels of magnesium sulfate when it is used as an anticonvulsant?
41. Prepare a list of assessments that should be implemented during the administration of magnesium sulfate to detect toxicity.
42. Explain the rationale for monitoring urine output during magnesium sulfate therapy.
43. What methods are used to assess deep tendon reflexes and what specific findings would require notification of the physician?

31. May cause hyperglycemia because of stimulation of the sympathetic system, resulting in an increase in glycogenolysis. Continuous, long-term infusions of terbutaline may also cause hypokalemia. Monitor serum electrolytes periodically.
32. Obtain baseline vital signs and weight. Monitor maternal and fetal heart rates. Perform baseline mental status assessment (e.g., alertness, orientation, anxiety level, muscle strength, tremors). Monitor diabetic patients for hyperglycemia.
33. Serum glucose, chloride, sodium, potassium, hematocrit, and carbon dioxide before initiation of therapy.
34. Neonatal adverse effects include hyperglycemia followed by hypoglycemia, hypotension, hypocalcemia, and paralytic ileus.
35. It is used to induce ovulation in women who are not ovulating because of reduced circulating estrogen levels.
36. A complete physical exam must rule out other pathologic causes for lack of ovulation.
37. See a health care provider for an eye exam. Avoid tasks requiring visual acuity (e.g., driving or operating power machinery). Visual disturbances usually subside in a few days to weeks following discontinuation of the medication.
38. Usually 6–10 days after the last dose of medication.
39. It depresses the central nervous system (CNS) and blocks peripheral nerve transmission, causing muscle relaxation.
40. 4–8 mEq/L.
41. Deep tendon reflexes: Patellar reflex qh (IV), or before every dose (IM). Hourly urine output: report output of less than 30 mL/hour or less than 100 mL/4 hours. Vital signs: take every15–30 minutes. Respirations must be at least 16/minute before further doses are administered. If blood pressure drops, do not administer another dose.
Fetal distress: do not administer. Mental status: check orientation and alertness before initiating therapy.
42. With reduced urine output, toxicity is more likely to occur.

44. Identify treatment for magnesium sulfate toxicity.
45. Describe specific procedures and precautions needed during the intravenous administration of magnesium sulfate.
46. What nursing assessments are needed to monitor infants born to mothers receiving magnesium sulfate?
47. What emergency supplies should be available in the immediate vicinity during magnesium sulfate therapy?
48. What are the action and purpose of administration of RhoGAM?
49. Identify the specific dosage, administration precautions, and proper timing of the administration of RhoGAM.
50. State the appropriate treatment of fever, arthralgia, and generalized aches and pains that can be anticipated following RhoGAM administration.
51. What is the purpose of erythromycin ophthalmic ointment?
52. Describe the specific procedures used to instill erythromycin ophthalmic ointment.
53. What is the causative organism of ophthalmia neonatorum?
54. Explain the rationale for administering phytonadione to the neonate.
55. What is the preferred site for intramuscular administration of vitamin K to a neonate?
56. Review the anatomical structures associated with the administration of intramuscular medications in an infant.
57. What side effects to report are associated with phytonadione therapy?

43. See text on Deep Tendon Reflex, p. 649.
44. Administer calcium gluconate 10%. Stop magnesium infusion.
45. Use an infusion pump. Periodic neurologic exam, I & O, fetal assessment, vital signs.
46. Monitor for hyporeflexia and respiratory depression. May also be hypotensive.
47. Calcium gluconate 10% solution ready for IV administration. Ambu bag, in case of respiratory depression. Discontinue the IV infusion.
48. It is used to prevent Rh immunization of the Rh– patient exposed to Rh+ blood as a result of a transfusion accident, during termination of pregnancy, or as a result of a delivery of an Rh+ infant. Action: prevents Rh hemolytic disease in subsequent delivery. Also used in the treatment of idiopathic thrombocytopenic purpura.
49. See drug monograph, pp. 653-654.
50. Use acetaminophen, not aspirin or other anti-inflammatory agents.
51. Used prophylactically to prevent ophthalmia neonatorum caused by *Neisseria gonorrhoeae* or *Chlamydia trachomatis.*
52. See Therapeutic Outcomes, textbook p. 654.
53. *Neisseria gonorrhoeae* or *Chlamydia trachomatis.*
54. Newborns are often deficient in bacteria to produce vitamin K. They are also deficient in clotting factors and are more susceptible to hemorrhagic disease.
55. Lateral aspect of the thigh.
56. See Parenteral Medications and Administration: Intradermal, Subcutaneous, and Intramuscular Routes in Chapter 11.
57. Bruising, hemorrhage, petechiae, bleeding from any site or orifice.

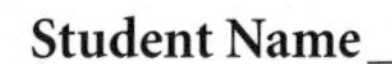

Student Name ______________________________

CHAPTER 40

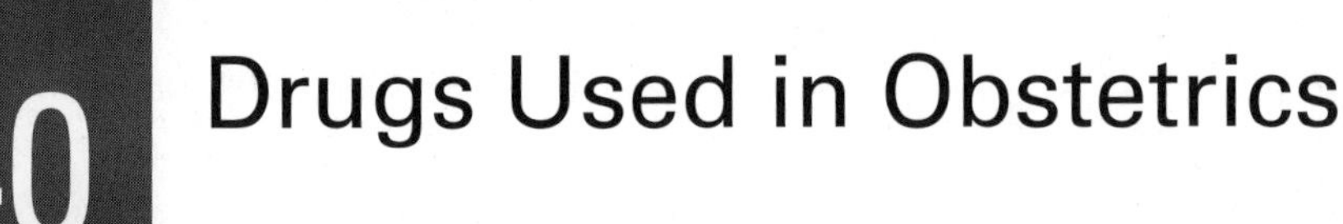

Drugs Used in Obstetrics

Learning Activities

FILL-IN-THE-BLANK

Finish each of the following statements using the correct term.

1. ______________ ______________ is the term used to describe persistent severe vomiting associated with pregnancy.

2. The health status of the neonate is estimated at 1 minute and 5 minutes after delivery using the ____________________ rating system.

3. An Rh-negative mother may receive Rho(D) immune globulin within __________ hours of the completion of the pregnancy.

4. On delivery, the breasts secrete a thin yellow fluid called ____________________.

5. ____________________ is a hormone produced in the hypothalamus and stored in the pituitary that when released, it stimulates the smooth muscle of the uterus, blood vessels, and the mammary glands.

6. Oxytocin infusions should be monitored by both a ____________________ (an instrument that measures uterine contractions) and a fetal heart monitor.

7. Normal fetal heart rate is between __________ to __________ beats per minute.

8. ____________________ is the most common electrolyte imbalance associated with terbutaline sulfate therapy.

9. RhoGAM is given to an Rh-________________ mother.

10. An adverse effect of ____________________ is water intoxication.

MATCHING

Match the generic drug name with its corresponding brand name. Each option will be used only once.

_____ 11. ergonovine maleate

_____ 12. oxytocin

_____ 13. terbutaline sulfate

_____ 14. clomiphene citrate

_____ 15. phytonadione

a. Pitocin
b. Clomid
c. Methergine
d. AquaMEPHYTON
e. Brethine

TRUE OR FALSE

Mark "T" for true and "F" for false for each statement. Correct all false statements.

_____ 16. Treatment of preterm labor often includes administration of uterine relaxants such as terbutaline and magnesium sulfate.

_____ 17. It is a legal requirement that every newborn baby's eyes be treated prophylactically for *Neisseria gonorrhoeae.*

_____ 18. In general, oxytocin should not be used to hasten labor.

_____ 19. Temperature elevations to approximately 38°C (100.6°F) occurring within 15 to 45 minutes and continuing for up to 6 hours are expected side effects of dinoprostone therapy.

_____ 20. Ergonovine therapy plays an active role in cervical softening and dilation unrelated to uterine muscle stimulation.

_____ 21. Methylergonovine is used for the induction of labor.

_____ 22. Ergonovine should not be used in patients who wish to breastfeed.

_____ 23. Oxytocin is the drug of choice for inducing labor at term and for augmenting uterine contractions during the first and second stages of labor.

DRUG ACTION/SIDE EFFECTS

24. *State the action and side effects of oxytocin.*

	Actions	Side Effects
OXYTOCIN		

CHAPTER 40

Student Name____

Drugs Used in Obstetrics

Practice Questions for the NCLEX Examination

_____ 1. A patient in her third trimester of pregnancy at 36 weeks gestation is ordered to receive dinoprostone transvaginally to continue cervical ripening. Which of the following practices should the nurse follow when administering this medication?
1. Place dinoprostone in the anterior fornix of the vagina.
2. Remove the dinoprostone at the onset of labor.
3. Warm the dinoprostone to body temperature before insertion.
4. Have the patient remain supine for 15 minutes after insertion of the dinoprostone and then have her ambulate.

_____ 2. Ms. A. is receiving an infusion of oxytocin to induce labor. Upon assessing Ms. A. and the fetal monitor, the nurse determines the infant is in distress. Which of the following actions should the nurse take? (Select all that apply.)
1. Turn Ms. A. to the right lateral position.
2. Notify the primary health care provider immediately.
3. Reduce the oxytocin infusion to the slowest possible rate according to hospital policy.
4. Administer oxygen by nasal cannula or face mask.

_____ 3. Which of the following activities should the nurse perform to administer Pitocin for the induction of labor?
1. Position the patient in the lithotomy position for ease of insertion.
2. Prepare the patient for general anesthesia.
3. Set up an IV pole to administer the Pitocin via gravity drip.
4. Administer Pitocin via a constant infusion pump to control the rate of administration.

_____ 4. When working with patients receiving oxytocin therapy, the nurse must assess for the development of water intoxication because oxytocin therapy causes:
1. extreme thirst in patients.
2. hypocalcemia.
3. stimulation of antidiuretic hormone.
4. hypertension.

_____ 5. A patient received oxytocin to induce labor and delivered a healthy baby. The nurse should ascertain whether the patient received __________ during the labor and delivery process in order to assess for possible complications.
1. antibiotics
2. a local anesthetic containing epinephrine
3. a Foley catheter
4. solid food

_____ 6. Which of the following side effects should the nurse assess for in a preterm neonate whose mother received terbutaline sulfate for treatment of preterm labor? (Select all that apply.)
1. Paralytic ileus
2. Hypoglycemia
3. Hyperglycemia
4. Hyperkalemia

_____ 7. A patient is receiving magnesium sulfate to inhibit preterm labor. The nurse should have which one of the following drugs readily available if magnesium intoxication should occur?
1. Atropine
2. Epinephrine
3. Calcium gluconate
4. Potassium chloride

_____ 8. A patient has been ordered Rho(D) immune globulin after delivery of her baby boy. Which of the following actions should the nurse take?
1. Confirm that the mother is Rh negative.
2. Administer the Rho(D) immune globulin to the baby and mother.
3. Ensure that the mother is not allergic to eggs.
4. Administer IGIM full-dose intravenously to the mother.

_____ 9. Which of the following statements about erythromycin ophthalmic ointment use in the care of the neonate is true?
1. Administer the ointment from the outside of the eye in towards the nose.
2. Instill a ribbon of the ointment along the upper conjunctival surface.
3. Administer the ointment within 2 hours of birth.
4. Irrigate the eyes after instillation.

_____ 10. Phytonadione is administered to the newborn via which route?
1. Intravenous
2. Intramuscular
3. Subcutaneous
4. Oral

_____ 11. Which of the following is considered to be a clinical indication for the use of uterine stimulants? (Select all that apply.)
1. Induction or augmentation of labor
2. Control of postpartum atony and hemorrhage
3. Control of postsurgical hemorrhage, as in cesarean birth
4. Induction of therapeutic abortion

_____ 12. A baby whose mother received magnesium sulfate is at risk for the development of which of the following complications? (Select all that apply.)
1. Hyperglycemia
2. Hypotension
3. Hyporeflexia
4. Respiratory depression

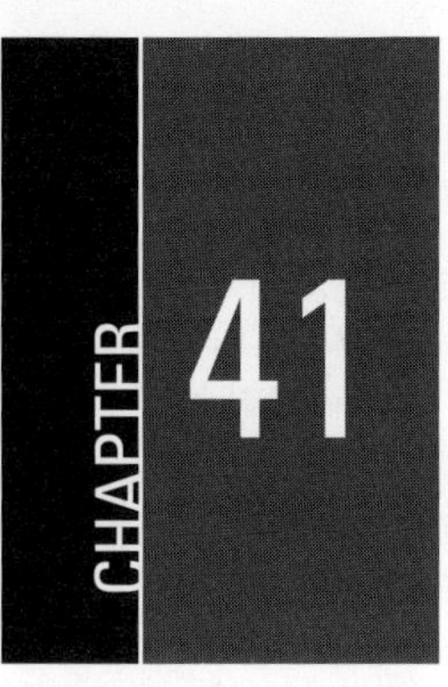

Drugs Used in Men's and Women's Health

Review Sheet

The QUESTION column and the ANSWER column have been offset so that you can cover the answers while reading the questions, allowing you to assess your knowledge.

Question

1. Define *leukorrhea.*
2. What types of infection are known to develop in the mouth, gastrointestinal tract, or vagina with the use of broad-spectrum antibiotics?
3. List the diseases collectively known as sexually transmitted diseases (STDs).
4. Identify the components of a female and/or male reproductive history.
5. What history of drug use would be of significance in a medication history and should be reported to the health care provider?
6. List laboratory studies used to detect infection in the male or female reproductive system.
7. Identify basic hygiene measures that should be taught to men and women.
8. Explain in detail the proper method of applying vaginal medications topically or intravaginally and discuss medication regimens used for both partners in a sexual relationship.
9. How is a psychosocial assessment that focuses on obtaining data related to STDs completed?
10. Compare the active ingredients of combination and progestin-only oral contraceptive agents.
11. Differentiate between the actions and the benefits of the combination pill and the minipill oral contraceptives.

Answer

1. Leukorrhea is an abnormal, usually whitish, vaginal discharge.
2. *C. albicans* and others, listed in Table 41-2.
3. See Box 41-1, p. 658.
4. See textbook, pp. 658-660.
5. Steroids, antibiotics, illegal drugs, allergies, and previous drug treatment of the same condition.
6. See textbook, p. 660.
7. See textbook, pp. 661-662.
8. See Patient Education and Health Promotion, Medications, textbook, p. 662.
9. See textbook, p. 660.
10. See textbook, pp. 662-663.

12. Describe the major adverse effects of and contraindications for the use of oral contraceptives.
13. Develop a specific education plan for teaching patients about oral contraceptives.
14. What medications, when combined with oral contraceptive therapy, require the use of an alternate form of contraceptive therapy?
15. What herbal product may reduce the effectiveness of oral contraceptives?
16. Explain how the transdermal contraceptive, ethinyl estradiol/norelgestromin (Ortho-Evra) is applied and the patient teaching that should be done regarding its use.
17. What drugs are contained in the vaginal ring (NuvaRing)?
18. Describe the procedure for insertion of the NuvaRing.
19. Explain the health teaching that should be initiated when the NuvaRing is prescribed.
20. What side effects need to be reported with the use of the NuvaRing?
21. Differentiate between the symptoms of obstructive and irritative benign prostatic hypertrophy (BPH).
22. Describe the medical treatment of BPH.

11. The combination pill prevents conception by inhibiting ovulation, making the cervical mucus thick and inhibiting sperm migration, and impairing implantation of the fertilized ovum. A new form of combination oral contraceptive was marketed in 2005 under the brand name Seasonale. Seasonale reduces the number of yearly menstrual periods from 13 to 4, so women menstruate only once every season. The minipill prevents conception through progestin activity on cervical mucus, uterine and fallopian transport, and implantation. Other mechanisms also contribute to preventing implantation.
12. Diseases that may be aggravated by oral contraceptive therapy include hypertension, gallbladder disease, diabetes mellitus, severe varicose veins, seizure disorders, oligomenorrhea or amenorrhea, and rheumatic heart disease. Side effects common with oral contraceptive therapy are nausea, headache, weight gain, spotting, depression, fatigue, chloasma, yeast infections, vaginal itching or discharge, and changes in libido.
13. See textbook, Nursing Process for Oral Contraceptives: Instructions for Using Combination Oral Contraceptives, pp. 663-667.
14. See textbook, pp. 668-669.
15. St. John's wort.
16. See textbook, pp. 669-670. Patients should be advised that in November 2005, the FDA issued a cautionary note about greater exposure to estrogens from the patch compared to taking a similar oral contraceptive tablet product. In general, increased estrogen exposure may increase the risk of blood clots.
17. Ethinyl estradiol (an estrogen) and norelestromin (a progestin) are contained in the NuvaRing.
18. See textbook, pp. 671-672.
19. See textbook, pp. 671-672.
20. Vaginal discharge, breakthrough bleeding, yeast infection, blurred vision, severe headaches, dizziness, leg pain, chest pain, shortness of breath, or acute abdominal pain.
21. See Table 41-6, p. 673.

23. What is androgenetic alopecia?
24. What premedication assessments should be made prior to administering $alpha_1$-adrenergic blocking agents and antiandrogen agents?
25. Define *erectile dysfunction* and differentiate between vascular, neurologic, and psychologic causative factors.
26. Why is it important to check for a history of cardiovascular disease before initiating sildenafil (Viagra) therapy?
27. What is the time of onset and duration of action of sildenafil?

22. $Alpha_1$-adrenergic blocking agents and alfuzosin or tamsulosin are used to relax the smooth muscle of the bladder and prostate. Antiandrogen agents such as finasteride and dutasteride selectively block androgens at the prostate cellular level and cause the prostate gland to shrink. Recent studies indicate that a combination of an alpha blocker with a 5-alpha reductase inhibitor is more effective in slowing the progression of BPH than either agent alone.
23. Male pattern baldness. Elevated dihydrotestosterone (DHT) induces androgenetic alopecia.
24. See textbook, pp. 673-675.
25. See textbook, p. 676.
26. Sildenafil can cause fatal interactions with nitroglycerin or isosorbide. Always check with the physician if a patient has any history of cardiovascular disease before initiating therapy.
27. Take 30 minutes to 4 hours before sexual activity; erectile function lasts for an hour or more, but is highly variable and dependent on a number of factors.

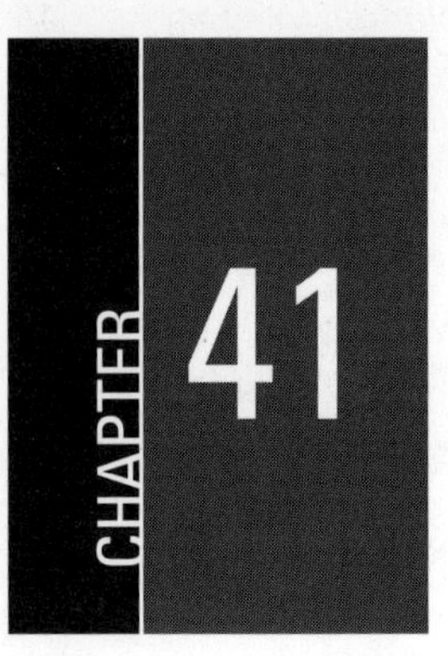

Student Name____

Drugs Used in Men's and Women's Health

Learning Activities

FILL-IN-THE-BLANK

Finish each of the following statements using the correct term.

1. ____________________ is usually an excessive whitish vaginal discharge that may occur at any age affecting almost all females at some time in their lives.

2. Men having homosexual relationships and people who inject drugs should be vaccinated for hepatitis ____________________.

3. ____________________ is manifested by irregular periods, infrequent periods, and spotting between periods.

4. St. John's wort may ____________________ the liver's metabolism of oral contraceptive hormones, possibly resulting in a ____________________ in contraceptive effect.

5. A condition called enlarged prostate, ____________________, or BPH is common in later life, affecting more than half of men in their 60s and as much as 90% of men in their 70s and 80s.

MATCHING

Match the generic drug name with its corresponding brand name. Each option will be used only once.

_____ 6. cefixime

_____ 7. acyclovir

_____ 8. metronidazole

_____ 9. doxycycline

_____ 10. miconazole

_____ 11. levofloxacin

a. Levaquin
b. Flagyl
c. Suprax
d. Micatin
e. Vibramycin
f. Zovirax

TRUE OR FALSE

Mark "T" for true and "F" for false for each statement. Correct all false statements.

_____ 12. The consistent use of male latex condoms significantly reduces the risk of HIV infection in men and women and of gonorrhea in men, but male condoms may be less effective in protecting against STDs that are transmitted by skin-to-skin contact because the infected areas may not be covered by the condom.

_____ 13. The reporting requirements to the health department of individual cases of syphilis, gonorrhea, and Chlamydia vary from state to state.

_____ 14. Many of the adverse effects of combination-type contraceptives are caused by the estrogen component of the tablet.

_____ 15. Because of a possibility of birth defects, the pill should be discontinued for one month before attempting pregnancy.

_____ 16. There is a higher incidence of ectopic pregnancy with the minipill because it does not inhibit ovulation in all women.

_____ 17. Erectile dysfunction is an inevitable outcome of aging.

DRUG ACTION/SIDE EFFECTS

18. *State the action and side effects of sildenafil.*

	Actions	Side Effects
SILDENAFIL		

CHAPTER 41

Student Name______________________________

Drugs Used in Men's and Women's Health

Practice Questions for the NCLEX Examination

_____ 1. After insertion of a vaginal medication (cream or suppository) the nurse should instruct the woman to remain in a recumbent position for at least _____ minutes to allow time for drug absorption.
1. 5
2. 10
3. 20
4. 30

_____ 2. Which patient statement regarding the use of combination oral contraceptives indicates that patient education has been effective?
1. "I will start the first pill on the first day my period begins."
2. "I will use another form of birth control during the first month."
3. "If I miss one pill, I will take two pills as soon as I remember and two the next day."
4. "I will take one pill in the morning one day, and the next day I will take the pill in the evening to rotate times the pill is taken."

_____ 3. In teaching a patient about the use of norelgestromin-ethinyl estradiol transdermal system, the nurse should include which of the following statements? (Select all that apply.)
1. "Trim the patch to best fit the area where you wish to apply it."
2. "Do not place the patch on your breast."
3. "Avoid lotions or creams in the areas of the skin where the patch is applied because the patch may not adhere properly."
4. "If the patch is partially detached for less than 24 hours, try to reapply it in the same place or replace it with a new patch immediately."

_____ 4. Which of the following statements about tamsulosin therapy is true?
1. The initial doses of tamsulosin may cause hypertension.
2. To decrease adverse effects of initial tamsulosin therapy, the drug should be given without food.
3. Initial doses of tamsulosin should be 4 mg.
4. Patients may experience dizziness, tachycardia, and fainting with initial doses of tamsulosin.

_____ 5. The primary action of tamsulosin in the treatment of benign prosthetic hyperplasia is:
1. blockage of beta stimulation.
2. inhibition of testosterone synthesis.
3. muscle relaxation of the bladder neck allowing greater urinary outflow.
4. reduction in prostate size.

_____ 6. Which of the following statements about sildenafil therapy is true?
1. If a patient is taking sildenafil, he should not take nitroglycerin therapy for the treatment of angina.
2. Nitrates from food sources react with sildenafil.
3. Higher doses of sildenafil therapy may be necessary with concurrent use of cimetidine.
4. Sildenafil therapy often causes patients to develop glaucoma.

Drugs Used to Treat Disorders of the Urinary System

Review Sheet

The QUESTION column and the ANSWER column have been offset so that you can cover the answers while reading the questions, allowing you to assess your knowledge.

Question

1. Differentiate among pyelonephritis, cystitis, prostatitis, and urethritis.
2. Identify the components of an assessment of the urinary tract.
3. Why is the use of strict aseptic technique needed with indwelling catheters?
4. In older adults, what is a common sign of a UTI?
5. Study Table 42-1 to identify details found on a routine urinalysis report.
6. What measures should be taught to prevent UTIs?
7. Should a urine specimen for bacterial culture and sensitivity be collected before or after starting antimicrobial therapy?
8. What health teaching should be completed when a patient has a UTI?
9. What is the action of a urinary antimicrobial agent?
10. What criteria are used to select a urinary antimicrobial agent?
11. What is the mechanism of action of fosfomycin (Monurol)?

Answer

1. Pyelonephritis is kidney infection, cystitis is bladder infection, prostatitis is prostate gland infection, and urethritis is infection of the urethra.
2. See textbook, p. 681.
3. To prevent urinary tract infections (UTIs).
4. Confusion.
5. See Table 42-1, textbook p. 682.
6. Personal hygiene measures—wiping front to back in females, keeping perineal area clean, avoiding nylon underwear and constrictive clothing in perineal area, avoiding scented bubble bath products and colored toilet paper, washing the perineal area immediately before and after intercourse, and urinating after intercourse.
7. Before giving the first dose of an antimicrobial agent.
8. Force fluids, 2000 mL or more per day. Continue medication for the entire course of treatment, even if symptoms have subsided fairly rapidly. Return for urine culture when scheduled. Have patient report perineal itching, vaginal discharge, or breakdown of tissue. Teach the patient ways to prevent future infections.
9. It is an antimicrobial agent that, if sufficiently concentrated in the urine, has an antiseptic effect on the urine and the urinary tract.
10. Identification of the specific pathogen by gram stain or urine culture and sensitivity.

12. What are the desired therapeutic outcomes of therapy with quinolone-type drugs?
13. Why are some urinary antimicrobial agents prescribed to be taken after the urine culture is sterile?
14. What drug class is approved for one-dose treatment of UTIs?
15. Identify premedication assessments used for quinolone therapy.
16. How is fosfomycin (Monurol) administered?
17. What are the major advantages of norfloxacin over other quinolones for the treatment of UTIs?
18. What type of anemia precludes the use of quinolone antibiotics?
19. Why must the urine be acidic during the administration of methenamine mandelate (Mandelamine)?
20. Urine pH should be maintained below what value for optimal results from methenamine mandelate therapy?
21. How is urinary tract acidification accomplished?
22. What drugs cause alkalinization of the urine?
23. What color change in the urine may occur with nitrofurantoin therapy?
24. Which urinary antimicrobial agent is more likely to cause photosensitivity?
25. Name two medicines that may be used in nonobstructive urinary retention (e.g., postoperatively, during postpartum period).
26. What drug should be readily available for treatment of serious adverse effects of bethanechol?
27. What is oxybutynin chloride (Ditropan) used to treat?
28. Name a urinary analgesic and describe its action.
29. What changes in urine color can often occur following the administration of phenazopyridine?

11. Inhibits bacterial cell wall synthesis and reduces adherence of bacteria to epithelial cells of urinary tract.
12. Resolution of the urinary tract infection.
13. To prevent recurrence of a urinary tract infection.
14. Fosfomycin antibiotics (Monurol).
15. See textbook, p. 685.
16. Empty entire contents of single-dose packet into 3–4 oz of water (not hot), stir to dissolve, and ingest immediately.
17. It is broad-spectrum with activity against gram-positive and -negative microorganisms. It also can be administered orally to patients.
18. Glucose-6-phosphate dehydrogenase deficiency.
19. For methenamine mandelate (Mandelamine) to be effective it must be converted to formaldehyde to suppress the growth of bacteria. The urine has to be acidic for this reaction to occur. Therefore, the patient may have vitamin C prescribed simultaneously for this purpose.
20. When the pH is above 5.5, methenamine is less likely to be converted to formaldehyde. Therefore, pH needs to be maintained at 5.5 or below.
21. Vitamin C.
22. Acetazolamide and sodium bicarbonate.
23. Urine may become tinted yellow to rust-brown.
24. Nalidixic acid (NegGram)
25. Bethanechol chloride (Urecholine) and neostigmine (Prostigmin).
26. Atropine sulfate.
27. Ditropan is a bladder antispasmodic.
28. Phenazopyridine hydrochloride (Pyridium) acts as a local anesthetic on the mucosa of the ureters and bladder, reducing spasm.

30. What are the three primary symptoms of overactive bladder syndrome?
31. What class of drugs are used to treat overactive bladder syndrome?
32. What is the action of the anticholinergic agents used in the treatment of overactive bladder syndrome?

29. Reddish-orange urine. Inform the patient not to be alarmed.
30. Frequency, urgency, and urinary incontinence.
31. Anticholinergic agents are the drugs of choice.
32. The anticholinergic agents are also known as *urinary antispasmodic agents.* They block the cholinergic receptors of the detrusor muscle of the bladder causing relaxation. They decrease involuntary contractions of the detrusor muscle and improve bladder volume capacity.

CHAPTER 42

Student Name ______________________

Drugs Used to Treat Disorders of the Urinary System

Learning Activities

FILL-IN-THE-BLANK

Finish each of the following statements using the correct term.

1. The normal amount of protein expected in a urinalysis is _____ to _____.

2. Oxybutynin chloride is a(n) ____________________ agent that acts directly on the smooth muscle of the bladder.

3. ____________________ is the first antibiotic agent to be approved as a single-dose treatment for urinary tract infections.

4. Patients taking phenazopyridine hydrochloride should be cautioned that their urine will become ____________________ in color.

5. The organism ____________________ accounts for about 80% of noninstitutionally acquired uncomplicated urinary tract infections.

6. In the presence of acidic urine, methenamine mandelate (Mandelamine) forms ____________________.

7. In order for methenamine mandelate (Mandelamine) to be active, the urine must be at a pH of _____ or below.

8. Oxybutynin chloride (Ditropan) is used to treat bladder ____________________.

MATCHING

Match the generic drug name with its corresponding brand name. Each option will be used only once.

_____ 9. fosfomycin

_____ 10. bethanechol chloride

_____ 11. phenazopyridine hydrochloride

_____ 12. oxybutynin

_____ 13. tolterodine

a. Ditropan
b. Urecholine
c. Detrol
d. Pyridium
e. Monurol

TRUE OR FALSE

Mark "T" for true and "F" for false for each statement. Correct all false statements.

_____ 14. The incidence of urinary tract infections in women is approximately 10 times higher than in men.

_____ 15. Patients with pyelonephritis have an infection of the bladder.

_____ 16. Phenazopyridine relieves burning, pain, urgency, and frequency associated with urinary tract infections.

_____ 17. Nitrofurantoin is an antibiotic that is not effective against microorganisms in the blood or in tissues outside the urinary tract.

_____ 18. Urinary tract infections are second only to upper respiratory infections as a cause of morbidity from infection.

_____ 19. Nitrofurantoin is an effective antibiotic for systemic infections.

DRUG ACTION/SIDE EFFECTS

20. *State the action and side effects of tolterodine.*

	Actions	Side Effects
TOLTERODINE		

CHAPTER 42

Student Name______________________________

Drugs Used to Treat Disorders of the Urinary System

Practice Questions for the NCLEX Examination

_____1. Which of the following statements should the nurse include when teaching a patient about fosfomycin therapy?
1. "This medication will treat bladder and kidney infections."
2. "If you should experience nausea after taking the fosfomycin, notify your health care provider at once."
3. "Dissolve the fosfomycin in 3 to 4 ounces of water and drink immediately."
4. "To consume the fosfomycin, sprinkle the contents of the packet on dry toast or cereal and take it in its dry form."

_____2. A patient has a history of diabetes mellitus which requires him to have Clinitest to measure urine glucose, a duodenal ulcer requiring sucralfate therapy, and he is on warfarin therapy for a recent mechanical mitral valve replacement due to rheumatic heart disease. The health care provider has just ordered a nalidixic acid for the treatment of a urinary tract infection which the patient has developed. When working with this patient, the nurse should:
1. administer the sucralfate with the quinolone antibiotic.
2. encourage the patient to drink eight to twelve 8-oz glasses of water daily.
3. be aware that nalidixic acid may produce false-negative Clinitest results.
4. assess for clotting problems, as the nalidixic acid will most likely decrease the anticoagulant effects of warfarin.

_____3. Which of the following patients would most likely be a candidate for tolterodine therapy?
1. 45-year-old with a history of ulcerative colitis
2. 73-year-old with prostatitis
3. 60-year-old with narrow-angle glaucoma
4. 50-year-old with asthma

_____4. A patient is experiencing burning, frequency, pain, and urgency associated with a urinary tract infection. The nurse would expect the health care provider to order which one of the following medications to treat these symptoms?
1. Phenazopyridine hydrochloride
2. Oxybutynin chloride
3. Methenamine mandelate
4. Nitrofurantoin

_____5. A postpartum patient who had a complicated vaginal delivery of a baby boy 9 hours ago is unable to void despite multiple nonpharmacologic interventions by the nurse. The nurse would expect the health care provider to order which drug to facilitate bladder tone and urination?
1. Bethanechol chloride
2. Neostigmine
3. Oxybutynin chloride
4. Tolterodine

_____ 6. Which of the following patients would be considered to have a urinary tract infection? (Select all that apply.)
1. Male with pyelonephritis
2. Female diagnosed with cystitis
3. Male with prostatitis
4. 4-year-old male with urethritis

_____ 7. Which of the following statements about phenazopyridine hydrochloride (Pyridium) for the treatment of patients with urinary tract infections is correct? (Select all that apply.)
1. Pyridium produces a local anesthetic effect on the mucosa of the ureters and bladder.
2. Pyridium is most effective against gram-negative bacterial urinary tract infections.
3. Pyridium relieves burning, pain, urgency, and frequency associated with urinary tract infections.
4. Pyridium reduces bladder spasms.
5. Pyridium causes the color of urine to become reddish-orange.

_____ 8. Oxybutin chloride (Ditropan) should be avoided for use in patients who have which of the following conditions? (Select all that apply.)
1. Allergy to penicillin
2. Glaucoma
3. Myasthenia gravis
4. Ulcerative colitis
5. Prostatitis

_____ 9. Which of the following statements about methenamine mandelate (Mandelamine) are correct? (Select all that apply.)
1. Mandelamine tablets should not be crushed, as this will allow the formation of formaldehyde in the stomach.
2. Mandelamine should not be administered with sodium bicarbonate.
3. Mandelamine will become inactive if administered with ascorbic acid (vitamin C).
4. Mandelamine should not be discontinued if nausea, vomiting, and belching develops without first consulting the health care provider.
5. Mandelamine is used in patients susceptible to chronic, recurrent urinary tract infections.

_____ 10. Which of the following statements about overactive bladder syndrome (OAB) are correct? (Select all that apply.)
1. The first line of pharmacologic treatment of OAB is the anticholinergic agents.
2. OAB cannot be cured.
3. Patients with OAB should be instructed to avoid caffeine.
4. The goals of therapy for OAB are to decrease frequency by increasing voided volume, decrease urgency, and reduce incidents of urinary urge incontinence.

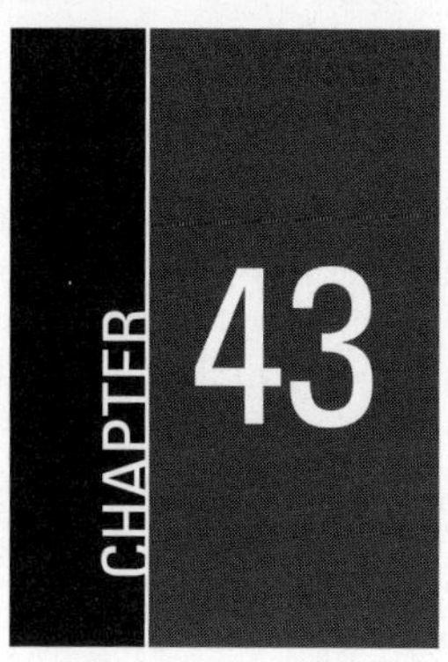

Drugs Used to Treat Glaucoma and Other Eye Disorders

Review Sheet

The QUESTION column and the ANSWER column have been offset so that you can cover the answers while reading the questions, allowing you to assess your knowledge.

Question

1. Identify the major structures of the eye (e.g., cornea, pupil, iris, canal of Schlemm).
2. Define: *miosis, mydriasis, cycloplegia, intraocular pressure,* and *glaucoma.*
3. Explain the normal drainage system of the eye.
4. What are the symptoms of acute closed-angle glaucoma?
5. What is the principal treatment of open-angle glaucoma?
6. Identify the normal intraocular pressure (IOP) reading when taken with a tonometer.
7. Compare the mechanisms of action of drugs used to lower IOP.

Answer

1. Refer to the textbook for a review of the basic structure and function of the eye. In particular, examine the location of the canal of Schlemm, Fig. 43-3. Note that dilation of the iris could result in a blockage of the canal of Schlemm.
2. Miosis: contraction of the iris sphincter muscle causing narrowing of the pupil of the eye. Mydriasis: contraction of the dilator muscle and relaxation of the sphincter muscle causing dilation of the pupil of the eye. Cycloplegia: paralysis of the ciliary muscles. IOP results from the excessive production of the aqueous humor or from decreased fluid outflow. Glaucoma: an eye disorder characterized by an increase in the IOP.
3. Aqueous humor flows between the lens and the iris into the anterior chamber of the eye. It drains through channels located near the junction of the cornea and the sclera through mesh-work into the canal of Schlemm and then into the venous system of the eye.
4. Gradual onset of intermittent symptoms, especially when the pupil is dilated. Symptoms include blurred vision, halos around white lights, frontal headache, and eye pain.
5. Historically, miotic agents (e.g., pilocarpine) were commonly used to increase outflow of aqueous humor; recently beta-adrenergic blocking agents (e.g., timolol maleate) are the initial drugs of choice. Other agents used are sympathomimetic agents (e.g., epinephrine), the carbonic anhydrase inhibitors (e.g., acetazolamide), and the cholinesterase inhibitors (e.g., echothiophate iodide).
6. 10–21 mm Hg.

8. Describe the actions of drugs known as mydriatic agents and miotic agents.
9. What should the nurse look for when performing an assessment of the pupil?
10. What action does an osmotic diuretic have on the IOP?
11. What are side effects from osmotic agents that can be anticipated?
12. Osmotic agents may produce fluid overload or heart failure. What are the signs and symptoms of this?
13. Describe the nursing assessments needed during the administration of osmotic agents.
14. Explain the administration techniques involved with osmotic agents.
15. Before administering a carbonic anhydrase inhibitor, the nurse should check the patient's chart for __________.

7. Osmotic agents: elevate osmotic pressure of the plasma, causing fluid from the extravascular spaces to be drawn into the blood, thereby reducing IOP.

   Carbonic anhydrase inhibitors: inhibit the enzyme carbonic anhydrase resulting in a decrease of aqueous humor production, thereby lowering IOP.

   Cholinergic agents: produce contraction of the iris (miosis) and ciliary body musculature (accommodation), thereby permitting outflow of aqueous humor by widening the filtration angle, thus decreasing IOP.

   Cholinesterase inhibitors: prevent destruction of acetylcholine, the cholinergic neurotransmitter within the eye. This results in increased cholinergic activity, and because of miosis the IOP is reduced.

   Adrenergic agents: have several uses in ophthalmology. These agents cause pupil dilation, increased outflow of aqueous humor, vasoconstriction, relaxation of ciliary muscle, and decreased formation of aqueous humor.

   Beta-adrenergic blocking agents: thought to reduce production of aqueous humor.

   Prostaglandin agonists: increase outflow of aqueous humor.
8. Mydriatic agents dilate the pupil and miotic agents constrict the pupil.
9. Pupil size, shape, and accommodation when exposed to light.
10. Osmotic agents reduce the volume of intraocular fluid present.
11. Thirst, nausea, dehydration, electrolyte imbalance (potassium, sodium, and chloride), headache, and circulatory overload.
12. Fluid overload/pulmonary edema; apprehension; cyanosis; diaphoresis; rapid pulse; dyspnea; and moist, gurgling-type respirations. Patients may also develop a productive cough with frothy, pink-tinged sputum.
13. Check urinary output frequently and record the amount accurately. An indwelling catheter is usually inserted, depending on the circumstances. Assess the intravenous site every 15 minutes, and take vital signs every 15 minutes, or more frequently, as ordered. Check the rate of infusion at least every 30 minutes.
14. See textbook, pp. 700-701.

16. Cholinergic agents cause the pupil to ____________.
17. List common side effects of cholinergic agents.
18. Explain how the systemic effects of cholinergic agents can be minimized.
19. Cholinesterase inhibitors block the destruction of what neurotransmitter, causing prolonged cholinergic activity and resulting in miosis and decreased IOP?
20. An overdose of a cholinesterase inhibitor will cause what symptoms?
21. What actions should be taken when cholinesterase inhibitors are used by farmers handling insecticides and pesticides?
22. Adrenergic agents cause pupil _______, and a _______ in formation of _______.
23. Adrenergic-blocking agents __________ IOP.
24. What premedication assessments should be made with adrenergic agents?
25. What types of patients should not receive beta-adrenergic blocking agents?
26. What are beta-adrenergic blocking agents used to treat?
27. What are some advantages of using beta-adrenergic blocking agents to reduce IOP?
28. When should beta-adrenergic blocking agents be withheld?
29. What is the action of a prostaglandin agonist on the eye?
30. Explain the precautions for instilling ophthalmic prostaglandin agonist medications to a person who wears contacts.
31. The class of drugs that produces both mydriasis and cycloplegia is _______.

15. A history of allergy to sulfonamides, whether the patient is pregnant; contact lenses are removed (before dorzolamide drops); gastric symptoms, and IOP value.
16. Constrict; this increases or widens the filtration angle near the canal of Schlemm, permitting outflow of the aqueous humor.
17. Reduced visual acuity, conjunctival irritation, headache, pain, and discomfort.
18. To reduce systemic absorption from the highly vascular nasal tissues, block the inner canthus of the eye for 1–2 minutes immediately after instilling the eye drop(s).
19. Acetylcholine.
20. Systemic toxicity manifested by sweating, salivation, vomiting, abdominal cramping, urinary incontinence, diarrhea, bronchospasms, dysrhythmias, and bradycardia.
21. Added absorption of insecticides and pesticides may occur through the skin and respiratory tract. Respiratory masks and frequent washing and clothing changes are advisable.
22. Dilation; decrease; aqueous humor.
23. Reduce IOP; also may reduce production of aqueous humor.
24. Vital signs including blood pressure, visual acuity, and IOP.
25. Patients with a respiratory condition (e.g., bronchitis, emphysema, and asthma) because beta blockers may produce severe bronchoconstriction. Use in patients with heart failure should be limited to those people whose disease is under control because hypotension, bradycardia, and/or heart failure may develop with use of these agents.
26. In ophthalmology, beta-adrenergic blockers are used to reduce elevated IOP in chronic open-angle glaucoma or ocular hypertension.
27. Beta-adrenergic blocking agents do not blur the vision and have little or no effect on pupil size or visual acuity.
28. Withhold the beta-adrenergic blocking agent and notify the health care provider if bradycardia, hypertension, or respiratory disorders are present.
29. Decrease IOP and increase outflow of aqueous humor.
30. Remove contact lenses, instill medication, and wait 15 minutes to reinsert the contact lenses.

32. What effect does the use of an anticholinergic agent have on IOP?
33. When mydriatic agents are administered, what patient reaction to bright lights is observed?
34. What specific medication is used to treat an ophthalmic fungal infection?
35. Antiviral agents may produce what adverse effects?
36. What is the major use of corticosteroid therapy in the eye?
37. What eye complications can occur with the long-term use of corticosteroids?
38. What is the desired action of an antihistamine on eye disorders?
39. The drug sodium fluorescein is used for what purpose?
40. When are artificial tears used?
41. Summarize macular degeneration and its cause and treatment.

31. Anticholinergic agents.
32. Increases IOP.
33. Squinting because of excessive dilation; reduced visual acuity.
34. Natamycin (Natacyn).
35. Sensitivity to bright lights, visual haze, lacrimation, redness, and burning.
36. For allergic reactions of the eye and other acute, noninfectious inflammatory conditions of the eye.
37. Increased IOP, glaucoma, and cataracts. Do not use with bacterial, fungal, or viral infections of the eye because corticosteroids decrease defense mechanisms and reduce resistance to pathologic organisms.
38. Antihistamines relieve signs and symptoms and prevent itching associated with allergic conjunctivitis.
39. Fitting hard contact lenses and as diagnostic aid to identify foreign bodies in the eye or corneal abrasions.
40. Artificial tear solutions are products made to mimic natural secretions of the eye. They provide lubrication for dry eyes and for artificial eyes. They are also used to prevent drying when a person has lost the blink reflex such as during surgery or when comatose.
41. Macular degeneration is a deterioration of the macula, a small area in the retina at the back of the eye that is required to see fine details clearly or to judge distances such as when driving an automobile. Central vision is affected by blurriness, dark areas, and distortion. Peripheral vision is usually not affected. Pegaptanib (Macugen) is a selective vascular endothelial growth factor (VEGF) antagonist. It is secreted and binds to its receptors located primarily on the surface of endothelial cells of blood vessels. VEGF induces new blood vessel growth and increases vascular permeability and inflammation, all of which are thought to contribute to the progression of the wet form of age-related macular degeneration. Pegaptanib is an antagonist that binds to extracellular VEGF, preventing it from binding to VEGF receptors, thus preventing it from forming new blood vessels. It is injected into the vitreous humor of the affected eye once every six weeks.

Student Name______________________________

Drugs Used to Treat Glaucoma and Other Eye Disorders

Learning Activities

FILL-IN-THE-BLANK

Finish each of the following statements using the correct term.

1. ____________________ is contraction of the iris sphincter muscle, which causes the pupil to narrow.

2. ____________________ is contraction of the dilator muscle and relaxation of the sphincter muscle, which causes the pupil to dilate.

3. Paralysis of the ciliary muscle is termed ____________________.

4. ____________________ is an eye disease characterized by abnormally elevated intraocular pressure, which may result from excessive production of the aqueous humor or from diminished ocular fluid outflow.

5. ______________ ______________ is used in fitting hard contact lenses and as a diagnostic aid in identifying foreign bodies in the eye and abraded or ulcerated areas of the cornea.

6. Before the administration of mannitol intravenously, the nurse should check the solution for ____________________.

7. Carbonic anhydrase inhibitors should not be administered to a patient who is allergic to ____________________.

MATCHING

Match the generic drug name with its corresponding brand name. Each option will be used only once.

_____ 8. ganciclovir

_____ 9. levofloxacin

_____ 10. tropicamide

_____ 11. carteolol

_____ 12. dipivefrin hydrochloride

_____ 13. acetazolamide

a. Quixin
b. Ocupress
c. Diamox
d. Vitrasert
e. Mydriacyl
f. Propine

TRUE OR FALSE

Mark "T" for true and "F" for false for each statement. Correct all false statements.

_____ 14. The lens is a transparent, gelatinous mass of fibers encased in an elastic capsule situated behind the iris.

_____ 15. The cornea, the eye's white portion, is contiguous with the iris and is nontransparent.

_____ 16. One of the greatest challenges in the care of chronic eye disorders such as glaucoma is convincing the patient of the need for long-term treatment and adherence to the therapeutic regimen.

_____ 17. Postoperative positioning of the patient after eye surgery usually requires having the patient lie on his or her back or on the nonoperative side.

_____ 18. Natamycin is an antibacterial agent used to treat infections of the eye.

_____ 19. If infiltration occurs with administration of intravenous mannitol, the nurse should stop the infusion, report, and then elevate the extremity and follow hospital protocol for extravasation.

DRUG ACTION/SIDE EFFECTS

20. *State the action and side effects of carbonic anhydrase inhibitors in the treatment of increased intraocular pressure.*

	Actions	Side Effects
CARBONIC ANHYDRASE INHIBITORS		

CHAPTER 43

Student Name ______________________________

Drugs Used to Treat Glaucoma and Other Eye Disorders

Practice Questions for the NCLEX Examination

_____ 1. Patients may receive osmotic agents to reduce intraocular pressure by which of the following routes? (Select all that apply.)
1. Intravenously
2. Orally
3. Topically
4. Intramuscularly

_____ 2. A patient receiving osmotic agents to reduce intraocular pressure is also taking lithium for the treatment of bipolar disorder. When working with this patient, the nurse knows that:
1. headache is an indication of cerebral dehydration.
2. the most common electrolyte imbalance to assess the patient for is hypomagnesemia.
3. the patient should be assessed for high lithium levels due to the mannitol treatment.
4. headache can be minimized by keeping the patient in a prone position.

_____ 3. The nurse should assess a patient for an allergy to which of the following before administering acetazolamide, a carbonic anhydrase inhibitor?
1. Penicillin
2. Eggs
3. Sulfonamides
4. Nuts

_____ 4. To prevent systemic effects by preventing absorption via the nasolacrimal duct, the nurse should carefully block the inner canthus of the eye for how long after instilling a cholinergic agent?
1. 1-2 minutes
2. 4-6 minutes
3. 8-10 minutes
4. 12-14 minutes

_____ 5. A patient with ______ is least at risk for developing complications related to adrenergic agents.
1. hypertension
2. diabetes mellitus
3. renal failure
4. hyperthyroidism

_____ 6. Which of the following patient statements indicates that teaching about ophthalmic antiviral agents has been effective?
1. "I will not exceed 7 days of continuous therapy because more than that will cause ocular toxicity."
2. "If transient tearing occurs upon instillation of the medication, I will rub my eyes to stop the tearing."
3. "I will discontinue treatment immediately if redness of the sclera develops after instilling the medication."
4. "I will use sunglasses to help reduce the brightness of light after instilling the medication."

_____ 7. Which of the following statements should the nurse include when teaching a patient about health promotion after eye surgery? (Select all that apply.)
1. "Avoid bending at the waist."
2. "Avoid any straining with stool."
3. "Report any pain not relieved by prescribed medications."
4. "Use aseptic technique when instilling eye medications."

_____ 8. Which of the following are actions of adrenergic agents in the treatment of glaucoma and other eye disorders? (Select all that apply.)
1. Increased outflow of aqueous humor
2. Vasodilatation
3. Constriction of the ciliary muscle
4. Decreased formation of aqueous humor

Drugs Affecting Neoplasms

Review Sheet

The QUESTION column and the ANSWER column have been offset so that you can cover the answers while reading the questions, allowing you to assess your knowledge.

Question

1. Define *cancer*.
2. What is apoptosis?
3. What are the phases of the cell cycle?
4. What are the major groups of chemotherapeutic agents currently used?
5. What are the targeted anticancer agents?
6. What are chemoprotective agents?

Answer

1. Cancer is a disorder of cellular growth, lifespan, and death. It is a group of abnormal cells that generally proliferate (multiply) more rapidly than do normal cells, lose the ability to perform specialized functions, invade surrounding tissue, and develop growth in other tissues distant to the site of original growth (metastasis).
2. Normal cells have a genetically programmed lifecycle that includes cell death known as *apoptosis*. Many types of cancer cells also lose the ability to die properly as part of their normal lifecycle.
3. See textbook, p. 714.
4. The major groups of chemotherapeutic agents currently used are classified as alkylating agents, antimetabolites, natural products, antineoplastic antibiotics, hormones, targeted anticancer agents, chemoprotective agents, and bone marrow stimulants.
5. The targeted anticancer agents have evolved from research that indicates that cell membrane receptors control cell proliferation, cell migration, angiogenesis, and cell death that are integral to the growth and spread of cancer. Targeted anticancer agents are noncytotoxic drugs that target the key pathways that provide growth and survival advantages for cancer cells. Because these pathways are relatively specific for cancer cells, theoretically, targeted agents are not associated with toxicities common with cytotoxic chemotherapy.

7. What do the bone marrow stimulants do in the treatment of cancer?
8. What is combination therapy?
9. State baseline assessments needed during the initiation of cancer therapy.
10. Cite the goals of chemotherapy and specific factors affecting the patient dosage, drug identification, drug preparation, and drug administration.
11. State the nursing interventions needed for people experiencing adverse effects from chemotherapy.
12. State the five classes of antineoplastic agents.
13. Define *cell cycle-specific* and *cell cycle-nonspecific* antineoplastic agents.
14. When is chemotherapy most effective?

6. Chemoprotective agents help reduce the toxicity of chemotherapeutic agents to normal cells.
7. Bone marrow stimulants trigger the recovery of bone marrow cells several days earlier than would be the natural course of recovery from treatment with chemotherapy which kills cancer cells and bone marrow cells. The major benefit of this earlier recovery is that the patient's immune system is able to respond to and stop infections from being so pathological, and patients are able to be released from the isolation room several days earlier.
8. Using both a cell cycle-specific and cell cycle-nonspecific agent at the same time for treatment of cancer.
9. The type of cancer being treated; the emotional status of the patient; the understanding the patient has of the diagnosis; the patient's usual methods of coping; the patient's degree of pain, usual eating pattern, and elimination pattern.
10. Control of growth of the cancer cells is the primary goal of treatment. See other goals, textbook, p. 716. Since many of the cancer drugs have similar spellings, it is imperative to check the drug name closely. Cancer drugs are given in a variety of forms: orally, intravenously, by bolus, and so forth. Therefore, the physician's order must be checked carefully. Many cancer drugs require reconstitution—follow directions precisely. When drugs are given IV, check the IV site carefully for extravasation. During oral administration, maintain an accurate record of the medication on the flow sheet and record any side effects experienced.
11. See textbook for adverse effects associated with chemotherapy. Monitor for nausea and vomiting, hydration, positioning, changes in bowel patterns, stomatitis, alopecia, neurotoxicity, musculoskeletal complaints, bone marrow depression, infection, thrombocytopenia, and activity intolerance.
12. Alkylating agents, antibiotics, antimetabolites, natural products, and hormones.
13. The action of cell cycle-specific antineoplastic agents occurs in a specific phase of the cell's growth. Cell cycle-nonspecific antineoplastics are active throughout the cell cycle.

15. Why is it difficult to kill tumor cells in the G_O phase?
16. What criteria are used to choose the type of chemotherapy to be administered?
17. What is/are the action(s) of trastuzumab (Herceptin)?
18. Discuss the three chemoprotective agents amifostine, dexrazoxane, and mesna. What are they primarily used for?
19. List questions that may be asked when taking a health history of the risk factors the individual has for development of cancer.
20. What are the common side effects to expect/report associated with chemotherapy?
21. Why is it sometimes advisable to discuss birth control and reproductive counseling prior to initiation of chemotherapy?
22. What type of oral hygiene measures should be instituted when chemotherapy is administered?
23. What are common signs and symptoms of bleeding the nurse should assess for, especially when platelet counts are decreased?
24. What is meant by "neutropenic precautions"?
25. When several courses of intravenously administered chemotherapy are planned, the antineoplastic agents are frequently administered via ________________.
26. What three types of emesis are associated with antineoplastic therapy?

14. When cells of the tumor are small in number and rapidly dividing.
15. Many chemotherapeutic agents kill cells when in the replication phase. Cells in the resting phase (G_0) of the cell cycle are not dividing and therefore are not susceptible to destruction by chemotherapeutic agents.
16. Type of tumor cells, the rate of growth, and size of the tumor.
17. Used in treatment of breast cancer with HER-2 positive tumors.
18. Examine Table 44-3 for detailed discussion.
19. See textbook, pp. 716, 724-726.
20. It depends on the type of chemotherapy drug administered. Generally, myelosuppression, anemia, bleeding, stomatitis, diarrhea or constipation, alopecia, anorexia, nausea, and vomiting are common symptoms. See a medical-surgical textbook for specific interventions for each of these side effects. Also read implementation and health promotion, pp. 726-729.
21. Reproductive abilities may be affected and agents may pass through the placental barrier; thus being potentially harmful to a fetus.
22. See Chapter 32.
23. Epistaxis, hematuria, bruises, petechiae, dark, tarry stools, "coffee ground emesis," blurred vision, excessive menstrual flow, hemoglobin, hematocrit.
24. Neutropenic precautions are designed to minimize the individual's exposure to microorganisms. Handwashing, avoiding exposure to individuals with infection, no fresh flowers or fruits and vegetables, no freestanding water (e.g., plants, flowers, humidifiers, denture cups). Avoid pets and people receiving immunizations.
25. Implantable vascular access devices.

27. Identify whether the following agents are cell cycle-specific or cell cycle-nonspecific: alkylating agents, antimetabolites, natural products, and antineoplastic antibiotics. What is the action of hormones?

26. Acute, delayed, and anticipatory emesis (see also Chapter 34).

27. Alkylating agents: cell cycle-nonspecific

    Antimetabolites: many are cell cycle-specific S phase

    Natural products: cell cycle-specific

    Antineoplastic antibiotics: act through various mechanisms to prevent replication as well as RNA synthesis. See drug class for discussion of specific antibiotic agents that are cell cycle-specific and cell cycle-nonspecific.

    Hormones: alter the hormone environment of the cell.

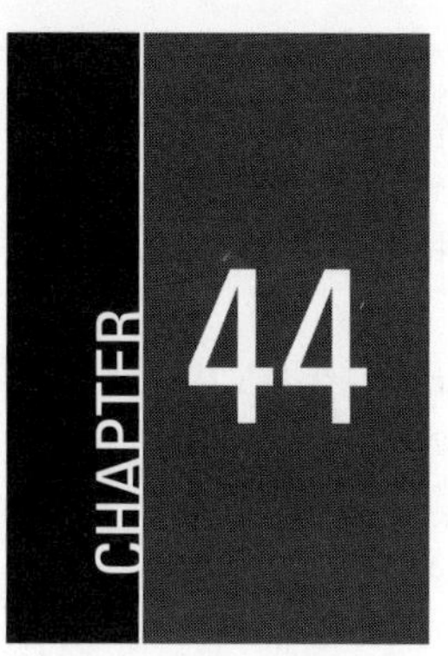

Student Name ______________________________

Drugs Affecting Neoplasms

Learning Activities

FILL-IN-THE-BLANK

Finish each of the following statements using the correct term.

1. When a cancer is beyond control, the goal of treatment may be ____________________, or the alleviation of symptoms.

2. In cancer treatment, the ____________________ are a group of medicines that help reduce the toxicity of chemotherapeutic agents to normal cells.

3. The ability of a malignant tumor to invade surrounding tissue and develop growths in other tissues distant to the site of original growth is referred to as ____________________.

4. ____________________ is the phase of cellular proliferation in which the cell divides into two equal daughter cells.

5. ____________________ and ____________________ are natural derivatives of the periwinkle plant that are used in the treatment of neoplasms.

MATCHING

Match the generic drug name with its corresponding brand name. Each option will be used only once.

_____ 6. busulfan

_____ 7. cyclophosphamide

_____ 8. streptozocin

_____ 9. plicamycin

_____ 10. epoetin alfa

_____ 11. filgrastim

a. Zanosar
b. Neupogen
c. Cytoxan
d. Procrit
e. Myleran
f. Mithracin

TRUE OR FALSE

Mark "T" for true and "F" for false for each statement. Correct all false statements.

_____ 12. The overall goal of cancer chemotherapy is to give a dose large enough to be lethal to the cancer cells, but small enough to be tolerable for normal cells.

_____ 13. Chemotherapy is most effective when the tumor is large and the cell replication is slow.

_____ 14. Combination therapy in the treatment of cancer, using cell cycle-specific and cell cycle-nonspecific agents, is superior in therapeutic effects than the use of single-agent chemotherapy.

_____ 15. Treatment of cancer often requires a combination of surgery, radiation, chemotherapy, and immunotherapy.

_____ 16. Cell cycle-nonspecific drugs are active throughout the cell cycle and may be more effective against slowly proliferating neoplastic tissue.

DRUG ACTION/SIDE EFFECTS

17. *State the action, acute and delayed toxicity, and major indications for of the following cancer chemotherapeutic agents.*

	Action	Acute Toxicity	Delayed Toxicity	Major Indications
CYTOXAN				
ONCOVIN				
ADRIAMYCIN				

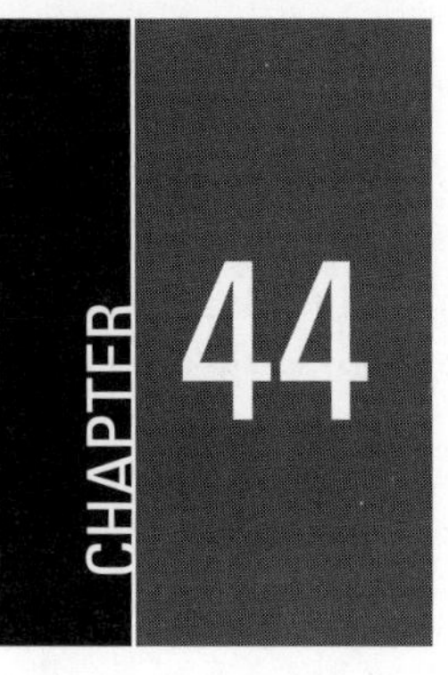

Student Name____

Drugs Affecting Neoplasms

Practice Questions for the NCLEX Examination

_____ 1. A patient has severe lesions in his mouth as a side effect of chemotherapy. It is most appropriate for the nurse to schedule oral hygiene measures using prescribed local anesthetic and antimicrobial solutions:
1. in the morning when he awakens and before bed.
2. after each meal.
3. once every eight hours.
4. hourly while he is awake.

_____ 2. Which of the following statements about hydration and chemotherapy are correct? (Select all that apply.)
1. Some chemotherapeutic agents require prehydration to prevent damage to the kidneys.
2. Some chemotherapeutic agents require prehydration to prevent damage to the bladder.
3. Prehydration prevents hair loss.
4. Prehydration will prevent dehydration from vomiting in highly emotogenic chemotherapy.

_____ 3. The nurse is teaching a patient how to manage his chemotherapy-induced diarrhea upon discharge from the outpatient cancer center. The nurse concludes that teaching was successful when the patient makes which of the following comments?
1. "I will decrease my fluid consumption to two 8-ounce glasses of liquid a day to keep my stool from being liquid."
2. "I will eliminate spicy foods from my diet."
3. "I will eat a diet high in fat to make up for lost calories."
4. "I will eat foods low in protein to prevent diarrhea from developing."

_____ 4. The nurse is teaching a patient measures he should initiate to minimize the chance of infection due to chemotherapy-induced neutropenia. Which of the following patient statements indicates that more teaching is needed?
1. "I will wash my hands at frequent intervals."
2. "I will avoid being around people who are known to have an infection."
3. "I will eat fresh fruit and vegetables to be sure to get an adequate source of vitamins on a daily basis."
4. "I will avoid being around my grandchildren when they have recently received their immunizations."

_____ 5. When teaching patients with cancer about pain relief measures, the nurse should include which of the following statements? (Select all that apply.)
1. "Pain is a normal response of the body to cancer; you will get used to it."
2. "Pain medications should be taken at prescribed intervals to obtain maximum relief."
3. "Start stool softeners and take them regularly to prevent constipation when morphine or codeine therapy is used."
4. "Spinal morphine may be delivered effectively via epidural or intrathecal catheters when oral and rectal forms of pain management no longer suffice."

_____ 6. Which of the following drugs are used to treat chemotherapy-induced anemia?
1. Sargramostim
2. Rituximab
3. Filgrastim
4. Epoetin alfa

_____ 7. Which of the following cancer chemotherapeutic antibiotics is most likely to cause cardiotoxicity as a delayed toxicity?
1. Dactinomycin
2. Bleomycin
3. Doxorubicin
4. Plicamycin

_____ 8. It is most important for the nurse to assess which of the following electrolytes before beginning tamoxifen therapy in a patient?
1. Sodium
2. Potassium
3. Magnesium
4. Calcium

_____ 9. Which of the following statements about Aranasep are true? (Select all that apply.)
1. Aranasep is used to stimulate erythropoiesis.
2. Aranasep is administered via subcutaneous injection.
3. Aranasep is used to reduce the neutropenia interval in bone marrow transplantation.
4. Aranasep is used to stimulate erythropoiesis.

_____ 10. When teaching a group of patients who are being treated for cancer about the use of steroids in cancer therapy, which of the following statements should the nurse include? (Select all that apply.)
1. "Steroids can also help reduce edema secondary to radiation therapy."
2. "Steroids can be used to restore some degree of a sense of well-being in critically ill patients."
3. "Steroids can be used as palliative therapy in temporarily suppressing fever."
4. "Steroids can be used to reduce diaphoresis."

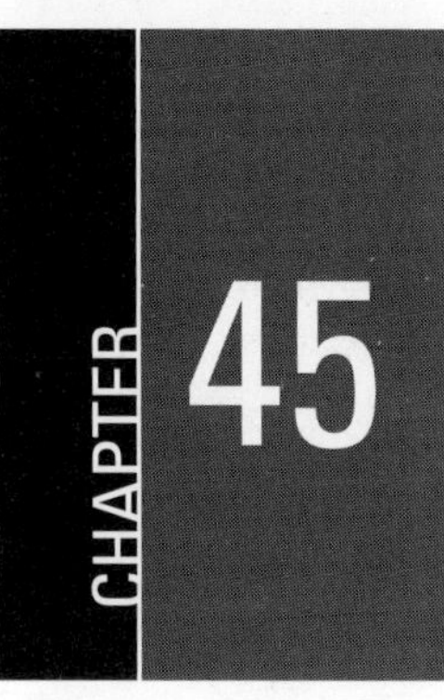

Drugs Used to Treat the Muscular System

Review Sheet

The QUESTION column and the ANSWER column have been offset so that you can cover the answers while reading the questions, allowing you to assess your knowledge.

Question

1. Describe the nursing assessments needed to evaluate a patient with a skeletal muscle disorder.
2. What adjustments are usually required during the initial phase when treating an individual with muscle spasms and pain?
3. What nursing measures can be implemented to alleviate lower back pain?
4. Immediately following a muscle injury _____ ___ packs will reduce the swelling.
5. To decrease swelling following an injury, how should the affected part be treated?
6. What two classes of drugs are used to relieve pain and inflammation associated with musculoskeletal disorders?
7. Compare the site of action of centrally acting and direct-acting muscle relaxants.
8. Both centrally acting and direct-acting skeletal muscle relaxants can produce hepatotoxicity. What are the signs and symptoms of this toxicity?
9. What premedication assessments should be made before administering centrally acting skeletal muscle relaxants?
10. Which class of muscle relaxants can cause photosensitivity?
11. What are the primary uses of baclofen?

Answer

1. See textbook, pp. 735-736.
2. Immobilize and elevate the affected part; range-of-motion exercises may be prescribed to prevent muscle atrophy and contractures.
3. Maintain proper body alignment; elevate the head of the bed 15 to 20 degrees and flex the knees slightly. Give prescribed analgesics and muscle relaxants.
4. Ice
5. Elevated and immobilized
6. Analgesic agents are used for pain and anti-inflammatory agents are used to reduce the inflammatory response.
7. Centrally acting muscle relaxants depress the central nervous system. Their major benefit may be their sedative effects. Direct-acting skeletal muscle relaxants act directly on the skeletal muscle producing generalized, mild weakness of skeletal muscles.
8. Anorexia, nausea, vomiting, jaundice, hepatomegaly, splenomegaly, and abnormal liver function tests (e.g., AST, ALT, LDH)
9. Baseline vital signs, mental status assessment, laboratory studies as ordered (e.g., liver function, complete blood count).
10. Direct-acting skeletal muscle relaxants.

12. Describe the signs of respiratory depression.
13. What laboratory values would be used to confirm hypoxia and hypercapnia?
14. Why are centrally acting muscle relaxants not given to people with long-term muscle spasticity?
15. What are the uses of dantrolene (Dantrium)?
16. Explain when and why neuromuscular blocking agents are administered.
17. What effect do neuromuscular blocking agents have on consciousness?
18. What nursing assessments should be made when a neuromuscular blocking agent has been administered?
19. Review the drug interactions that enhance therapeutic and toxic effects of neuromuscular blocking agents and identify the three classes of drugs commonly administered that may interact with neuromuscular blocking agents.
20. Where in the patient's chart is administration of a neuromuscular blocking agent recorded?
21. Name common neuromuscular blocking agents by their generic and brand names.
22. What premedication assessments should be done prior to the administration of a neuromuscular blocking agent?
23. Explain the treatment of overdose of neuromuscular blocking agents.

11. Baclofen is used to manage muscle spasticity resulting from multiple sclerosis, spinal cord injuries, and other spinal cord diseases.
12. Early signs: restlessness; anxiety; decreased mental alertness; headache; increase in heart rate, blood pressure, and respiratory rate. Later signs: heart rate increases; blood pressure decreases; cyanosis; use of accessory chest, abdominal, and neck muscles in respiratory effort; flaring nostrils. Changes in mental status: confusion progressing to coma.
13. Hypercapnia (elevated pCO_2), hypoxemia (decreased pO_2), and decreased oxygen saturation (SaO_2).
14. They would further reduce the functioning of the individual by reducing the overall strength of the remaining active muscle fibers.
15. Control spasticity of chronic disorders (e.g., cerebral palsy, multiple sclerosis, spinal cord injury, stroke syndrome). Dantrolene is also used to treat neuroleptic malignant syndrome.
16. To provide muscle relaxation during anesthesia, facilitate endotracheal intubation and prevent laryngospasm, decrease muscular activity in electroshock therapy, and aid in reducing muscle spasms associated with tetanus.
17. No effects. Unless anesthetized, the patient is fully conscious but unable to respond due to neuromuscular blockade.
18. Patent, adequate airway, check lung sounds bilaterally. Residual effects may be apparent for up to 72 hours especially in neonates and infants—watch for respiratory depression. Check cough reflex and ability to swallow. Question any antibiotic orders that prescribe aminoglycosides or tetracycline when neuromuscular blockers have been used.
19. Aminoglycoside antibiotics, beta-adrenergic blocking agents, and diuretics that cause potassium depletion.
20. Anesthesiologist's record.
21. See Table 45-2.
22. See textbook, p. 741.
23. See textbook, p. 742.

CHAPTER 45

Student Name ____________________

Drugs Used to Treat the Muscular System

Learning Activities

FILL-IN-THE-BLANK

Finish each of the following statements using the correct term.

1. Neuromuscular blocking agents may cause patients to experience an increase in salivation due to release of ____________________.

2. Antibiotic orders that prescribe ____________________ and ____________________ should be questioned in patients who have received neuromuscular blockers, as these drugs may potentiate the neuromuscular blocking activity.

3. In treating patients who have overdosed on neuromuscular blocking agents, ______________ ______________ is usually administered with neostigmine or pyridostigmine to block bradycardia, hypotension, and salivation induced by these agents.

4. Analgesics, sedatives, and tranquilizers, in combination with muscle relaxants, may potentiate respiratory depression. This may occur _______ hours or more after drug administration.

MATCHING

Match the generic drug name with its corresponding brand name. Each option will be used only once.

_____ 5. vecuronium bromide

_____ 6. pancuronium bromide

_____ 7. succinylcholine

_____ 8. dantrolene

_____ 9. baclofen

a. Liorseal
b. Norcuron
c. Pavulon
d. Dantrium
e. Anectine

TRUE OR FALSE

Mark "T" for true and "F" for false for each statement. Correct all false statements.

_____ 10. Assessment of the patient's vital signs, mental status, and particularly respiratory function is mandatory for people receiving neuromuscular blocking agents.

_____ 11. The development of cyanosis is an early sign of respiratory complications associated with the administration of neuromuscular blocking agents.

_____ 12. In the immediate period after muscle injury, heat packs are applied to alleviate swelling, and later in the course of treatment, ice packs are used to provide comfort.

_____ 13. Immediately after muscular trauma, immobilization of the affected part will decrease muscle spasms and therefore decrease pain.

_____ 14. Patients receiving neuromuscular blocking agents usually experience a decrease in the amount of saliva produced.

DRUG ACTION/SIDE EFFECTS

15. *State the action and side effects of neuromuscular blocking agents.*

	Actions	Side Effects
NEUROMUSCULAR BLOCKING AGENTS		

CHAPTER 45

Student Name______________________________

Drugs Used to Treat the Muscular System

Practice Questions for the NCLEX Examination

_____ 1. Which of the following statements about centrally acting skeletal muscle relaxants is true?
1. These agents directly relax the muscles by suppressing nerve conduction at the myoneural junction.
2. Centrally acting skeletal muscle relaxants do not produce sedation in patients receiving them.
3. These agents should not be used in the treatment of muscle spasticity associated with cerebral or spinal cord disease.
4. Centrally acting skeletal muscle relaxants produce their therapeutic effect by stimulating the central nervous system.

_____ 2. Which of the following statements by a patient taking dantrolene for treatment of muscle spasticity of stroke syndrome indicates that he is in need of more teaching?
1. "I will avoid exposure to the sun but I can still use a tanning lamp."
2. "If I develop side effects from this medication, I will not discontinue treatment until I notify my health care provider."
3. "I will notify my health care provider if my skin turns yellow."
4. "I know that it might take up to a week for me to see any response to this drug."

_____ 3. Which of the following drugs are antidotes for neuromuscular blocking agents? (Select all that apply.)
1. Edrophonium chloride
2. Pyridostigmine bromide
3. Naloxone
4. Neostigmine methylsulfate

_____ 4. Patients receiving neuromuscular blocking agents:
1. are at risk for the development of bronchospasm, edema, and urticaria.
2. do not experience pain.
3. have an enhanced cough reflex.
4. experience a decrease in salivation.

_____ 5. Which of the following drugs would be considered the safest to administer to a patient who has received a neuromuscular blocking agent?
1. General anesthetics
2. Furosemide
3. Cortocosteroids
4. Insulin

_____ 6. Which of the following statements about the effects of neuromuscular blocking agents in patients with muscular disorders are true? (Select all that apply.)
1. Neuromuscular blocking agents have no effect on consciousness.
2. Neuromuscular blocking agents have no effect on memory.
3. Neuromuscular blocking agents have no effect on pain threshold.
4. Patients receiving neuromuscular blocking agents may not receive pain medications.

_____ 7. Immediate treatment of a musculoskeletal injury would include:
1. application of heat.
2. thromboembolic deterrent hose (TED).
3. application of ice.
4. exercise of the affected part.

_____ 8. The primary use of centrally acting skeletal muscle relaxants is to:
1. treat muscle spasticity.
2. strengthen remaining active muscles.
3. provide analgesia.
4. relieve muscle spasms.

_____ 9. Centrally acting skeletal muscle relaxants may cause: (Select all that apply.)
1. blood dyscrasias.
2. electrolyte imbalance.
3. hepatotoxicity.
4. nephrotoxicity.
5. cardiac complications.

_____ 10. A 5-year-old patient receiving a neuromuscular blocking agent as part of her anesthesia for abdominal surgery is now complaining of pain. What additional data are essential to collect before giving the prescribed analgesic?
1. Laboratory results for CBC and electrolytes
2. Vital signs
3. Family history
4. Estimated time of discharge

Antimicrobial Agents

Review Sheet

The QUESTION column and the ANSWER column have been offset so that you can cover the answers while reading the questions, allowing you to assess your knowledge.

Question

1. What criteria are used to select an antimicrobial agent?
2. Describe the signs and symptoms of the common side effects seen with antimicrobial therapy.
3. Differentiate between gram-negative (Gm–) and gram-positive (Gm+) microorganisms, and anaerobic and aerobic properties of microorganisms.
4. Describe basic principles of patient care that can be implemented to enhance an individual's therapeutic response during an infection.

Answer

1. The HCP must choose an antimicrobial agent that will be effective against the type of organism present and one that will not be too toxic to the patient.
2. Allergy: rash or skin reaction (e.g., hives with or without dyspnea, laryngeal edema, shock, stridor, and sternal retractions). Direct tissue damage: hepatotoxicity (liver damage) as noted by an elevation of AST, ALT, GGT, and alkaline phosphatase. Ototoxicity: dizziness, tinnitus, and progressive hearing loss. Nephrotoxicity [renal damage: as noted by an increase in serum creatinine, BUN, and by alterations in the urine (e.g., decrease in specific gravity, casts, or protein in the urine, and an excess of RBCs over 0–3)]. Secondary infection: stomatitis, glossitis, itching, vulvovaginitis, cold sores, or canker sores. See textbook, p. 749, Blood Dyscrasias, and p. 748, Nausea, Vomiting, and Diarrhea.
3. Classification of microorganisms as *gram-positive* or *gram-negative* refers to the type of staining properties of a bacterium. Cells with a cell wall retain stain and are referred to as *gram-positive* cells. Cells without a cell wall do not retain the gram stain, and are referred to as *gram-negative* cells. Broad-spectrum antibiotics are effective against many gram-positive and gram-negative organisms. Anaerobic bacteria grow in the absence of oxygen; aerobic bacteria require oxygen to reproduce.

5. Review components of a baseline assessment to evaluate a patient's hydration status and assessments needed to detect renal or hepatic toxicity.
6. Identify significant data in a patient's history that could alert the medical team that the patient is more likely to experience an allergic reaction.
7. Describe the usual management of nausea, vomiting, and diarrhea when they occur in conjunction with antimicrobial therapy.
8. State the signs and symptoms of a secondary infection and actions that can be taken to minimize these effects.
9. Review techniques and procedures for parenteral administration and vaginal insertion of drugs.
10. Identify significant information relating to patient education when caring for a person receiving an antibiotic.
11. Cite the primary uses of aminoglycosides and the serious side effects that require close monitoring of the patient.

4. Adequate rest, hydration, and nutrients. Teach personal hygiene measures (e.g., handwashing, proper techniques for changing dressings).
5. Hydration: skin turgor, intake and output, inspect mucous membranes for moisture or dryness, check firmness of eyeballs, check specific gravity of urine (see Table 42-1). Renal toxicity: decreasing urine output, increasing BUN and/or serum creatinine; check for presence of protein, blood, or casts in the urine. Hepatic toxicity: anorexia, nausea, vomiting, jaundice, hepatomegaly, splenomegaly, and abnormal (elevated) liver function tests (AST, ALT, LDH, GGT, alkaline phosphatase).
6. Before administering any antibiotic, check for any prior allergies to medications or foods or the presence of asthma. If the patient is allergic to anything, get details regarding the symptoms and previous treatment of the allergy.
7. Gather data relative to the patient's usual pattern of elimination (e.g., number of stools per day, consistency) and compare this information with the current data. Read individual drug monographs to identify antimicrobials that may cause diarrhea, nausea, or vomiting. Report these to the physician.
8. Be particularly alert for secondary infection in patients receiving broad-spectrum antibiotics and those patients who are immunosuppressed. Assess for white patches in the mouth, cold sores, canker sores, vaginal itching, diarrhea, and recurrent fever.
9. See Chapter 8, Percutaneous Administration; Chapter 10, Parenteral Administration: Safe Preparation of Parenteral Medications; Chapter 11, Parenteral Administration: Intradermal, Subcutaneous, and Intramuscular Routes; and Chapter 12, Parenteral Administration: Intravenous Route.
10. With the instructor's assistance, identify significant points relating to the prescribed drug therapy that should be taught to the patient for each class of antimicrobials ordered.

12. Identify precautions needed to prevent incompatibilities between aminoglycosides and other medications.
13. State the mechanism of action of aminoglycosides on the bacterial cell.
14. What premedication assessments should be made before aminoglycoside therapy?
15. What is the mechanism of action of carbapenems?
16. Prior to administration of a carbapenem, what premedication assessments should be performed?
17. Why is it essential to report the occurrence of severe diarrhea with antibiotic therapy?
18. Explain the admixture compatibility of carbapenems.
19. Cite the effectiveness of cephalosporins, according to generation, against gram-positive and gram-negative microorganisms.

11. Aminoglycosides are used to treat gram-negative bacteria causing meningitis, wound infections, chronic urinary tract infections, and life-threatening septicemia. Monitor the patient closely for ototoxicity and nephrotoxicity. If the patient has had anesthesia within 48–72 hours that included the administration of a skeletal muscle relaxant, withhold aminoglycoside and ask health care provider for further instructions.
12. Do not mix aminoglycosides in the same syringe or infuse these drugs simultaneously with other medications. Tag the chart of any patient going to surgery who is receiving an aminoglycoside. Respiratory depression may occur when these agents are combined with skeletal muscle relaxants.
13. Aminoglycosides inhibit protein synthesis of bacteria.
14. Baseline assessment of allergies, presenting symptoms, T, P, R, BP, and hydration status. Check for any hearing disorders or deficits or renal disease. If present, hold drug and notify physician. Check for patient having received any skeletal muscle relaxants within the past 72 hours. If taking aminoglycosides, check serum level. Check for laboratory results ordered by the health care provider (e.g., CBC with differential).
15. Carbapenems inhibit bacterial cell wall synthesis.
16. Check T, P, R, BP, and hydration status for preexisting gastric symptoms and any allergies (specifically to penicillin and cephalosporins), obtain laboratory studies, check for history of seizures and assess basic mental status and symptoms present.
17. Severe diarrhea with any antibiotic may indicate drug-induced pseudomembranous colitis.
18. See textbook, p. 754.

20. What premedication assessments should be performed before therapy with cephalosporins?
21. State the mechanism of action of cephalosporins on the cell wall.
22. What types of infections can be treated effectively using cephalosporins?
23. What side effects from cephalosporins should be reported?
24. Why may hypoprothrombinemia occur with cephalosporin therapy?
25. What are the signs and symptoms of thrombophlebitis, which may occur with cephalosporin therapy?
26. What precautions should be instituted when cephalosporins are combined with probenecid or alcohol?
27. What is the difference between bacteriostatic and bactericidal?

19. The first-generation cephalosporins have good activity against gram-positive bacteria and mild activity against gram-negative bacteria. The second-generation cephalosporins have somewhat increased activity against gram-negative bacteria but are much less active than the third-generation agents. The-third generation agents are less active than first-generation agents against gram-positive cocci. Some of the third-generation agents are also active against *Pseudomonas aeruginosa*, a very potent gram-negative microorganism. The third-generation cephalosporins have greater activity against gram-positive penicillinase-producing bacteria than first-generation cephalosporins. Fourth-generation cephalosporins are considered broad-spectrum, with both gram-negative and gram-positive coverage.
20. Baseline assessment of allergies, presenting symptoms, T, P, R, BP, and hydration status, symptoms of renal disease or bleeding disorder (hold drug and notify physician if present), and laboratory studies as ordered by physician (e.g., CBC with differential).
21. Interferes with synthesis of bacterial cell wall.
22. Respiratory, urinary, gastrointestinal, skin, and soft-tissue infections, septicemia, meningitis, osteomyelitis, and certain sexually transmitted diseases.
23. Diarrhea, secondary infections, abnormal liver and renal function tests.
24. Although rare, hypoprothrombinemia may develop in the older adult, debilitated, or otherwise compromised patient with borderline vitamin K deficiency. Treatment with broad-spectrum antibiotics eliminates enough gastrointestinal flora to cause a further reduction in vitamin K synthesis.
25. Report redness, warmth, tenderness to touch, or edema in the affected part. Homans' sign in lower extremities.
26. Probenecid with cephalosporins may increase likelihood of toxicity. When combined with alcohol, cephalosporins may produce flushing, dyspnea, tachycardia, and hypotension. Do not ingest alcohol within 72 hours of taking cephalosporins.

28. What effect do cephalosporins have on oral contraceptives?

29. What is the action of the glycylines (Tigecycline)?

30. How is telithromycin used?

31. Identify the uses of macrolides.

32. State the actions of penicillins on the bacterial cell.

33. Identify the clinical uses of penicillins.

34. For what types of adverse effects should a patient taking penicillin be monitored?

35. Cite questions that should be asked to screen a patient for a penicillin allergy before administration of the agent.

27. Bactericidal agents kill the microorganism; bacteriostatic agents weaken the microorganism. Whether an agent is bacteriostatic or bactericidal depends on the organism and concentration of medication present.

28. Cephalosporins may interfere with the contraceptive activity of oral contraceptives. Oral contraceptives should not be discontinued, but counseling regarding use of additional methods of contraception should be planned.

29. Tigecycline is chemically related to the tetracyclines, but is not susceptible to the mechanisms that cause resistance to the tetracyclines. Its acts by binding to the 30S ribosome, preventing protein synthesis. It is a bacteriostatic antibiotic effective against a broad spectrum of gram-positive, gram-negative, and anaerobic microorganisms. It is not effective against viruses.

30. Telithromycin is used to treat acute bacterial sinusitis, bronchitis, and pneumonia caused by susceptible strains of gram-positive bacteria. In an effort to slow the development of strains of bacteria resistant to telithromycin, it should be used only when the pathogen is resistant to other available antibiotics.

31. Macrolides are used for respiratory, gastrointestinal tract, skin and soft-tissue infections, and STDs, especially when penicillins, cephalosporins, and tetracyclines cannot be used.

32. Penicillins act by interfering with the synthesis of the bacterial cell wall. They are most effective against bacteria that are multiplying.

33. Treatment of middle ear infection, pneumonia, meningitis, urinary tract infections, syphilis, and gonorrhea; and as a prophylactic antibiotic before surgery or dental procedures for patients with a history of rheumatic fever.

34. Watch for diarrhea, abnormal liver and renal function tests, thrombophlebitis, and electrolyte imbalances from sodium or potassium types of penicillin. Older adult or debilitated patients with impaired renal function are more likely to develop adverse effects.

36. Identify precautions necessary to prevent an incompatibility between penicillin and other medications given intramuscularly or intravenously.
37. Briefly describe the mechanisms of action of the quinolones and fluoroquinolones.
38. Review the multiple uses of quinolones and fluoroquinolones.
39. Why are the quinolones not used in children under the age of 12 years?
40. What premedication assessments should be made prior to beginning quinolone therapy?
41. Describe the effects of antacids, iron, and sucralfate on quinolones and the adaptations in scheduling required if both agents are prescribed concurrently.
42. Identify the drug interactions that may occur when quinolones are combined with concurrent use of NSAIDs or sparfloxacin.
43. What is the mechanism of action of the new class of antibiotics known as *streptogramins*?
44. What are the uses of streptogramins?
45. What precautions need to be used when reconstituting streptogramins or administering them IV?
46. Cite the mechanism of action of sulfonamides and the importance of monitoring following administration.
47. State the effect of sulfonamides on people taking sulfonylurea oral hypoglycemic agents.

35. "Have you ever taken an antibiotic before?" "Do you have any known allergies to foods or medications?" If so, obtain further details, such as: "When you got sick while taking the medication, what symptoms did you have?" "What did the doctor tell you to do when this occurred?" "Do you have hay fever or asthma?"
36. Do not mix penicillin with other drugs in the same syringe or infuse together with other drugs.
37. Quinolones act by interfering with replication of bacterial DNA. Quinolones are effective against gram-negative and gram-positive bacteria, including anaerobes. Fluoroquinolones act by inhibiting activity of DNA gyrase, an enzyme essential for the replication of bacterial DNA.
38. See textbook, p. 762.
39. Quinolones may cause permanent damage to cartilage in a pediatric patient.
40. Baseline assessment of allergies, presenting symptoms, T, P, R, BP, and hydration status, gastric symptoms present, baseline laboratory studies as ordered, check for pregnancy. Warn about possible photosensitivity with lomefloxacin.
41. Antacids, iron-containing products, and sucralfate may decrease the absorption of quinolones. The antibiotic should be scheduled 4 hours before or 4 hours after taking any of these medications.
42. See textbook, p. 764.
43. Streptogramins (quinupristin, dalfopristin) act by inhibiting protein synthesis in bacterial cell wall.
44. These agents should be reserved for treatment of serious or life-threatening infections associated with vancomycin resistance.
45. See textbook, p. 764.
46. Sulfonamides inhibit bacterial biosynthesis of folic acid, leading to inadequate metabolism and cell death. People taking sulfonamides for 14 days or more need periodic monitoring of RBC and WBC (with differential) counts. All patients receiving sulfonamides need adequate hydration and should be encouraged to drink eight 12-oz glasses of water daily.

48. State the mechanism of action of tetracyclines.
49. List a minimum of two types of antibiotics that may cause photosensitivity.
50. Identify the effects of administering tetracyclines during pregnancy and at the age of tooth development.
51. Describe the dosage and administration considerations when tetracycline is prescribed.
52. Identify the causative organism and mode of transfer of tuberculosis.
53. Describe factors that need consideration to enhance a patient's response to antitubercular therapy.
54. Develop a teaching plan for patients receiving antitubercular agents.
55. Compare the mechanisms of action of ethambutol, isoniazid, and rifampin.
56. Identify the effects of rifampin on body secretions (e.g., urine, feces, saliva, and sputum).
57. What drug interaction does rifampin have with oral contraceptives?
58. What is the mechanism of action of monobactams?

47. Sulfonamides may displace sulfonylurea oral hypoglycemic agents from their protein binding sites, potentially resulting in hypoglycemia. Have patients taking these two agents concurrently test their blood glucose 1/2 hour ac and hs to detect the development of a problem.
48. Tetracyclines inhibit protein synthesis by bacterial cells.
49. Quinolones, tetracyclines, sulfonamides, and griseofulvin may cause photosensitivity. Patients taking these antibiotics should be cautioned to avoid exposure to sunlight and ultraviolet lights. Discourage the use of artificial tanning lights and instruct patients to wear clothing that provides adequate coverage of the body when in the sunlight.
50. Do not administer tetracycline during the last half of pregnancy or to children through 8 years of age because it may cause enamel hypoplasia and permanent staining of the teeth. Do not administer to nursing mothers because it is secreted in breast milk.
51. Take medication 1 hour before or 2 hours after ingesting antacids; milk; dairy products; or products containing calcium, aluminum, magnesium (antacids), or iron (vitamins). Exception: doxycycline is not affected by food or milk.
52. *Mycobacterium tuberculosis* is spread by airborne droplets from the cough or sneeze of a person infected with the organism.
53. Personal hygiene, nutritional status, and stress reduction are factors that must be considered during the treatment of tuberculosis.
54. Review your teaching plan with the course instructor.
55. Ethambutol inhibits TB bacterial growth by altering cellular RNA synthesis and phosphate metabolism. The mechanism of action of isoniazid is unknown. It appears to disrupt the *M. tuberculosis* cell wall and inhibit replication. Rifampin acts against enzymes in the bacterial cell required to produce DNA.
56. Rifampin may tinge urine, feces, saliva, sweat, and tears a reddish-orange color.
57. Rifampin interferes with the contraceptive activity of birth control pills. Alternate methods of birth control should be used during rifampin therapy.

59. What is the mechanism of action of chloramphenicol?
60. State specific limitations for the use of chloramphenicol.
61. Identify specific nursing assessments needed to detect possible serious hematologic effects from chloramphenicol.
62. What is the mechanism of action of clindamycin?
63. Describe effective treatment for diarrhea associated with clindamycin therapy.
64. State the primary clinical uses for metronidazole.
65. What premedication assessments should be done whenever metronidazole (Flagyl) is to be administered?
66. What is the mechanism of action of spectinomycin?
67. Identify the effectiveness of spectinomycin against gonorrhea and syphilis.
68. Cite specific recommendations for intramuscular administration of spectinomycin.
69. Why should serology testing for syphilis be done prior to initiating therapy using spectinomycin?
70. What is the primary therapeutic outcome expected from tinidazole therapy?
71. What is the mechanism of action of vancomycin?
72. Describe nursing assessments that may be used to detect ototoxicity.
73. Describe "red man syndrome" and identify the drug is associated with its occurrence.

58. Monobactams are a new class of synthetic, bactericidal antibiotics that act by inhibiting cell wall synthesis.
59. Chloramphenicol acts by inhibiting bacterial protein synthesis.
60. Use only for serious infections; it is particularly effective in treating rickettsial infections, meningitis, and typhoid fever.
61. Check for sore throat, feelings of fatigue, elevated temperature, small petechial hemorrhages, and bruises of the skin. Report any of these symptoms immediately to the physician. Routine laboratory studies including RBC, WBC, and differential counts are scheduled for patients taking chloramphenicol 14 days or longer.
62. Clindamycin acts by inhibiting protein synthesis.
63. Do not self-treat diarrhea. (Kaopectate for persistent diarrhea from clindamycin therapy is used since it absorbs clindamycin. Do not use diphenoxylate, loperamide, or paregoric.) Patients should be instructed to contact the physician for specific directions.
64. Metronidazole is used to treat trichomoniasis, giardiasis, amebic dysentery, amebic liver abscess, and anaerobic bacterial infections.
65. See textbook, pp. 773-774.
66. Spectinomycin acts by inhibiting protein synthesis.
67. Spectinomycin is used to treat gonorrhea in both males and females. It is not effective in treatment of syphilis.
68. Use a 20-gauge needle, and inject into upper outer quadrant of gluteal muscle. Causes pain at injection site.
69. This drug masks symptoms of syphilis.
70. Elimination of parasitic infection.
71. Vancomycin acts by preventing synthesis of bacterial cell walls.
72. Dizziness, tinnitus, and progressive hearing loss (e.g., turns the TV on louder, has to have conversation repeated).

74. What type of dressings should be avoided with topical antifungal medications and what type of precautions should be taken to prevent accidental pregnancy when these drugs are administered intravaginally?
75. What is the mechanism of action of amphotericin B?
76. Cite the primary uses of amphotericin B.
77. Describe the systemic side effects seen with intravenous administration of amphotericin B.
78. Identify the monitoring parameters used to detect nephrotoxicity.
79. Cite specific dosage and administration characteristics associated with the use of amphotericin B.
80. Review procedures used to administer topical medications to the skin.
81. Describe the uses of fluconazole (Diflucan) and flucytosine (Ancobon, Ancotil).
82. Compare the premedication assessments needed for flucytosine (Ancobon), griseofulvin (Fulvicin, Grifulvin), itraconazole (Sporanox), ketoconazole (Nizoral), and terbinafine (Lamisil).
83. What action prohibits the administration of itraconazole to a patient with heart failure?
84. What are the therapeutic outcomes from administration of abacavir (Ziagen)?
85. Describe the mechanisms of action and uses of griseofulvin (Fulvicin, Grifulvin).
86. State laboratory tests needed periodically to monitor renal, hepatic, and hematopoietic function when griseofulvin is administered.

73. "Red man syndrome" or "redneck syndrome" is caused by rapid IV infusion of vancomycin; symptoms include sudden hypotension with or without maculopapular rash over face, neck, upper chest, and extremities.
74. Avoid occlusive dressings. Alternative forms of birth control should also be used when antifungal ointments are instilled intravaginally. Diaphragms and condoms may deteriorate with prolonged contact with petroleum-based ointment.
75. Amphotericin B disrupts the cell membrane of fungal cells resulting in loss of cellular content and death of the cell.
76. Amphotericin B is used to treat systemic fungal infections and meningitis.
77. Nephrotoxicity, electrolyte imbalances, chills, fever, malaise, headache, nausea and vomiting, and thrombophlebitis.
78. Nephrotoxicity is indicated by increased excretion of uric acid, magnesium, oliguria, granular casts in urine, proteinuria, increased BUN, and serum creatinine. Report decrease in daily urine volume or changes in visual appearance of the urine.
79. See textbook, p. 780.
80. See Chapter 8, Percutaneous Administration.
81. Fluconazole is used for cryptococcal meningitis and oropharyngeal, esophageal, vulvovaginal, or systemic candidiasis. Flucytosine is effective against susceptible candidal septicemia, endocarditis, urinary tract infections, cryptococcal meningitis, and pulmonary infections.
82. See textbook, pp. 781-785.
83. Itraconazole has the action of being a negative inotropic agent and may seriously aggravate a patient with heart failure.
84. Abacavir slows clinical progression of HIV-1 infection and reduces the frequency of opportunistic secondary infections.
85. Griseofulvin acts by stopping cell division and new cell growth and is used to treat ringworm of scalp, body, nails, and feet.

87. State the mechanisms of action and types of fungal infections for which itraconazole, ketoconazole, miconazole, and terbinafine are used.
88. What are the therapeutic outcomes of abacavir (Ziagen), efavirenz (Sustiva), and lamivudine (Epivir)?
89. Identify the mechanism of action of acyclovir (Zovirax), didanosine (Videx), famciclovir (Famvir), and valacyclovir (Valtrex).
90. Cite the potential effects of acyclovir on renal function.
91. Identify the first antiviral agent that is effective against respiratory viruses.
92. What is the drug lamivudine (Epivir) used to treat?
93. What is oseltamivir (Tamiflu) used to treat?
94. Explain the administration of aerosol ribavirin powder using a small-particle aerosol generator (SPAG-2).
95. What is valacyclovir (Valtrex) used to treat?
96. Does zanamivir (Relenza) reduce the transmission of influenza to others?
97. Cite the clinical limitations of zidovudine in the treatment of human immunodeficiency virus (HIV).
98. Identify the hematologic tests that should be completed periodically during the use of zidovudine.

86. Hepatotoxicity (liver damage) is noted by an elevation in AST, ALT, GGT, and alkaline phosphatase. Nephrotoxicity (renal damage) is indicated by an increase in serum creatinine, BUN, and by alterations in the urine (e.g., decrease in specific gravity, casts or protein in the urine, and an excess of RBCs over 0–3). Hematologic: monitor for the development of sore throat, fever, purpura, jaundice, or excessive progressive weakness; check RBC, WBC, and differential counts.
87. Ketoconazole, itraconazole, and miconazole act by interfering with cell wall synthesis, causing leakage of cellular contents. (Itraconazole, see textbook, p. 783.) Ketoconazole is used orally to treat candidiasis, chronic mucocutaneous candidiasis, oral thrush, coccidioidomycosis, histoplasmosis, chromomycosis, and paracoccidioidomycosis. Miconazole is used parenterally to treat similar fungal infections. Terbinafine is used to treat onychomycosis of the toenail or fingernail due to dermatophytes. (Terbinafine, see textbook, p. 785.)
88. Abacavir (Ziagen), efavirenz (Sustiva), and lamivudine (Epivir) slow the progression of HIV-1 infection and reduce the frequency of opportunistic secondary infections.
89. These antiviral agents act by inhibiting the viral cell wall replication.
90. Transient elevation of serum creatinine. Patients who are poorly hydrated, have low renal function, or who receive acyclovir by a bolus are susceptible to renal tubular damage.
91. Ribavirin (Virazole).
92. Lamivudine (Epivir) is combined with zidovudine in treating HIV-1 infection.
93. See textbook, p. 795.
94. See textbook, pp. 796-797.
95. Acute herpes simplex virus (shingles).
96. No.
97. It prolongs the lives of AIDS and AIDS-related complex (ARC) patients, reduces the risk and severity of opportunistic infections, and improves immune status. Zidovudine does not cure acquired immunodeficiency.

99. Describe the effect of zidovudine and amprenavir on transmission of HIV to others through sexual contact or blood contamination.
100. Describe the proper schedule for administering zidovudine and essential health teaching needed.
101. Review current Centers for Disease Control recommendations for handling body secretions and blood for all patients.
102. Which of the antiviral agents may reduce pulmonary function?
103. Which antiviral agent may reduce the effectiveness of oral contraceptives?
104. Which antiviral agents may produce peripheral neuropathy?
105. What are the drugs emtricitabine, stavudine, and enfuvirtide used for?
106. Study the antibiotic tables throughout the chapter and identify common endings in the generic names of the antimicrobial agents.

98. Monitor CBC with differential, platelets, hemoglobin, hematocrit, amylase, and liver function tests.
99. This drug does not reduce the risk of transmitting HIV to others through sexual contact or blood contamination.
100. Oral medication is taken every 4 hours around the clock even though it interrupts normal sleep. Do not share with other people.
101. Check with your instructor to obtain the latest recommendations or research the information on the CDC website.
102. Both ribavirin and zanamivir may affect pulmonary function.
103. Amprenavir.
104. Didanosine, lamivudine, zidovudine.
105. Emtricitabine, stavudine, and enfuvirtide are used in combination with other antiviral agents for the treatment of HIV-1 infection.
106. See textbook Tables 46-1 through 46-9. Note: Because of the number of drugs included in these tables, ask the instructor to identify the more common drugs that will be encountered in the clinical site(s) where you are assigned.

CHAPTER 46

Student Name ______________________________

Antimicrobial Agents

Learning Activities

FILL-IN-THE-BLANK

Finish each of the following statements using the correct term.

1. Antimicrobial agents that are derived from other living microorganisms are called ____________________.

2. Damage to the eighth cranial nerve, or ____________________, can occur from drug therapy, particularly from aminoglycosides.

3. Examples of antimicrobial agents that are potentially nephrotoxic include ____________________, ____________________, and ____________________.

4. When hypoprothrombinemia is present, the usual treatment is administration of vitamin ____________________.

5. Unless contraindicated by coexisting disease, patients taking antimicrobial agents should be encouraged to have an adequate fluid intake of __________ to __________ mL per 24 hours.

6. ____________________ were the first true antibiotics to be grown and used against pathogenic bacteria in human beings.

7. The ____________________ class of antibiotics should not be administered during the last half of pregnancy or while breastfeeding; do not administer to children until permanent teeth are in place (usually by age 8 years).

8. When antibiotics are described as "broad spectrum" in their clinical activity, it means that the antibiotic is generally effective against both ____________________ and ____________________ bacteria.

9. The ____________________ class is not considered a true antibiotic; its action is to inhibit biosynthesis of folic acid, which results in bacterial cell death.

10. The ____________________ class of antimicrobials is reserved for serious life-threatening infections that are vancomycin-resistant.

11. ____________________ is required for aerobic bacteria growth.

12. In general, a person who is allergic to sulfonamides should not take ______________ oral hypoglycemic agents.

13. ____________________ agents kill bacterial pathogens.

14. Two major side effects associated with aminoglycoside antibiotics are ______________ and ______________.

MATCHING

Match the definition with the term that it best describes.

_____ 15. A microorganism that is able to grow and function without oxygen

_____ 16. Causing destruction or death of bacteria

_____ 17. A microorganism that lives and grows with oxygen present

_____ 18. Restrains or reduces the development or reproduction of bacteria

a. Bacteriostatic
b. Anaerobic
c. Bactericidal
d. Aerobic
e. Bacteremia

Match the definition with the term that it best describes.

_____ 19. Overgrowth of organisms resistant to current antibiotic therapy

_____ 20. Causes elevation in AST, ALT, LDH, and alkaline phosphatase

_____ 21. Causes increase in serum creatinine and BUN

_____ 22. Causes dizziness, tinnitus, and progressive hearing loss

a. Ototoxicity
b. Nephrotoxicity
c. Secondary infection
d. Pathogenic
e. Hepatotoxicity

Match the definition with the term that it best describes.

_____ 23. An inflammation of a vein

_____ 24. Reduction in formation and excretion of urine

_____ 25. Characterized by poor blood clotting

_____ 26. Increased albumin in urine

a. Thrombus
b. Phlebitis
c. Oliguria
d. Proteinuria
e. Hypoprothrombinemia

Match the generic drug name with its corresponding brand name. Each option will be used only once.

_____ 27. tolnaftate

_____ 28. oxfloxacin

_____ 29. ampicillin

_____ 30. clarithromycin

_____ 31. azithromycin

_____ 32. cephalexin

_____ 33. cefixime

_____ 34. cefadroxil

_____ 35. ertapenem

_____ 36. neomycin

a. Zithromax
b. Invanz
c. Floxin
d. Suprax
e. Neo-Fradin
f. Tinactin
g. Biaxin
h. Keflex
i. Principen
j. Duricef

TRUE OR FALSE

Mark "T" for true and "F" for false for each statement. Correct all false statements.

_____ 37. The selection of the antimicrobial agent must be based on the sensitivity of the pathogen and the possible toxicity to the patient.

_____ 38. Antibiotics are usually given at even intervals over 24 hours to maintain cyclical blood levels of the medication.

_____ 39. Tetracyclines may be given with antacids, milk, and other dairy products or products containing calcium, magnesium, aluminum, magnesium, or iron.

_____ 40. Drugs such as sulfonamides require forcing fluids unless contraindicated by coexisting medical conditions.

_____ 41. Although serious reactions may occur with the first administration of a drug, repeated exposures to a previous sensitized substance can be fatal.

_____ 42. Patients with a sexually transmitted disease who are being treated with antimicrobial agents should be instructed to refrain from sexual intercourse during therapy.

_____ 43. Nursing mothers should remind their health care provider that they are breastfeeding so that antibiotics may be selected that will have no effect on the infant.

_____ 44. The sulfonamides are not true antibiotics because they are not synthesized by microorganisms.

_____ 45. Cephalosporins may be used as an alternative to penicillins for people allergic to penicillin.

_____ 46. Aminoglycosides cause hepatotoxicity.

_____ 47. Tetracyclines (except doxycycline) should not be taken concurrently with iron- or calcium-containing foods.

_____ 48. Patients receiving aminoglycosides should have a warning sign placed on the front of the chart before a procedure requiring a general anesthetic.

_____ 49. Diarrhea may be a symptom of secondary infection.

_____ 50. Chloramphenicol may cause fatal bone marrow depression.

_____ 51. Patient education for people taking antibiotics should stress taking all the prescribed medication.

_____ 52. Only drugs ending in "-mycin" are classified as macrolides.

_____ 53. Sulfonamides, when given to a patient taking sulfonylurea oral hypoglycemic agents, may cause hypoglycemia.

DRUG ACTION/SIDE EFFECTS

54. *State the action and side effects of penicillin.*

	Actions	Side Effects
PENICILLIN		

CHAPTER 46

Student Name ____________________

Antimicrobial Agents

Practice Questions for the NCLEX Examination

_____ 1. Neomycin has been ordered for a patient who is scheduled for a colon resection. When the patient asks the nurse why he is getting an antibiotic before surgery, the nurse replies that this is necessary because:
1. all patients requiring colon surgery are considered infectious.
2. this drug will reduce the normal flora content of the intestine.
3. he will develop an infection as soon as the surgeon opens the colon in the operating room.
4. any patient undergoing anesthesia must take neomycin.

_____ 2. When administering aminoglycoside drugs to patients, which of the following must be assessed by the nurse? (Select all that apply.)
1. Anesthesia administration to the patient within the past 48 to 72 hours
2. Development of dizziness, tinnitus, and progressive hearing loss
3. Allergy to penicillin, because patients allergic to penicillin are allergic to aminoglycosides
4. History of renal disease

_____ 3. A patient taking an anticonvulsant for a seizure disorder has also been ordered a carbapenem antibiotic for an intra-abdominal infection. Which of the following patient statements indicates that more teaching about this drug is necessary?
1. "If I should have blood and mucus in my stool, I should contact my health care provider."
2. "I should report any severe diarrhea to my health care provider and withhold the next dose of the antibiotic until I have approval to continue taking this drug."
3. "I should sit down if I feel dizzy until that feeling goes away."
4. "I should stop taking the anticonvulsant drug while taking my carbapenem antibiotic."

_____ 4. A patient has been ordered a cephalosporin for a respiratory tract infection. It is now 0900. The patient received his prescribed antacid at 0800. When would be the earliest time the nurse should administer the cephalosporin?
1. 0900
2. 1000
3. 1100
4. 1200

_____ 5. The most common side effect of oral macrolide therapy is:
1. diarrhea, nausea, and vomiting.
2. hypoprothrombinemia.
3. electrolyte imbalance.
4. rash.

_____ 6. Which of the following statements regarding bacterial resistance to penicillin are true? (Select all that apply.)
1. Bacteria that become resistant to penicillin produce a protein called *penicil* that affects the antibacterial activity of penicillins.
2. Penicillinase-resistant penicillins have been developed to maintain the antimicrobial activity of penicillin.
3. Many bacteria that are initially sensitive to penicillin develop a protective mechanism and become resistant to penicillin therapy.
4. The cause of resistance to penicillin is the bacteria's ability to secrete penicillinase which inactivates the penicillin antibiotics by splitting open the beta-lactam ring of the penicillin molecule.

_____ 7. Which of the following is the drug of ch oice for treating patients exposed to anthrax?
1. Penicillin
2. Streptogramins
3. Quinolones
4. Tetracyclines

_____ 8. Which of the following statements about tetracyclines are true? (Select all that apply.)
1. They are often used in patients allergic to penicillins.
2. They are particularly effective against acne.
3. Tetracyclines administered during the ages of tooth development may cause enamel hypoplasia and permanent yellow, gray, or brown staining of the teeth.
4. Tetracyclines do not enter the breast milk of lactating women, so nursing mothers on tetracycline therapy are encouraged to continue to breastfeed their infants.

_____ 9. Which of the following is the drug of choice for tuberculosis prophylaxis?
1. Ethambutol
2. Isoniazid
3. Rifampin
4. Pyridoxine

_____ 10. Which of the following statements by a patient who has been ordered isoniazid therapy for the treatment of active tuberculosis indicates that patient teaching has been effective?
1. "It is important that I take the pyridoxine pill with this drug."
2. "I will take this pill with food."
3. "If I develop tingling and numbness of my hands and feet, I will immediately discontinue treatment with this drug and discard any remaining pills I have, because this is a sign of an extreme allergic reaction."
4. "If I develop nausea and vomiting, I will immediately stop use of this drug."

_____ 11. When providing patient teaching to a 23-year-old woman who has been prescribed rifampin, the nurse would include which of the following statements? (Select all that apply.)
1. "You should use an alternative method of birth control if you are currently taking oral contraceptives."
2. "If you wear soft contact lenses, they may become permanently discolored due to rifampin use."
3. "You may expect your urine to turn green because of the side effects of rifampin."
4. "You may experience nausea, vomiting, anorexia, and abdominal cramps when taking rifampin, but these symptoms will usually be mild and resolve with continued therapy."

_____ 12. Which of the following should the nurse be aware of in relation to administration of vancomycin?
1. Rapid intravenous administration may result in a severe hypertensive episode.
2. Patients receiving intravenous vancomycin may develop red man syndrome.
3. Patients receiving vancomycin must be placed on continuous electrocardiographic monitoring.
4. Vancomycin may only be administered intravenously.

_____ 13. When teaching a patient about proper administration and use of a topical antifungal agent for treatment of a vaginal yeast infection, which of the following statements should the nurse include? (Select all that apply.)
1. "Wash the applicator after each use."
2. "Use a pad to protect your clothing."
3. "Discontinue use of the intravaginal antifungal if menstruation begins."
4. "You should use contraception other than a diaphragm or condom while you are using the intravaginal antifungal."

_____ 14. Patients receiving which one of the following antiviral agents are most at risk for the development of "cushingoid appearance"?
1. Acyclovir
2. Amantadine hydrochloride
3. Amprenavir
4. Didanosine

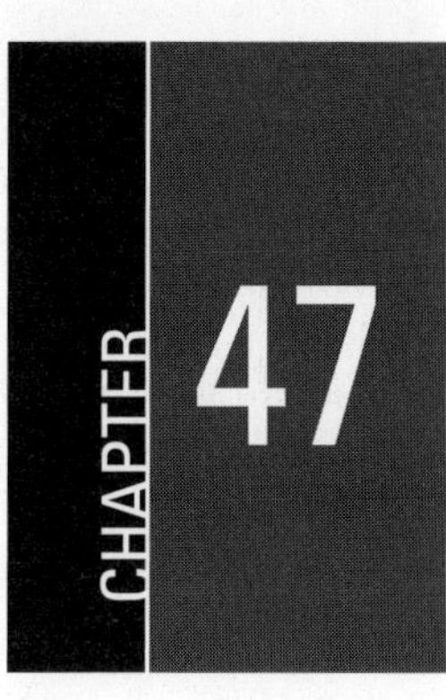

Nutrition

Review Sheet

The QUESTION column and the ANSWER column have been offset so that you can cover the answers while reading the questions, allowing you to assess your knowledge.

Question

1. What factors affect one's nutritional requirements?
2. Summarize information related to nutrition on the MyPyramid guidelines.
3. What do the new guidelines recommend concerning fat consumption?
4. What do the new guidelines recommend for dairy product consumption?
5. What are the Dietary Reference Intakes (DRIs)?
6. What are the Estimated Average Requirements (EAR) and Recommended Dietary Allowances (RDAs)?
7. What is the unit of measurement of energy requirements?
8. What are other names for simple carbohydrates?

Answer

1. See textbook, pp. 803-804.
2. The pyramid recommends eating a variety of foods per day to receive the necessary nutrients while consuming an appropriate amount of calories to maintain health and weight. Daily servings of food groups are recommended along with reminders of the importance of physical activity. The new guidelines stress the importance of controlling weight.
3. Research indicates that monounsaturated and polyunsaturated fats have some health benefits. The latest guidelines recommend getting between 20% and 35% of daily calories from fats, and recognizes the potential health benefits of monounsaturated and polyunsaturated fats. Saturated fats should continue to be limited.
4. The new guidelines recommend drinking three glasses of low-fat milk or eating three servings of other dairy products per day to prevent osteoporosis. Calcium supplements have been shown to reduce the incidence of osteoporosis and do not add calories to the diet.
5. The DRIs are a series of tables that provide quantitative estimates of nutrient intakes to be used in planning and assessing diets for healthy people.
6. The EAR is a nutrient intake value that is estimated to meet the requirements of half of the healthy individuals in a group. The most well-known component of the DRIs is the RDA.
7. Kilocalories (kcal).

9. What percent of calories of the total daily dietary intake of an adult is recommended to come from carbohydrates?
10. Carbohydrates supply _____ kilocalories of energy per gram, fats supply _____ kilocalories of energy per gram, and proteins supply _____ kilocalories of energy per gram.
11. What are the end products of protein metabolism?
12. How many water-soluble and fat-soluble vitamins are there to date?
13. Why are minerals essential to life?
14. Name three forms of malnutrition.
15. What laboratory studies can be used to assess lean body mass?
16. Differentiate between enteral and parenteral nutrition.
17. Explain components of a nutritional assessment.
18. What physical changes are related to a malnourished state?
19. What are the general routines used for checking tube placement and residuals?
20. When is the use of enteral nutrition contraindicated?
21. What premedication assessments should be performed prior to administering enteral nutrition?
22. Differentiate among bolus, intermittent, and continuous feedings.
23. How should prescribed medications be administered via a feeding tube?
24. List side effects of enteral feedings that should be reported to the physician.
25. Review the drug monograph for enteral nutrition and note drugs that interact with grapefruit juice.
26. What is the difference between peripheral parenteral nutrition solutions (PPN), and total parenteral nutrition (TPN) solutions?

8. Simple carbohydrates are known as *monosaccharides* and *disaccharides*.
9. 45% to 65%.
10. Carbohydrates supply 4 kilocalories, fats supply 9 kilocalories, and proteins supply 4 kilocalories.
11. Nitrogenous products such as urea, uric acid, ammonia, carbon dioxide, and water.
12. Thirteen total vitamins; 9 water-soluble; 4 fat-soluble.
13. See textbook, p. 814.
14. Marasmus, kwashiorkor, and mixed kwashiorkor-marasmus.
15. Albumin, pre-albumin, retinol-binding protein, transferrin.
16. Enteral nutrition is administered orally; parenteral nutrition is given via venous access and implantable vascular access devices.
17. See textbook, pp. 817-818.
18. Height, weight, muscle circumference, skin fold thickness, skin integrity, cardiovascular, respiratory, neurological alteration, thyroid function, gastrointestinal symptoms.
19. See textbook, pp. 822-823.
20. Enteral nutrition is contraindicated when the individual has intractable vomiting, a paralyzed ileum, or certain types of fistulas.
21. See textbook, pp. 822-823.
22. See textbook, p. 823.
23. See textbook, p. 823.
24. Pulmonary complications (aspiration), diarrhea, constipation, nausea, vomiting, increased residual volume, rash, chills, fever, and respiratory difficulty.
25. See textbook, p. 824.

27. List premedication assessments that should be performed before administering TPN or PPN.
28. List side effects of parenteral feedings that should be reported to the physician.
29. List key signs and symptoms of fat-soluble and water-soluble vitamin deficiencies.

26. PPN solutions consist of 2%–5% crystalline amino acid preparations and 5%–10% dextrose with electrolytes and vitamins. TPN consists of 15%–25% glucose, amino acids (3.5%–15%), fat emulsion (10%–20%), electrolytes, vitamins, and minerals. Due to high osmolality (see Chapter 12), TPN solutions must be administered through a central venous access line.
27. See textbook, pp. 824-825.
28. Hypoglycemia, hyperglycemia, fluid imbalance, rash, chills, fever, respiratory difficulty, electrolyte imbalances, and hepatotoxicity.
29. See textbook, p. 825.

Student Name____

Nutrition

Learning Activities

FILL-IN-THE-BLANK

Finish each of the following statements using the correct term.

1. ____________________ are the only sugars capable of being used directly to produce energy for the body.
2. Complex carbohydrates such as starch, dextrin, and fiber are also known as ____________________.
3. ____________________ is a protein deficiency that develops when the patient receives adequate fats and carbohydrates in the diet, but little or no protein.
4. The equipment used to administer tube feedings are changed in accordance with the clinical facility's policy, which is usually every _____ hours.
5. Deficiencies of vitamin _____ are often associated with neurologic alterations.
6. Carbohydrates and proteins supply approximately _____ kilocalories of energy per gram.
7. Edema of the abdomen and subcutaneous tissue is a possible sign of ____________________ deficiency.
8. A ____________________ deficiency can increase the heart rate and heart size.
9. A pyridoxine deficiency can result in ____________________.
10. Vitamin _____ deficiency can result in anemia, depression, and delayed wound healing.

MATCHING

Match the generic drug name with its corresponding brand name. Each option will be used only once.

_____ 11. oral supplements

_____ 12. standard isotonic formulas

_____ 13. pediatric formulas

_____ 14. specialized formulas

a. Isocal
b. Boost
c. Glucerna
d. Similac

TRUE OR FALSE

Mark "T" for true and "F" for false for each statement. Correct all false statements.

_____ 15. Fiber is recognized as a macronutrient, a separate factor necessary for complete nutrition and wellness.

_____ 16. Essential fatty acids (EFAs) are produced by the body.

_____ 17. Parenteral feedings are administered orally, either by drinking or instillation into the stomach by way of a feeding tube or feeding gastrostomy port.

_____ 18. Total parenteral nutrition (TPN) orders are formulated daily based on the patient's status, weight, and fluid and electrolyte balance.

_____ 19. Vitamins, whose name originally derived from the term "vital amines," are a specific set of chemical molecules that regulate human metabolism necessary to maintain health.

DRUG ACTION/SIDE EFFECTS

20. *State the action and side effects of parenteral nutrition.*

	Actions	Side Effects
PARENTERAL NUTRITION		

CHAPTER 47

Student Name________________________________

Nutrition

Practice Questions for the NCLEX Examination

_____ 1. Advantages of enteral nutrition over parenteral nutrition include which of the following? (Select all that apply.)
1. Enteral nutrition provides gastrointestinal stimulation.
2. Enteral nutrition has less chance of infection associated with its use.
3. Enteral feedings are more expensive.
4. Enteral nutrition is more physiologic.

_____ 2. When administering drugs to a patient receiving a tube feeding, the nurse should:
1. crush enteric-coated tables before administration via the feeding tube.
2. crush slow-release tablets before administration via the feeding tube.
3. combine all drugs together and administer at the same time.
4. administer the medicines on an empty stomach.

_____ 3. Patients taking calcium channel blockers should not drink:
1. milk.
2. orange juice.
3. grapefruit juice.
4. carbonated soft drinks.

_____ 4. A patient is receiving total parenteral nutrition at a rate of 80 mL per hour, which is due to be changed at 0800. It is 0930 when the nurse first assesses the patient and finds 300 mL of the TPN fluid remaining in the bag. The nurse should:
1. continue the infusion of the current rate until it is complete.
2. increase the rate of the TPN to 150 mL per hour to use up the remainder of fluid in the least amount of time.
3. hang an intravenous bag of normal saline if the next bag of TPN is not readily available.
4. discard any TPN remaining in the current bag and hang a new bag of TPN.

_____ 5. A patient admitted with a diagnosis of malnutrition has been ordered TPN. At the start of his therapy, it is most important for the nurse to assess for the development of:
1. hyperglycemia.
2. rash.
3. diarrhea.
4. abdominal cramping.

_____ 6. Which of the following statements about kwashiorkor are true? (Select all that apply.)
1. It is a fat deficiency.
2. Patients with this condition are often difficult to recognize because they appear to be well-nourished.
3. Patients with this condition receive adequate carbohydrates in the diet.
4. Patients with this condition receive adequate fats in the diet.

_____ 7. Which of the following routes may be used for administering formulas for the provision of enteral nutrition? (Select all that apply.)
1. Orally
2. Nasogastric
3. Nasoduodenal
4. Nasojejunal
5. Needle-catheter jejunostomy

_____ 8. Patients taking monoamine oxidase inhibitors should be taught to avoid which of the following foods? (Select all that apply.)
1. Figs
2. Fava beans
3. Pickled herring
4. Sauerkraut
5. Chicken livers

Herbal and Dietary Supplement Therapy

Review Sheet

The QUESTION column and the ANSWER column have been offset so that you can cover the answers while reading the questions, allowing you to assess your knowledge.

Question	Answer
1. Define the key terms associated with this chapter.	
2. Describe the role of the Food and Drug Administration (FDA) in the regulation of herbal products.	1. See textbook, pp. 828 and 830.
3. What factors should be considered when recommending herbal products?	2. The FDA has no direct role in regulation of herbal products. The Dietary Supplement Health and Education Act (DSHEA) of 1994 governs the use of herbal medicines, vitamins, minerals, and amino acids. Under this Act, almost all herbal medicines, vitamins, minerals, amino acids, and other supplemental chemicals used for health were reclassified legally as dietary supplements, a food category. The labels and advertisements from the manufacturer must contain a statement that the product has not yet been evaluated by the FDA for treating, curing, or preventing any disease. The law does not prevent other people from making claims (founded or unfounded) about the therapeutic effects of supplement ingredients. The end result of the new law is that dietary supplements are not required to be safe and effective and unfounded claims of therapeutic benefit abound. There are now hundreds of herbal medicines and other dietary supplements being marketed in the United States as single- and multiple-ingredient products for an extremely wide variety of uses, all implying that they will improve one's health. The vast majority of the popular claims made for herbal medicines and dietary supplements are unproven. There are also no standardized manufacturing practices that control the manufacture of most of these products as there are with medicines approved by the FDA.

4. Prepare a list of herbal products listed in the chapter and insert the corresponding popular uses by lay people of these herbal products.
5. What questions as part of a medication history should elicit information regarding the use of herbal products and other alternative medicines?
6. What potential drug interactions may occur with each herbal product listed?
7. What is the common use for aloe?
8. What is the most common drug interaction with aloe?
9. What is the common use for black cohosh?
10. When should black cohosh not be used?
11. What is the common use for chamomile?

3. See Box 48-1, p. 829.
4.

Herbal Product:	*Use(s):*
Aloe	See p. 830.
Black cohosh	See p. 831.
Chamomile	See p. 831.
Echinacea	See p. 832.
Ephedra	See p. 832.
Feverfew	See p. 833.
Garlic	See p. 833.
Ginger	See p. 834.
Ginkgo	See p. 835.
Ginseng	See p. 835.
Goldenseal	See p. 836.
Green tea	See p. 836.
Saw palmetto	See p. 837.
St. John's wort	See p. 837.
Valerian	See p. 838.
Other Dietary Supplements:	
Coenzyme Q_{10}	See p. 838.
Creatine	See p. 839.
Gamma-hydroxybutyrate (GHB)	See p. 840.
Lycopene	See p. 840.
Melatonin	See p. 841.
Policosanol	See p. 841.
S-adenosylmethionine (SAM-e)	See p. 842.

5. Consult with your instructor for assistance.
6. Review individual monographs throughout chapter.
7. Aloe has been used for arthritis, colitis, common cold, hemorrhoids, seizures, and glaucoma. Most recently, aloe gel has been marketed for topical use to treat pain, inflammation, and itching, and as a healing agent for sunburn, skin ulcers, psoriasis, and frostbite.
8. Patients who are diabetic should have their blood glucose monitored because there have been claims that when taken orally, aloe may have hypoglycemic effects.
9. Black cohosh is used to reduce symptoms of premenstrual syndrome (PMS), dysmenorrhea, and menopause.
10. Black cohosh should not be used in the first two trimesters of pregnancy because of its uterine relaxing effects.

12. What is echinacea commonly used for?

11. Chamomile is used as a digestive agent for bloating, an antispasmodic and an antiinflammatory in the gastrointestinal tract, an antispasmodic for menstrual cramps, an anti-inflammatory for skin irritation, and a mouthwash for minor mouth irritation or gum infections.

13. What is ephedra commonly used for?

12. Echinacea is a nonspecific immunostimulant that may prevent or treat viral respiratory tract infections such as the common cold or flu. It may be used to treat urinary tract infections and may be applied externally to difficult-to-heal superficial wounds.

14. When is the use of ephedra contraindicated?

13. Ephedra is used as a bronchodilator for asthma, a nasal decongestant, and a central nervous system (CNS) stimulant.

15. What are the side effects of ephedra?

14. Ephedra is contraindicated in patients with heart conditions, hypertension, diabetes, and thyroid disease.

16. What is feverfew commonly used for?

15. Ephedra elevates systolic and diastolic blood pressure and heart rate, causing palpitations. It also causes nervousness, headache, insomnia, and dizziness.

17. What is garlic commonly used for?

16. Feverfew is used to reduce the frequency and severity of migraine headaches. Its antiinflammatory effects have also been used to treat rheumatoid arthritis.

18. What is ginger commonly used for?

17. The most frequent use of garlic supported by scientific literature is in reducing cholesterol and triglycerides. It has demonstrated antiplatelet activity similar to aspirin, and may also modestly lower blood pressure.

19. What is ginkgo commonly used for?

18. Ginger has been used for centuries to alleviate nausea and vomiting. It has also been found to be modestly effective in reducing inflammation associated with rheumatoid arthritis and muscle discomfort.

20. What is ginseng commonly used for?

19. Ginkgo biloba extract is used primarily to increase cerebral blood flow, particularly in geriatric patients. Other uses include improved walking distance in patients with intermittent claudication, improvement in erectile dysfunction secondary to antidepressant therapy, improved peripheral blood flow in patients with diabetes mellitus, and improved hearing in patients with hearing impairment due to poor circulation to the ears.

21. What is goldenseal commonly used for?

20. Ginseng is not used as a cure for disease, but as an "adaptogen" in maintaining health.

22. When should goldenseal not be taken?
23. What is green tea commonly used for?
24. What is saw palmetto commonly used for?
25. What drug should not be used with saw palmetto?
26. What is St. John's wort commonly used for?
27. What are the side effects of St. John's wort?
28. What syndrome is use of St. John's wort associated with?
29. What is valerian commonly used for?
30. What is coenzyme Q_{10} commonly used for?
31. What is creatine commonly used for?
32. What is gamma-hydroxybutyrate commonly used for?
33. What are the adverse effects of GHB?

21. Goldenseal is used topically as a tea for treatment of canker sores, sore mouth, and cracked and bleeding lips. It may help fight viral upper respiratory infections such as cold or flu. There is a common myth that goldenseal will mask assays for street drugs.
22. Goldenseal in high doses may have a uterine stimulant effect, so it should not be taken during pregnancy.
23. Green tea is used to improve cognitive performance. It raises blood pressure, heart rate, and contractility, and acts as a diuretic. It has been shown to lower cholesterol, triglycerides, and low-density lipoprotein, and raise high-density lipoprotein. There is some evidence that green tea might reduce the risk of bladder, esophageal, and pancreatic cancer, and reduce or prevent the onset of parkinsonism. Green tea is also used to treat diarrhea.
24. Saw palmetto is used to treat the symptoms associated with benign prostatic hyperplasia (BPH), to reduce the risks associated with urinary retention, and to minimize the need for surgery associated with BPH.
25. Finasteride.
26. St. John's wort is used to treat mild depression and to heal wounds.
27. St. John's wort may cause photosensitivity.
28. Serotonin syndrome.
29. Valerian is used for restlessness and may promote sleep.
30. CoQ_{10} is primarily used as an adjunct therapy for chronic heart failure. It may also be used to treat other cardiovascular diseases, cancer, muscular dystrophy, periodontal disease, and AIDS.
31. Creatine supplementation is thought to enhance muscle performance for short periods of intense exercise. Patients with heart failure and muscular dystrophy might benefit from creatine supplementation.
32. Despite the FDA ban of GHB in 1990, GHB continues to be marketed as a dietary supplement "growth hormone stimulator." GHB is usually abused for its intoxicating, sedative, and euphoric properties, particularly at rave parties where it is used as a "date rape" drug. It is available as a prescription product for treating patients with narcolepsy.

34. What is lycopene commonly used for?

35. What is melatonin commonly used for?

36. What is policosanol commonly used for?

37. What is SAM-e commonly used for?

33. The adverse effects of GHB are highly individualized; however, those that are potentially life-threatening include vomiting with aspiration to the lungs, respiratory depression, bradycardia, and hypotension.
34. There is some evidence to suggest that diets high in lycopene may reduce risk of prostate cancer. It has antioxidant properties that may lower LDL-cholesterol, thus protecting against heart attack and stroke. Lycopene may also protect against macular degeneration and cataracts.
35. Melatonin is best known as a sleep aid and treatment for jet lag. It may also be helpful in patients withdrawing from benzodiazepine therapy.
36. Policosanol is used to treat dyslipidemia. It is also used as a platelet inhibitor for the treatment of intermittent claudication. Policosanol is also used to treat myocardial ischemia in patients with coronary artery disease.
37. SAM-e is used for the treatment of depression, osteoarthritis, and fibromyalgia.

Student Name________________________________

Herbal and Dietary Supplement Therapy

Learning Activities

FILL-IN-THE-BLANK

Finish each of the following statements using the correct term.

1. ____________________ medicines are defined as natural substances derived from botanical or plant origin.

2. Concurrent consumption of large quantities of green tea with warfarin may ____________________ the anticoagulant effects of warfarin.

3. The most common use of ginger is to alleviate ____________________ and ____________________.

4. Most individuals using St. John's wort do so for its supposed ability to treat mild ____________________ and to heal ____________________.

5. There is some evidence to suggest that diets high in ____________________ may reduce the risk of prostate cancer.

MATCHING

Match each herb to the other name it is known by. Each option will be used only once.

_____ 6. valerian

_____ 7. St. John's wort

_____ 8. ginkgo

_____ 9. black cohosh

_____ 10. echinacea

_____ 11. aloe

_____ 12. goldenseal

a. squawroot
b. klamath weed
c. burn plant
d. maidenhair tree
e. amantilla
f. purple coneflower
g. yellow root

TRUE OR FALSE

Mark "T" for true and "F" for false for each statement. Correct all false statements.

_____ 13. Under the Dietary Supplement Health and Education Act (DSHEA) of 1994, almost all herbal medicines, vitamins, minerals, amino acids, and other supplemental chemicals used for health were reclassified legally as dietary supplements, a food category.

_____ 14. Diet supplements should not be recommended for use by pregnant women, lactating mothers, infants, or young children without approval from the patient's primary care health provider.

_____ 15. Homeopathy employs the use of therapeutic doses of botanical drugs.

_____ 16. It is reported that SAM-e may reduce some of the side effects of levodopa used to treat parkinsonism, but it is also thought that SAM-e may reduce the beneficial effects of levodopa in the treatment of parkinsonism over time.

_____ 17. Ginseng has been shown to lower insulin levels in laboratory animals.

_____ 18. Chamomile has been shown to be an effective antidepressant.

_____ 19. Echinacea is a bacteriostatic and bactericidal agent.

_____ 20. There are essentially no drug interactions with ephedra.

_____ 21. Feverfew is used as an antiplatelet and antihypertensive agent.

_____ 22. Garlic affects platelet aggregation and therefore should be used with caution for clients taking antiplatelet medications.

_____ 23. Saw palmetto is used to treat symptoms of benign prostatic hyperplasia.

_____ 24. Ginseng may cause hyperglycemia.

_____ 25. Valerian is used as a sleep aid and as a mild tranquilizer.

DRUG ACTION/SIDE EFFECTS

26. *State the action and side effects of ginkgo.*

	Actions	**Side Effects**
GINKGO		

CHAPTER 48

Student Name ____________________

Herbal and Dietary Supplement Therapy

Practice Questions for the NCLEX Examination

_____ 1. A 62-year-old woman is on hormone replacement therapy to treat symptoms associated with menopause and to prevent osteoporosis. She also takes medication to control high blood pressure. She is interested in taking black cohosh and asks the nurse about it. What is the most appropriate response by the nurse?
1. "Studies have found that black cohosh is an excellent herb for women to treat symptoms of menopause that are not controlled by hormone replacement therapy."
2. "High blood pressure will be lowered with the use of black cohosh, so you won't need to take your high blood pressure pills any longer."
3. "Black cohosh works by stimulating the body to produce its own natural testosterone."
4. "Black cohosh may cause added antihypertensive effects when taken with medication to lower blood pressure. Consult your health care provider before adding black cohosh to your treatment regimen."

_____ 2. The herb most commonly used in the treatment of asthma is:
1. ephedra.
2. echinacea.
3. chamomile.
4. goldenseal.

_____ 3. Which of the following statements should the nurse include when teaching a patient about St. John's wort? (Select all that apply.)
1. "The active ingredients of St. John's wort are unknown."
2. "St. John's wort may cause photosensitivity, so individuals using it should avoid overexposure to the sun."
3. "Patients who take other serotonin stimulants should not take St. John's wort without consulting their health care provider."
4. "St. John's wort is a safe alternative to other medications for anyone with depression."

_____ 4. SAM-e has been proposed for the treatment of: (Select all that apply.)
1. depression.
2. osteoarthritis.
3. diabetes mellitus.
4. fibromyalgia.

_____ 5. The herb most commonly used for treating symptoms associated with benign prostatic hypertrophy is:
1. valerian.
2. feverfew.
3. saw palmetto.
4. ginseng.

Substance Abuse

Review Sheet

The QUESTION column and the ANSWER column have been offset so that you can cover the answers while reading the questions, allowing you to assess your knowledge.

Question	Answer
1. Define *substance-related disorders, substance abuse, impairment, dependence, addiction,* and *illicit substances.*	
2. Differentiate among the biological model, psychological theories, and sociocultural factors that are associated with substance abuse.	1. See textbook, pp. 844-845.
3. List sociological signs of impairment associated with substance abuse.	2. Biologic model: caused by person's genetic profile. Psychologic theory: sees alcoholism as occurring in an individual who is fixated in the oral stage of development and is seeking oral gratification. This theory also recognizes a link to depression, anxiety, antisocial personality, and dependent personality. Sociocultural: the individual is influenced by such things as attitudes, norms, values, nationality, religion, gender, family background, and social environment.
4. List four tests used to screen for alcohol and substance abuse.	3. Substance abuse first affects the family life, then social life, and finally results in physical and mental changes.
5. What is the prevalence of substance abuse by health care professionals?	4. See Table 49-2.
6. Cite legal considerations associated with substance abuse and dependence in health care providers.	5. See textbook, p. 849.
7. List three long-term goals of treatment of substance abuse as defined by the American Psychiatric Association.	6. See textbook, pp. 850-851; research laws governing nursing in the state where you are practicing.
8. Cite examples of organizations that promote the goals of abstinence from substance abuse.	7. Reduction or abstinence in use and effects of substances; reduction in frequency and severity of relapse; and improvement in psychological and social functioning.
9. Compare the effects on the body of acute and chronic use of alcohol.	8. AA, NA, and others.

10. Define *alcohol intoxication* and *alcohol withdrawal.*
11. What drugs are used to treat alcohol withdrawal symptoms?
12. Describe components of an alcohol relapse prevention program.
13. Name three medications used to promote abstinence from alcohol use.
14. List commonly abused opiates.
15. List the signs and symptoms of opioid intoxication and opioid withdrawal.
16. What limitations does naltrexone (ReVia) have in the treatment of opioid addiction?
17. Name two new dosage forms of buprenorphine approved for opioid maintenance programs.
18. What effect does cocaine have on the CNS?
19. What is the difference between "freebase" and "crack" cocaine?
20. Describe the signs and symptoms of cocaine intoxication and withdrawal from cocaine.
21. List the nursing assessments that should be used when substance abuse is suspected or diagnosed.
22. What laboratory tests are routinely ordered for drug screening?
23. Study Table 49-1 to identify drugs, usage forms, possible side effects, signs of overdose, and long-term effects of drugs classified as stimulants, depressants, narcotics, cannabis, hallucinogens, and inhalants.

9. See textbook, pp. 852-853.
10. See textbook, p. 852.
11. Benzodiazepines are used for detoxification. Long-acting chlordiazepoxide, diazepam, and clorazepate are the most commonly used protocol for alcohol withdrawal.
12. See textbook, p. 854.
13. Disulfiram (Antabuse), naltrexone (ReVia), and acamprosate (Campral).
14. Heroin, morphine, hydromorphone, codeine, oxycodone, and hydrocodone; opiate-like substances (e.g., meperidine, fentanyl, others).
15. See textbook, pp. 854-855.
16. Naltrexone does not block the desire to get "high;" it only blocks the "high" when an opioid is used.
17. Buprenorphine-only (Subutrex) and buprenorphine-naloxone (Suboxone).
18. Blocks metabolism of catecholamines in the brain, bringing on a sudden CNS stimulation with euphoria or a "rush."
19. "Freebase" is cocaine hydrochloride mixed with ammonia and dissolved in ether. As ether evaporates, it forms a powder residue that can be smoked for its "high." "Crack" cocaine is cocaine hydrochloride mixed with baking soda that is heated to form "rocks" which are then smoked.
20. See textbook, p. 856.
21. See textbook, pp. 856-858.
22. See textbook, p. 858.
23. See Table 49-1.

CHAPTER 49

Student Name______________________________

Substance Abuse

Learning Activities

FILL-IN-THE-BLANK

Finish each of the following statements using the correct term.

1. ______________ ______________ is defined as the periodic purposeful use of a substance that leads to clinically significant impairment.

2. If substance abuse behavior is not stopped, it leads to a more serious medical condition known as substance ____________________ or ____________________.

3. A(n) ____________________ substance is any chemical or mixture of chemicals that alters biologic function and is not required for the maintenance of health.

4. ____________________ is defined as the ingestion of ethanol to the point of clinically significant maladaptive behavioral or psychologic changes.

5. THC, hashish, and marijuana are classified as ____________________.

6. LSD and PCP are classified as ____________________.

7. Nicotine, caffeine, amphetamines, and cocaine are classified as ____________________.

8. Lack of coordination, sluggishness, slurred speech, and disorientation are possible side effects of the use of drugs classified as ____________________.

MATCHING

Match the common drug name with its corresponding medical name. Each option will be used only once.

_____ 9. sedatives

_____ 10. tranquilizers

_____ 11. opium

_____ 12. heroin

_____ 13. marijuana

a. valium
b. tetrahydrocanabinol
c. paregoric
d. phenobarbital
e. diacetylmorphine

TRUE OR FALSE

Mark "T" for true and "F" for false for each statement. Correct all false statements.

_____ 14. Even though substance abuse has been a condition of the human mind since prehistoric times, and very extensively studied, there is no one theory that accounts for why individuals abuse chemicals.

_____ 15. Substance abuse has been linked to several psychological traits, but there is no particular evidence that these traits cause the substance abuse.

_____ 16. The disease of substance impairment problems usually manifests first in social life then followed by family life.

_____ 17. There are twelve steps to the Alcoholics Anonymous program.

DRUG ACTION/SIDE EFFECTS

18. *State the actions and side effects of the following drug that affects substance abuse.*

	Actions	Side Effects
DIAZEPAM		

CHAPTER 49

Student Name______________________________

Substance Abuse

Practice Questions for the NCLEX Examination

_____ 1. A 21-year-old female is bought in to the emergency department for a suspected cocaine overdose. Which of the following symptoms would the nurse expect this patient to have? (Select all that apply.)
1. Pupillary constriction
2. Respiratory depression
3. Chest pain
4. Sweating or chills

_____ 2. Patients being treated for recovery from opioid addiction would likely receive which of the following drugs? (Select all that apply.)
1. Meperidine
2. Methadone
3. Levomethadyl acetate
4. Clonidine

_____ 3. The first step to the Twelve Steps of Alcoholics Anonymous is:
1. "Make a list of all people harmed by use of alcohol."
2. "Make a searching and fearless moral inventory of yourself."
3. "Become entirely ready to have God remove all defects of your character."
4. "Admit that you are powerless over alcohol and that your life has become unmanageable."

_____ 4. When working with a patient who has overdosed on amphetamines, the nurse would expect the patient to exhibit which of the following signs/symptoms? (Select all that apply.)
1. Agitation
2. Hallucinations
3. Decreased body temperature
4. Convulsions

_____ 5. When providing teaching about the effects of substance use and abuse with pregnancy, the nurse should include which of the following statements? (Select all that apply.)
1. "Using alcohol and drugs while pregnant has a strong likelihood of harming the baby after birth."
2. "Infants of drug addicts must be monitored closely for symptoms of withdrawal after delivery."
3. "Using alcohol and drugs during pregnancy has a high likelihood of causing the need for induction of pregnancy due to the fetus being post-term."
4. "Alcohol and drug use during pregnancy has been associated with potentially fatal bleeding disorders."

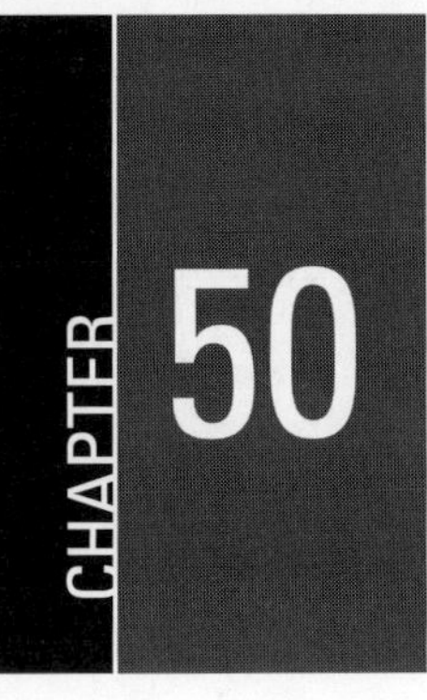

Miscellaneous Agents

Review Sheet

The QUESTION column and the ANSWER column have been offset so that you can cover the answers while reading the questions, allowing you to assess your knowledge.

Question

1. What is the therapeutic outcome of the use of acamprosate?
2. What are side effects to report with the use of acamprosate?
3. What is the action and primary use of allopurinol?
4. What are expected side effects of allopurinol therapy?
5. What is the primary therapeutic outcome of colchicine therapy?
6. In which patient groups should colchicine be used with extreme caution?
7. Via which routes should colchicine not be administered?
8. What is disulfiram used for?

Answer

1. The primary therapeutic outcome expected from acamprosate is improved adherence with an alcohol treatment program by abstinence from alcohol.
2. Monitor alcohol-dependent patients, including those patients being treated with acamprosate for the development of symptoms of negative thoughts, feelings, behaviors, depression, or suicidal thinking. Alert families and caregivers of patients being treated with acamprosate of the need to monitor for the emergent nature of these symptoms and to report such symptoms to the patient's health care provider.
3. Allopurinol blocks the terminal steps in uric acid formation by inhibiting the enzyme xanthine oxidase. This agent can be used to treat primary gout or gout secondary to antineoplastic therapy.
4. Patients should be told that the frequency of gout attacks may increase for the first few months of therapy. The patient should continue therapy without changing the dosage during the attacks. Nausea, vomiting, diarrhea, dizziness, and headache are usually mild and tend to resolve with continued therapy.
5. Elimination of joint pain secondary to acute gout attack.
6. Older adults or debilitated patients, and patients with impaired renal, cardiac, or gastrointestinal function should be extremely cautious with colchicine.
7. Subcutaneously or intramuscularly.

9. How is a disulfiram reaction manifested?
10. What is the therapeutic outcome of donepezil?
11. What are the side effects to report for patients taking donepezil therapy?
12. What is the action of lactulose?
13. What are the therapeutic outcomes of lactulose therapy?
14. What is the primary therapeutic outcome of memantine?
15. What are the drugs that interact with memantine?
16. What is the primary therapeutic outcome of probenicid?
17. Who should not receive probenicid therapy?
18. What is the action of tacrine?
19. What are the side effects to expect with tacrine therapy?

8. Disulfiram is used in alcohol rehabilitation programs for chronic alcohol patients who want to maintain sobriety.
9. Disulfiram reaction is manifested by nausea, severe vomiting, sweating, throbbing headache, dizziness, blurred vision, and confusion.
10. Improved cognitive skills.
11. The health care provider should be notified if the patient's heart rate is less than 60 beats per minute.
12. Lactulose is a sugar that acidifies the colon, thus preventing the absorption of ammonia.
13. Improved orientation to surroundings and a gentle laxative effect with formed stool.
14. Improved cognitive skills.
15. Acetazolamide and sodium bicarbonate.
16. The primary therapeutic outcome of probenicid is prevention of acute attacks of gouty arthritis.
17. Patients with histories of blood dyscrasias or uric acid kidney stones should not receive probenicid.
18. Tacrine is an acetylcholinesterase inhibitor that allows acetylcholine to accumulate at cholinergic synapses causing a prolonged and exaggerated cholinergic effect.
19. Nausea, vomiting, dyspepsia, and diarrhea.

CHAPTER 50

Student Name______________________________

Miscellaneous Agents

Learning Activities

FILL-IN-THE-BLANK

Finish each of the following statements using the correct term.

1. The primary therapeutic outcome expected from tacrine therapy is improved ____________________ skills.

2. Lactulose is a sugar that acidifies the colon, thus preventing the absorption of ____________________.

3. Tacrine is a(n) ____________________ inhibitor that allows acetycholine to accumulate at cholinergic synapses causing a prolonged and exaggerated cholinergic effect.

4. Cholinergic agents cause a(n) ____________________ of the heart rate.

MATCHING

Match the generic drug name with its corresponding brand name. Each option will be used only once.

_____ 5. tacrine

_____ 6. lactulose

_____ 7. disulfiram

_____ 8. allopurinol

_____ 9. acamprosate

_____ 10. donepezil

_____ 11. memantine

a. Cognex
b. Zyloprim
c. Cephulac
d. Antabuse
e. Campral
f. Aricept
g. Namenda

TRUE OR FALSE

Mark "T" for true and "F" for false for each statement. Correct all false statements.

_____ 12. Tacrine is used in the treatment of mild to moderate dementia to enhance cholinergic function.

_____ 13. Probenicid acts as an analgesic in the treatment of gout.

_____ 14. Lactulose is used to reduce formation of ammonia in the gut.

_____ 15. Allopurinol can be used to treat gout secondary to antineoplastic therapy.

_____ 16. Disulfiram is an agent that, when ingested before any form of alcohol consumed, produces a very unpleasant reaction to the alcohol.

DRUG ACTION/SIDE EFFECTS

17. *State the action and side effects of lactulose.*

	Actions	Side Effects
LACTULOSE		

CHAPTER 50

Student Name_______________

Miscellaneous Agents

Practice Questions for the NCLEX Examination

_____ 1. When teaching the family of an Alzheimer's patient about the side effects of tacrine, the nurse would include which of the following statements? (Select all that apply.)
1. "Patients taking tacrine are at a high risk for the development of increased heart rate."
2. "Notify the health care provider if the patient develops a yellow cast to his skin."
3. "Diarrhea is a common side effect of this drug."
4. "If nausea and vomiting develop, these effects are often reduced if the tacrine dose is lowered."

_____ 2. A patient has been ordered probenicid therapy for the treatment of hyperuricemia and chronic gouty arthritis. Which of the following statements by the patient indicates that more teaching is necessary?
1. "This drug works on the tissues of my great toe, where I usually get the gout, to get rid of the problem."
2. "I can expect that the incidence of gout attacks may increase for the first few months of therapy with this drug."
3. "I will tell my health care provider if I develop vomiting that looks like coffee grounds."
4. "If I develop a rash, I will tell my health care provider because this most likely means that I have an allergy to this drug."

_____ 3. It is most important for the nurse to assess a patient on lactulose therapy for which of the following electrolyte imbalances?
1. Hypocalcemia
2. Hypernatremia
3. Hypokalemia
4. Hypermagnesemia

_____ 4. Which of the following statements by a patient indicates that more teaching is needed about lactulose therapy?
1. "I can expect to have some distention of my abdomen."
2. "I will continue to take my daily laxative when on lactulose therapy."
3. "I should be aware of the possible development of diarrhea because this is a sign of overdosage that can be corrected by a dosage reduction."
4. "I will continue to take my weight and record it daily."

_____ 5. Which of the following statements by a patient indicates that more teaching is needed about disulfiram therapy and alcohol?
1. "I must look at the contents of any drug I take, including those that are over-the-counter, because any type of alcohol may produce a reaction when taken with disulfiram."
2. "I should continue with the behavioral therapy I am currently involved with while on disulfiram."
3. "I will call my health care provider if I develop a rash."
4. "Little sips of alcohol-containing drinks are allowed, because I must drink at least 8 ounces of an alcohol-containing substance for the disulfiram to cause a reaction."

_____ 6. The nurse identifies which of the following routes as appropriate for the administration of colchicine? (Select all that apply.)
1. Oral
2. Intravenous
3. Subcutaneous
4. Intramuscular

_____ 7. Which of the following actions should the nurse take when there is extravasation of colchicine? (Select all that apply.)
1. Flush the IV
2. Elevate the infiltrated area
3. Prepare to assist with administration of drugs to counteract the necrotizing effects
4. Massage the infiltrated area

_____ 8. Which of the following statements should the nurse include when teaching the patient and family about donepezil? (Select all that apply.)
1. "Notify your health care provider if your pulse is less than 60 beats per minute."
2. "Discontinue use of the drug if you should develop diarrhea early on in the treatment program."
3. "This drug will prevent your disease from getting worse."
4. "You may feel a little nauseated when first taking this medication, but this usually subsides after 2 to 3 weeks of therapy."